READINGS
ON
RESEARCH
IN
STUTTERING

READINGS ON RESEARCH IN STUTTERING

E. Charles Healey

UNIVERSITY OF NEBRASKA-LINCOLN

Longman

New York & London

Readings on Research in Stuttering

Longman, 95 Church Street, White Plains, N.Y. 10601

Associated companies:
Longman Group Ltd., London
Longman Cheshire Pty., Melbourne
Longman Paul Pty., Auckland
Copp Clark Pitman, Toronto

Executive editor: Raymond T. O'Connell
Production editor: Janice Baillie
Text design adaptation: Betty L. Sokol
Cover design: Lorraine Mullaney
Production supervisor: Kathleen M. Ryan

Library of Congress Cataloging in Publication Data

Readings on research in stuttering / [compiled by] E. Charles
Healey.
      p.   cm.
   Includes bibliographical references.
   1. Stuttering.   I. Healey, E. Charles.
RC424.R319   1990
616.85′54—dc20   90-31116
                                              CIP

ISBN: 0-8013-0410-5

ABCDEFGHIJ-AL-99 98 97 96 95 94 93 92 91 90

Contents

Preface

This work represents an update, a revision, and a new packaging of a book entitled *Readings in Stuttering,* published in 1986. Those familiar with the first edition will note that I have made a number of changes in this one. The changes include a new title, the removal of the glossary of terms, and the elimination of the unrelated photographs that accompanied some of the articles. Chapter titles and the introductions preceding the collection of articles in each chapter have also undergone substantial modifications.

Despite all of these changes, the intent of this book has remained the same. As with the first edition, my goal was to put together a collection of readings in stuttering that reflects major themes or trends in recent research in the area. The current book of readings is a representative sample of articles that have been published from a variety of sources over the last ten years.

Considering all the articles and book chapters written during this time period, it was difficult to know which readings to select for the revised edition. Those I have included reflect my perception of recent research that conveys an important message. Instructors who use this book for graduate courses in stuttering may disagree with my choice of readings as well as my perception of what the literature has to say. They may also find the arrangement and content of some chapters not suitable to their purposes. For these reasons, I have included a list of suggested additional readings at the end of each chapter so that other articles could be included, or could replace the ones in this book for a course reading list. The lists of suggested readings are also provided to give additional references to those who want to pursue a particular topic in greater detail.

All of the readings except two are from journal articles. This was deliberate for two reasons. First, I believe that it is important to make students aware of the journal literature and have them understand that our information about stuttering comes primarily from journals. Second, chapters from books or presentations that are reprinted in conference proceedings typically represent one author's opinion and interpretation of the literature. Many times opinions are not clearly separated from empirical observations. By contrast, journal articles undergo a peer review process that encourages authors to present the data from an unbiased point of view.

Given this perspective, I have kept my own editorial comments about each reading to a minimum. Most of my comments about an article in the chapter introductions summarize the major point(s) of the article. The key features of each reading are integrated into the content of the chapter "theme." Furthermore, each chapter introduction was written from the standpoint that a student would have only a minimal knowledge base about stuttering before reading this book. My intent was to introduce a topic and provide some background information about the readings included in a particular chapter.

The book begins with a collection of readings devoted to the nature of stuttering. The readings in Chapter 1 cover a variety of topics including some of the general "facts" about stuttering, two theoretical notions about stuttering, and two articles that address the genetic aspects of stuttering. Chapter 2 is concerned with recent behavioral and physiological research efforts with children who stutter. The readings in Chapter 3 provide an account of the renewed interests researchers have shown in stutterers' speech motor control processes during stutterers' disfluent and perceptually "fluent" moments. The articles in Chapter 4 present information about the diagnosis of stuttering in children and adults as well as some conceptual notions about the criteria that could be used in identifying individuals who stutter. Finally, the readings in Chapter 5 give the reader a general overview of some topics related to the treatment of stuttering in children and adults.

The completion of this book would not have been possible without the support of many people. I am grateful to the authors of the articles for allowing me to reprint their work. Clearly, this book would never have made it off the ground without their kindness and generosity. I would also like to thank Ray O'Connell and Richard Bretan at Longman for their encouragement and assistance throughout the revision process. I also want to express my appreciation to the three anonymous reviewers of the first edition of this book. Their insights and suggestions for this second edition were extremely helpful to me, particularly in terms of suggesting readings and pointing out some of the changes that would make the second edition more useful as a textbook. I would also like to recognize the support that I have received over the years from my parents and the late Evelyn O. Stephenson. Finally, I express my sincere appreciation to my wife, Connie, and my sons, Gavin and Nathan, for their patience and understanding during the preparation of this book.

CHAPTER ONE

The Nature of Stuttering

Of all the disorders of communication, stuttering would be considered by many to be one of the most perplexing problems that speech-language pathologists encounter. Even though a great deal of research and intensive study have been conducted, there is much that we still do not understand about the nature of the problem. However, from a vast number of research studies conducted over the past five decades it is possible to reach some general conclusions about the disorder. In this chapter, the articles that have been selected provide the reader with a description of information about stuttering that has been collected over the years as well as discussions of some issues that still remain unresolved.

In this chapter, the article by Smith and Weber presents a discussion of the controversy of whether stuttering stems from a physiological or psychological basis. Although both points of view have merit, Smith and Weber argue that the time has come to integrate these two concepts into a meaningful theory of stuttering that would explain the psychophysiological aspects of the disorder.

In the second article of this chapter, Andrews, Craig, Feyer, Hoddinott, Howie, and Neilson provide comprehensive reviews and analyses of past research in stuttering. Some of the basic "facts" about stuttering have been known for years and have provided us a basis of understanding of the nature of this speech disorder. One of those "facts" concerns the age of onset of the disorder. Stuttering typically begins between the ages of 2 and 5 with the mean around 4 years of age. The onset of stuttering can occur after the preschool age range but it becomes less common as the child gets older. Thus, it is somewhat unexpected to find the onset of stuttering in adolescents and adults but it does occasionally happen. Usually, the onset of stuttering in adults is related to some form of emotional or physical trauma. For example, the articles by Attanasio (1987) and Deal (1982) describe cases in which the onset of stuttering occurred in adult life.

We also know that stuttering is more commonly found in males than in females with a ratio of about three boys to every girl that stutters. The prevalence of stuttering is about 1 percent of any given population. Statistics supplied by the U.S. Department of Health and Human Services suggest that there are approximately 2 million stutterers in the United States and about 15 million worldwide. Stutterers can be found in most cultures. While the prevalence of stuttering may differ according to geographic and cultural background, we know that stuttering is a universal problem and has been for centuries.

Another interesting feature about the prevalence of stuttering is that the disorder tends to occur more in families of stutterers than in families of nonstutterers. Recent evidence strongly suggests this family pattern of stuttering is related to genetic and environmental factors. Identical twins are particularly susceptible to stuttering as noted in the article in this chapter by Howie. Interestingly, too, both the spontaneous recovery (i.e., the reduction or elimination of stuttering on its own accord) and persistence of stuttering into adulthood are related to families that have a history of stuttering. Unfortunately, at this time in history, we have no idea of exactly what is genetically or environmentally transmitted that increases the chances of someone becoming a stutterer. An excellent source of information on the genetic components of stuttering can be found in the chapter by Kidd (1984) cited in the references.

As stated previously, we know too that identical twins have a greater concordance for stuttering than do fraternal twins. However, current genetic models are not capable of showing why, in some cases, one monozygotic twin stutters and the other twin does not. In the article by Cox, it is suggested that what has been termed molecular genetics might provide some new insights into the genetics of stuttering. Cox shows that by following pieces of DNA (the basic material of life) in family members of stutterers, it might be possible to determine a link between DNA and the genes responsible for passing the disorder from one generation to the next.

The strong tendency for family members to recover spontaneously from stuttering has been summarized (Andrews et al. 1983). It is thought that spontaneous recovery could occur in approximately 80 percent of the cases. In reviewing past spontaneous recovery studies, Martin and Lindamood (1986) suggest that this percentage is probably too high. Their conclusion is based on an analysis of the manner in which the spontaneous recovery figures have been reported, the different ages upon which the data are collected, and the methodology employed. Given the vast differences in the way the spontaneous recovery data have been collected, Martin and Lindamood conclude that the commonly reported figure of 80 percent of these children recovering from stuttering is not supported by research.

Given the information gained from an analysis of the family history of stuttering and spontaneous recovery data, we could conclude that the environment and heredity are important factor(s) in the etiology of stuttering. Nonetheless, the specific cause of stuttering in all cases is still unknown and it may be that we will never discover the factors that cause stuttering. More than likely, there are different causes for stuttering. Researchers, theorists, and clinicians have long thought that stuttering is a multidimensional problem caused by a variety of physiological, psychosocial, and environmental factors.

Nonetheless, research has not been able to show conclusively that stuttering results from any one factor such as physiological deficits, psychological abnormalities, persistent anticipatory-struggle reactions, or aberrant classical and/or operant conditioning. Perhaps when we identify and categorize stutterers into subgroups, it will be possible to achieve a better understanding of the specific cause(s) of stuttering in certain individuals. Most recently, Adams (1988) has summarized various explanations by scientists who have speculated about the cause of stuttering. He discusses Kent's (1983) neuropsychological perspective on stuttering, the "Demands and Capacities" model, Yeudall's (1985) neurophysiological model of stuttering, and the central capacity hypothesis described in the Andrews et al. article.

Besides wanting to know what causes stuttering, most people are curious as to why stutterers have the ability to become fluent when speaking in a "novel" pattern. For many years it has been recognized that stutterers will be fluent when they speak in an unusual way such as when they sing, shout, whisper, speak in unison with another person, or speak in a foreign language. While there are exceptions to the rule, the consistency with which this phenomenon occurs is overwhelming. Researchers and clinicians have been intrigued by this feature of stuttering and have sought to unravel the mystery behind these various fluency-inducing conditions.

As seen in the article by Andrews, Howie, Dozsa, and Guitar at the end of this chapter, some of the more widely accepted explanations for the reduction of stuttering in these novel speaking conditions include a decrease in communicative pressure, distraction of attention away from the stuttering, and reduced complexity in the motor execution of the speech processes. Before we can accept or reject any of these explanations, additional research is needed about the nature of the changes in stutterer's fluency under a variety of novel speaking conditions.

REFERENCES

Adams, M. R. (1988). Five-year retrospective on stuttering theory, research, and therapy: 1982–1987. *Journal of Fluency Disorders, 13*, 399–406.

Attanasio, J. S. (1987). A case of late-onset or acquired stuttering in adult life. *Journal of Fluency Disorders, 12*, 287–290.

Deal, J. L. (1982). Sudden onset of stuttering: A case report. *Journal of Speech and Hearing Disorders, 47*, 301–304.

Kent, R. (1983). Facts about stuttering: Neuropsychologic perspectives. *Journal of Speech and Hearing Disorders, 48*, 249–254.

Kidd, K. K. (1984). Stuttering as a genetic disorder. In R. Curlee & W. Perkins. *Nature and treatment of stuttering: New Directions*. San Diego: College-Hill Press.

Martin, R., & Lindamood, L. (1986). Stuttering and spontaneous recovery: Implications for the speech-language pathologist. *Language, Speech, Hearing Services in Schools, 17*, 207–218.

Yeudall, L. A. (1985). A neuropsychological theory of stuttering. *Seminars in Speech and Hearing, 6*, 197–224.

The Need for an Integrated Perspective on Stuttering

Anne Smith
Christine Weber

In the January/February 1986 issue of the *Journal of Pediatric Ophthalmology and Strabismus*, an article titled "Stuttering as a Complication of Strabismus Surgery" appeared. It was written by Samuel Jones, an ophthalmologist in Kansas City. Two cases were reported in which children developed stuttering following "inappropriate or abusive treatment" by anesthesia departments. Jones stated, "High levels of anxiety can lead to regression in a child's mental development, including stuttering, which is a regression to an earlier speech pattern and failure to develop fluent speech" (p. 38). He suggested that this viewpoint was supported by statements made by a "speech therapist," who reportedly told the family that a frightening experience had probably caused the stuttering.

In considering our perspective on stuttering, we began by asking ourselves this question: how can a physician hold such a naive, uninformed, outdated, and narrow view of stuttering? The answer to that question, we believe, is that speech-language pathologists have not conveyed to other health professionals and the general public a well-reasoned, integrated view of the factors that contribute to the development and maintenance of stuttering. This failure reflects on those of us who do research, develop theories of stuttering, and train speech-language pathologists. We have failed to develop an integrated framework for the investigation of stuttering, and without such a framework, we cannot progress in our attempts to understand this disorder and educate others about it.

Our perspective on stuttering, then, is that there are too many perspectives on stuttering. The student trying to learn about stuttering is faced with lists: lists of facts and lists of theories. Each methodological approach is embedded within its own theory: electroencephalography (EEG) is used to test the notion that stuttering results from aberrant central processing; techniques of behavior modification are applied to stuttering "as a learned behavior"; results of auditory tests are interpreted as evidence that stuttering is a disorder of auditory feedback mechanisms; investigations of laryngeal behavior are used to suggest that the "core" of the disorder is faulty laryngeal control; and studies of the heritability of stuttering imply that it is a "genetic disorder." Each perspective or theory attempts to account for some of the experimental results on stuttering, but none has attempted to account for all of the research findings. Which of these fragmented theories captures students' minds and shapes their thinking about the nature of stuttering and its appropriate treatment will depend on which set of beliefs is held by their professor and what currency each point of view happens to have at the particular time.

The complexity, heterogeneity, and lability of stuttering have provided a fertile base for the proliferation of these diverse, fragmented theories. We would argue, however, that there has been only one essential and central controversy in stuttering: whether stuttering is a physiological or a psychological phenomenon. The debate has raged in many forms. One psychological point of view is embodied in Wendell Johnson's theory that stuttering grows out of listeners' critical responses to the normal disfluencies of early childhood. Other accounts of stuttering typically classified as "psychological" have been derived from learning theory and personality theory. Investigators using physiological measures, on the other hand, whether EEG, electromyography, or measures of laryngeal function, have argued that stuttering is essentially due to faulty physiology.

We are not able here to review all of the theories that fit into the "physiological" versus the "psychological" camps, but refer the reader to a recent article by Wingate (1986), which reviews this controversy. Wingate provides clear evidence that the controversy persists. His central message is that recent literature, particularly in the major journals of the field of stuttering, shows there is a trend toward considering stuttering to reflect some physiological aberration. He further states that this interest in the physiology of stuttering, which had a good start in the first decades of this century, "was subverted within a few years by the rapid development of an alternative interest—the psychological" (p. 49). In other words, Wingate says, the physiological view of stuttering was overtaken by the psychological from about 1920 to

Reprinted from *ASHA, 30*, no. 4, 30–32. Copyright © 1988 American Speech-Language-Hearing Association.

1970, but in recent years physiology has reemerged as champion.

The persistence of the physiological/psychological controversy in stuttering research and theory has impeded progress in developing a truly integrated theory of stuttering. We do not understand why this spurious debate continues because it is derived from a false dichotomy between physiological and psychological factors. Researchers in speech-language pathology have not incorporated into their thinking the fact that psychological factors such as emotions and learning have a physiological substrate. We may analyze different variables, some of which may seem to be more "psychological" and others more "physiological," but these different levels of analysis simply represent different levels of thinking about the same processes.

To illustrate this point, consider an experiment by Wolpaw, Braitman, and Seegal (1983). Using operant conditioning, they trained monkeys to maintain a certain angle of the elbow and a constant level of biceps muscle activity associated with this elbow position. In the first stage of their experiment, monkeys were rewarded with a squirt of juice simply for maintenance of these background conditions. After a period of training in which a consistent background was established, the monkey continued to perform the learned task while pulses were intermittently delivered to displace the arm and elicit a stretch reflex in the biceps. Wolpaw and his colleagues wanted to know if they could change the amplitude of the reflex response of the biceps muscle by rewarding only large reflex responses. Therefore, in the next stage of the experiment, the reflex response amplitude was measured on delivery of each displacement pulse. If it was larger than a criterion value, the monkey received a juice reward. Wolpaw and colleagues found that they could in fact change the reflex response amplitude. After a period of 5 to 10 days, the responses increased significantly and continued to increase over a period of weeks. In addition, when the reward contingency was changed so that only small responses were rewarded, the amplitude change was reversed, making the reflex response consistently smaller than the original response. Because the background muscle activity was always the same, Wolpaw and his colleagues could claim that the changes in reflex amplitude were due to changes in the monosynaptic reflex circuit itself.

This experiment is a convincing demonstration of the plasticity of the nervous system. Here in the most simple neural circuit, a reflex involving a sensory neuron, a motoneuron, and one synapse between them, we can see that learning produced changes in physiology. Wolpaw and his colleagues think the most likely explanation for the reflex amplitude change is either a change at the synapse or a change in the sensitivity of the sensory receptor. For our purposes, this experiment shows that "psychological" variables such as learning and memory have a neural substrate, that even simple neural pathways like reflexes can be altered by environmental conditions. In other words, in this example

change in the physiological processes mediating reflex response amplitude *is* learning. These phenomena cannot be understood within a perspective that dichotomizes learning, a "psychological" process, and physiological variables such as reflex amplitude; nor can stuttering be understood within such a perspective.

We suggest that it is time for those interested in stuttering to move beyond the physiological/psychological controversy and develop an integrated framework for investigating this complex human behavior. Gray's recent book, *The Neuropsychology of Anxiety,* develops an integrated theory of anxiety and its relation to functions of the septo-hippocampal system. Gray synthesizes knowledge derived from many different types of investigations: detailed behavioral studies of the effects of various reward contingencies on anxiety, pharmacological evidence concerning the effects of drugs that reduce anxiety, neuroanatomical mapping of the septo-hippocampal system (part of the limbic system), and neurophysiological studies, ranging from single unit recordings to EEG studies. In addition to reviewing a vast array of experimental evidence, other theories of anxiety and septo-hippocampal function are weighed for their success in accounting for all of the experimental findings. One of Gray's comments could well serve as a model for the integrated framework needed to investigate stuttering: "The theory presented here is truly neuropsychological, not a neural and psychological part glued together merely by statements of identity." An integrated theory of stuttering might be called a psychophysiological theory of stuttering.

What would the "bare bones" of such a theory be? To attempt to answer that question, we present a brief "status report" on stuttering, a summary of the factors that appear to play a significant role in stuttering. First, there is good experimental evidence that there is a genetic predisposition to stutter. In other words, stuttering runs in families. There is also clear evidence that stuttering involves a breakdown in speech motor processes. Even the apparently normal or "fluent" speech of those who stutter appears to be different from the normal speech of those who do not stutter. There is some evidence that people who stutter may have a deficient neural substrate for the performance of motor behaviors. This has been referred to as a reduced capacity for sensorimotor integration, which could be part of the inherited substrate for stuttering to develop. It is not clear whether this is a generalized reduction in sensorimotor organization or whether it is confined to the structures involved in speech production.

Genetic predisposition is an important determining factor in the development of stuttering, but learning and environmental factors also are critical in the development and continuation of stuttering. Fluency can be greatly affected by variables such as the situation in which speech occurs, communicative intent, and listeners' responses. It is also clear that emotional factors, or what we may want to call psychological "state" variables, play an important role in disfluent behavior. From a variety of sources, we know something about the physiological processes that accompany these psychological states, for example, the secretion of adrenal catecholamines during arousal. We know almost nothing about how the physiological processes associated with emotions can affect speech motor performance. In other words, how can emotional arousal contribute to the breakdowns in speech motor behavior that are characteristic of stuttering? This is an area in which research is greatly needed.

Finally, we would like to point out that the arguments presented in this article concerning the need for an integrated approach to research and theory on the nature of stuttering also apply to the practice of stuttering therapy. If stuttering is viewed solely as a psychological phenomenon, one-sided therapies will result, therapies that work only on changing environmental, personality, attitudinal, or emotional factors and ignore the benefit of teaching speech management techniques. If stuttering is viewed narrowly as a "physiological aberration," therapy may erroneously stress only motoric training without considering the client's emotional reactions to disfluency, attitudes about stuttering, or intellectual need to understand stuttering. Individual clients may need different amounts and kinds of effort in each of these realms, because the factors that produce stuttering are not equally weighted for every person who stutters. True, long-lasting success attributable to stuttering therapy is notoriously elusive. Until we have a better understanding of the nature of stuttering, it will be difficult to determine with any certainty the best treatment program for each client. In the meantime, each client will receive better treatment if the speech-language pathologist approaches the disorder with an integrated view of the factors that produce stuttering.

REFERENCES

Gray, J. A. (1982). *The neuropsychology of anxiety: An enquiry into the function of the septo-hippocampal system.* Oxford: Clarendon Press.

Jones, S. T. (1986). Stuttering as a complication of strabismus surgery. *Journal of Pediatric Ophthalmology and Strabismus, 23,* 38–40.

Wingate, M. (1986). Physiological and genetic factors. In Shames, G. H., & Rubin, H., *Stuttering then and now* (pps. 49–69). Columbus, OH: Charles E. Merrill.

Wolpaw, J. R., Braitman, D. J., & Seegal, R. F. (1983). Adaptive plasticity in primate spinal stretch reflex: Initial development. *Journal of Neurophysiology, 50,* 1296–1311.

Stuttering: A Review of Research Findings and Theories Circa 1982

Gavin Andrews
Ashley Craig
Anne-Marie Feyer
Susan Hoddinott
Pauline Howie
Megan Neilson

This paper is a record of a further attempt to discipline the available knowledge on stuttering into journal articles. In 1979 we (Andrews, Guitar, & Howie, 1980) used the empirical meta-analytic technique to organize the treatment literature; for the present task another quasi-empirical technique was developed. Given that there are some thousands of "findings" in the literature about stuttering it was decided to pay attention only to findings that had been replicated. It was considered that these had the most reasonable chance of being "facts," those stubborn, dependable relationships that regularly occur (Cook & Leviton, 1980).

Findings supported by two or more research studies were identified to determine the status of the discovered "fact" according to the following criteria: Class A facts are findings replicated in two or more research centers, there being no negative reports; Class B facts are findings replicated in two or more research centers, but challenged by a minority of conflicting reports; Class C facts are findings replicated by the same research center, there being no conflicting reports; and Class D facts are findings replicated by the same research center but challenged by a minority of conflicting reports. Sometimes when there were considerable numbers of conflicting findings, an attempt was made to account for the conflict, either in terms of insufficient power to reveal a positive association or in terms of the methods used in the experiments. Judgment of research quality is subjective and was not used as an inclusion criterion. Unpublished material is influential and was included when we had copies of the manuscript. These are listed as reference notes. Some areas of investigation are not amenable to experimental replication (e.g., prevalence rates), but in these the reliability of the data increases when a number of estimates return the same finding. In these cases no letter is used to classify the fact but the standard error of the mean (*SEM*) is quoted.

The material to be evaluated was obtained in the following manner. This laboratory has had an active interest in stuttering for 20 years and during that time some 1,500 research reports have been collected from journals, books, dissertations, and conferences. This collection was supplemented from three sources: a Medline search for the years covered by that data base up to July 1982, the bibliography of Bloodstein (1981), and preprints of forthcoming papers. As in any good laboratory, the available data base should be regarded as comprehensive but not exhaustive. Findings which do not appear to have been replicated are not reviewed. Some will have been replicated and we will have missed this; others will undoubtedly be true but must await replication before we will feel confident about them. Confirmed negative findings were usually ignored unless important to a current theoretical issue. In the first four parts of this review the authors have been conservative and not speculative, but above all we have tried to be impartial.

The field of stuttering was divided among the authors, the relevant literature read, and the facts identified then verified by the group of authors. In this paper statements embodying a fact are italicized and the class (see above descriptions) given in parenthesis. The dissenting reports are discussed where relevant. References given were usually selected to cover an early report and a major report. In B and D class facts references to negative findings may be given. Where possible the most recent report is also listed and the set of references given should, when their reference lists are used, allow readers to access the complete literature relevant to the fact. The aim of the review was to provide a guide to the literature for both students and researchers. In order to minimize presentation bias the information is largely organized in accord with the chapter outlines of Bloodstein

Reprinted from *Journal of Speech and Hearing Disorders, 48*, 3 (August 1983), 226–245. Copyright © 1983 American Speech-Language Hearing Association.

(1981) with the exception that discussion of theoretical issues is deferred to Part 5.

PART 1. NATURAL HISTORY: SYMPTOMS, PREVALENCE, INCIDENCE

Stuttering is defined in the International Classification of Diseases as "disorders in the rhythm of speech, in which the individual knows precisely what he wishes to say, but at the time is unable to say it because of an involuntary, repetitive prolongation or cessation of a sound" (World Health Organization, 1977, p. 202). This definition is virtually identical to that of Andrews and Harris (1964) which reads, "because of an involuntary repetition, prolongation or cessation of sound" (p. 1) and is in accord with Wingate's standard definition, in which the key elements of stuttering are repetitions and prolongations of sound and syllable whether audible or silent (Wingate, 1964). While this is not a fact there is a consensus that repetitions and prolongations are necessary and sufficient for the diagnosis of stuttering to be made.

Nonfluencies are a feature of the speech of preschool children. These tend to be word and phrase repetitions, interjections, and revisions. Part-word repetitions and prolongations (sometimes called dysrhythmic phonations) do occur but are less frequent. *In studies of young children's speech, stutterers show many times more part-word repetitions and prolongations than do children not regarded as stutterers* (A) (Johnson, 1955; Mann, 1955). *But this is probably best regarded as a dimensional and not a categorical difference* (B) since, in favor of the dimensional point of view, both Yairi and Clifton (1972) and Westby (1979) have presented profiles of the speech disfluencies of highly disfluent children regarded as normal speakers in which the disfluencies are comparable in frequency and nature to those of some stutterers. Conversely, in favor of stuttering being a category, others (Bjerkan, 1980; Floyd & Perkins, 1974) have found the speech of children regarded as stutterers to be qualitatively or quantitatively distinct from the range of utterances of normally speaking children. When these parameters are explored experimentally *the probability of speech being identified as stuttered depends both on the occurrence of audible prolongations and double unit repetitions and on the outright frequency of repetition or prolongation* (A) (Curran & Hood, 1977; Huffman & Perkins, 1974; Sander, 1961). Listeners can be trained to record the frequency and type of stuttering and intraobserver reliabilities greater than .95 are commonly attained for the total count (usually expressed as a frequency ratio), although reliabilities for individual subtypes of stuttering may be as low as .6 (Howie, 1981b) and agreement on loci of stuttering is also low (Curlee, 1981). *Repetitions are the first signs of stuttering noted in the majority of children* (A) (Andrews & Harris, 1964; Bloodstein, 1960a, b), and the additional speech signs,

accessory movements, and associated features then follow in those children who develop a persistent and severe stutter.

There is information about vocal tract physiology during the moment of stuttering but we could identify no replicated findings, probably because the precise manner of stuttering is unique to each individual. There are facts concerning vocal tract function during ostensibly nonstuttered speech of adult stutterers. Investigations of the rate of transition through a consonant-vowel-consonant (CVC) syllable have returned conflicting results, but it appears that *persistent stutterers' unvoiced plosive to vowel voice onset times are slower than those of nonstutterers* (B) (Agnello, 1975; Hillman & Gilbert, 1977; Metz, Conture, & Caruso, 1979; Zimmermann, 1980a). Furthermore, *segments of speech from normal speakers differ qualitatively from comparable nonstuttered segments of speech from severe untreated stutterers* (B) (Few & Lingwall, 1972; Healey, 1982; Healey & Adams, 1981b; Prosek & Runyan, 1982; Wendahl & Cole, 1961).

The average stutterer begins to stutter without any obvious cause; usually stuttering just develops. It might be helpful to call this idiopathic stuttering and contrast it to acquired stuttering. Acquired stuttering can begin in a previously fluent speaker after brain damage—usually of vascular or traumatic origin. The symptoms can include all those described by Wingate (1964) and the clinical picture can be indistinguishable from idiopathic stuttering. Recovery can occur spontaneously or following treatment for the stutter or even following removal of the focal lesion. *Acquired cases with onset in adult life are well documented* (A) (Donnan, 1979; Helm, Butler, & Benson, 1978; Quinn & Andrews, 1977; Rosenbek, Messert, Collins, & Wertz, 1978; Rosenfield, 1972). Some children undoubtedly acquire their stuttering after brain injury (Bohme, 1968), but as it is difficult to be certain in the individual child, such cases are confused with cases of idiopathic stuttering.

Idiopathic stuttering most commonly begins in childhood. To get information about the frequency of onset at various ages it is necessary either to study a group of children prospectively until an age when the risk of new cases is small, or alternatively, to assess retrospectively a representative sample of older stutterers to ascertain the age at which their stuttering began. Both strategies have been used and yield comparable results: *The vast majority of stutterers begin stuttering somewhere between the onset of speech and puberty, most between 2 and 5, the mean age of onset being about 5, the median about 4* (A) (Andrews & Harris, 1964; Berry, 1938; Meltzer, 1935). Thus, in at least half of the cases, speech development is well underway when stuttering begins. These age-of-onset data also allow calculation of the proportion of the risk of becoming a stutterer that is left behind with each birthday, information which is essential when processing family history and twin data for evidence of genetic transmission. If the varying age of onset is not taken into account in calculating family incidence patterns, then the data will be distorted, because young children who will later begin to stutter will have been confidently classified as nonstutterers. [See Andrews & Harris (1964) for use of this correction.]

There are many studies of the prevalence of stuttering, that is, the percentage of the population actually stuttering at any point in time. Bloodstein (1981) lists 13 studies of U.S. school children (mean prevalence .9%) and 18 studies of non-U.S. school children (mean prevalence 1.1%). These prevalence figures differ, but the differences could be accounted for by the high proportion of U.S. children remaining at school after puberty, because the prevalence seems to be constant from school entry to age 12 and declines slowly thereafter. Both Louttit and Halls (1936) and Andrews and Harris (1964) found the prevalence after puberty to be significantly less (.8%) than the prevalence before puberty, presumably because of the lack of new cases among teenagers and the gradual remission of established cases at this age. There are no prevalence studies of population samples of adults. In summary then, *the prevalence of stuttering in prepubertal school children is 1.0 percent (SEM = .1) but generally drops in postpubertal school children. The prevalence in the unselected adult population is unknown* (Andrews & Harris, 1964; Bloodstein, 1981; Louttit & Halls, 1936).

What is the lifetime risk or incidence of stuttering? If the risk of becoming a stutterer is mostly over by puberty, then estimates of the lifetime risk can be made by prospective studies finishing at puberty or retrospective studies of postpubertal populations. Bloodstein cites eight such studies in which *the mean lifetime expectation of ever being a stutterer was 4.2 percent (SEM = .6%) and the median was 4.9 percent* (Andrews & Harris, 1964; Bloodstein, 1981).

Some stutterers recover spontaneously, others recover after minimal therapy, and others require skilled and time-consuming treatment. Excluding the last category it should be possible to estimate the proportion who get better either spontaneously or with minimal therapy (i.e., <10 hours) by the following equation: Incidence 0–16 years (median 4.9%) minus prevalence at 16 (.8%) should equal the proportion recovered by 16 (4.9% − .8% = 4.1%). Thus 4.1/4.9 percent or 84 percent of children who have ever stuttered will have recovered by 16. Studies of recovery confirm such a figure. There are four retrospective studies of selected young adult populations (Bloodstein, 1981, p. 87); the percent reporting recovery vary from 60 to 82 percent, mean 71 percent. Of course, such studies are likely to be flawed by problems of selection and accuracy of recall. A better method of estimating the extent of recovery is to see a group of children who are stuttering and then review them a number of years later and discover how many still stutter. There is one prospective study that followed an unselected sample of children from onset to 15 years and found that 79 percent of the children no longer stuttered (Andrews & Harris, 1964). There are five other studies (Byrne, 1931; Fritzell, 1976; Johnson, 1955, two studies; Panelli, McFarlane, & Shipley, 1978) which have followed selected groups of children for

varying periods of time. In each instance we compared their data to those for age-matched children drawn from the Andrews and Harris study. There was no significant difference between the recovery rate calculated from these five reports (mean 49.6%) and the recovery rate found in the Andrews and Harris age-matched children (mean 50.4%) even though the recovery rate varied from a low of 23 percent to a high of 80 percent depending on the age span studied. Taken together these six prospective studies form a solid basis for estimating the probability of recovery. *Recovery in school-age children is common; the best estimate of the probability of recovery by 16 years is 78 percent (SEM = 4%).*

The above estimate of 78 percent is a cumulative figure and therapists need guidance when they see a child of a particular age group. When the probability of recovery is related to age the following data emerge as conservative estimates: At 16 years 75 percent of those stuttering at age 4 will be better, as will 50 percent of those stuttering at age 6 and 25 percent of those stuttering at age 10. These data are also of some value when counseling parents about the importance of treatment for the school-age child. There is one more important corollary to be derived from these data. If three quarters of those who begin to stutter recover by 16, then studies of differences between adult stutterers and nonstutterers may actually be studies of attributes that have inhibited the expected recovery, and not necessarily of attributes related to becoming a stutterer. It is important to realize that any attribute associated with persistent stuttering may not explain why one stutters, only why one did not recover. In other words, an attribute may be both a causative and a maintaining factor.

Three times as many boys as girls stutter and this disproportion increases with age (B) (Andrews & Harris, 1964; Bloodstein, 1981). As the age of onset appears to be the same for both sexes (Andrews & Harris, 1964), then it follows that girls must recover more quickly, and indeed recent evidence presented by Seider, Gladstien, and Kidd (in press) lends weight to this deduction. This suggests that environmental or genetic attributes which inhibit recovery should be more evident in the few women who continue to stutter.

Environmental factors can affect an organism at any time from conception to death. For example, thalidomide, clearly an environmental agent, produced abnormalities which were congenital but not inherited. Environmental factors are of great interest for they could both cause stuttering and inhibit its remission, thereby causing the stuttering to persist. Conversely, environmental factors could prevent stuttering occurring even in predisposed persons, or they could aid in remission. Perinatal brain damage is the only environmental event likely to be a cause of some idiopathic stuttering because it is associated with *epilepsy, cerebral palsy, and other neurological syndromes associated with higher-than-expected prevalence of stuttering* (B) (Bohme, 1968; Gens, 1950; Heltman & Peacher, 1943;

Ingram, 1963); conversely, *deafness is the only condition associated with a reduced prevalence of stuttering* (A) (Backus, 1938; Harms & Malone, 1939). There are no other established facts about the more obvious features in a stutterer's environment that might point to the cause or maintenance of stuttering, be they family structure, race, socio-cultural factors, or parental characteristics. Stutterers appear to come from the same environment as do nonstutterers, with one exception; they come from families with an excess of stuttering relatives.

There are seven studies which show that *the risk of stuttering among first-degree relatives of stutterers is more than three times the population risk* (A) (see Andrews & Harris, 1964; Johnson, 1959; Kidd, 1980). Both environmental and genetic explanations have been proposed to account for this fact; but whereas the environmental proposals are not supported by data, the genetic proposals are supported because the *risk of the relative stuttering varies by sex of relative and sex of proband* (A) (Andrews & Harris, 1964; Kidd, 1980). Male relatives of female stutterers are at greatest risk, having four times the risk of stuttering that female relatives of male stutterers have, and the other combinations occupy intermediate positions. This variation in risk can be accounted for by genetic models, but no environmental model has as yet been proposed that could account for these data. These data are valuable when a stutterer asks about the probability of his or her children becoming stutterers. By pooling the data from 725 families covered by the Andrews and Harris and the Kidd studies, the following risks emerge as the best estimates. For men who ever stuttered, 9 percent of their daughters and 22 percent of their sons will be stutterers; while for the fewer women who ever stuttered the risks are higher, as 17 percent of their daughters and 36 percent of their sons will be affected.

Twin studies have shown that monozygotic twins have a higher concordance for stuttering than do dizygotic same-sexed twins (B) (Howie, 1981a; Nelson, Hunter, & Walter, 1945). Another way of assessing the strength of a genetic relationship is to compare the corrected risk of stuttering in relatives of the index stutterer. If one pools the data from Howie (1981a), Kidd (1980), and Andrews and Harris (1964), a monozygotic co-twin has an estimated 77 percent chance of being a stutterer, a dizygotic same-sexed co-twin has a 32 percent chance of being a stutterer, while a same-sexed sibling has an 18 percent chance of being a stutterer. There is no simple way of accounting for these data on a nongenetic basis. Nevertheless, *discordant monozygotic twin pairs exist in whom zygosity determination has been precise* (A) (Godai, Tatarelli, & Bonanni, 1976; Howie, 1981a). Therefore, as genetically identical twins who are discordant for stuttering exist, then pre- or postnatal environmental factors must be important in some stutterers. Environmental factors have been looked for in discordant monozygotic twins, but as yet none has been identified.

Two models, the single major locus model and the multifactorial model, both including sex limitation, have been found to fit the familial risk data precisely (Kidd, 1980). Decisions that a certain condition is genetically determined are probability decisions based on the goodness of fit of specific models which may contain environmental parameters. On the basis of the established data the probability is high that the predisposition to stutter is controlled by genetic factors. It is interesting to speculate on what could be inherited. There are very few clues; even the *severity of stuttering is not related to the extent of the family history of stuttering* (B) (Andrews & Harris, 1964; Jameson, 1955; Kidd, Heimbuch, Records, Oehlert, & Webster, 1980).

PART 2. STUTTERER–NONSTUTTERER DIFFERENCES

Following Bloodstein's pattern we must next look at data on how stutterers differ from nonstutterers, bearing in mind that differences, if they are to be contributive in a causative sense, should be evident before or when the child begins to stutter. Differences found only in adults may simply be other evidence of factors inhibiting remission or even differences which are consequences of stuttering for a number of years.

Intelligence

There are four controlled investigations of samples of school children. *When stutterers (mean age 10) are compared with nonstutterers they are found to score significantly (half a standard deviation) lower on intelligence tests than nonstutterers* (A) (Andrews & Harris, 1964, 2 studies; Okasha, Bishry, Kamel, & Hassan, 1974; Schindler, 1955). This deficit is evident in both verbal and nonverbal intelligence tests and is unlikely to be due to performance on the tests being depressed by difficulties in communication because of stuttering. This appears to be a valid difference, not an artifact of test anxiety (Andrews & Harris, 1964), so two predictions can be derived. First, stutterers should show evidence of more educational difficulties than their classmates. *They do lag some 6 months behind their peers educationally* (A) (Conradi, 1912; Darley, 1955; McAllister, 1937; Schindler, 1955). Second, a half standard deviation reduction in intelligence in a disability group should mean that the prevalence of the disability under study would increase threefold in mentally retarded children. *The median prevalence of stuttering in mentally retarded children in the studies cited by Bloodstein (1981) is 3 percent.* In contrast, the intelligence and social class of stutterers in treatment is often found to be above average (Andrews & Harris, 1964; Cox, 1982). This finding may represent the influence of intelligence and social class on access to health care.

Personality Factors

When researchers used to consider stuttering a symptom of emotional disorder in childhood, there was considerable evidence collected about stutterers' personality attributes and their propensity to show anxiety or neurotic symptoms. *No differences in personality factors related to neuroticism have been demonstrated in controlled studies of unselected populations* (A). This conclusion is based on tests with the *Sarason General Anxiety Scale for Children* (Andrews & Harris, 1964), *Structured Psychiatric Interview* (Andrews & Harris, 1964), *Eysenck Personality Inventory* (Hegde, 1972), *California Test of Personality* (Prins, 1972), *Minnesota Multiphasic Personality Inventory* (Horlick & Miller, 1960; Lanyon, Goldsworthy, & Lanyon, 1978; Pizzat, 1951), and *Speilberger Anxiety Scales* (Molt & Guilford, 1979; Zenner & Shepherd, Note 1*). *Stutterers do show more difficulties than nonstutterers with social adjustment* (A) (Brown & Hull, 1942; Prins, 1972; Wingate, 1962), but this finding is probably a consequence rather than a cause of stuttering.

Speech and Language Development

If one were looking for stutterer-nonstutterer differences, logically one would begin by looking at speech development. *Stutterers are late in passing their speech milestones* (B). There are six positive studies (Andrews & Harris, 1964, two studies; Berry, 1938; Darley, 1955; Johnson, 1959; Morley, 1957), and one negative study (Johnson, 1955). The extent of the delay is probably about 6 months. This delayed acquisition of language is also reflected in performance on tests of language proficiency at a later age. There are eight studies that have shown that *stutterers perform more poorly than nonstutterers on some tests of language: the Peabody Picture Vocabulary Test, length and complexity of utterance, and some Illinois Test of Psycholinguistic Ability subtests* (A) (Murray & Reed, 1977; Perozzi & Kunze, 1969; Silverman & Williams, 1967; Stocker & Parker, 1977; Wall, 1980; Westby, 1979; Williams & Marks, 1972; Kline & Starkweather, Note 2). It would have been helpful if the effects of intelligence had been shown to be independent before drawing the conclusion that poorer language skills in these tests were a separate entity. Similar language skill defects have been reported in highly disfluent nonstuttering children (Westby, 1979).

There have been seven studies which found *stutterers to show three times greater risk of articulation disorder than nonstutterers* (B) (Andrews & Harris, 1964, 2 studies; Darley, 1955; Johnson, 1959; Morley, 1957; Schindler, 1955; Williams & Silverman, 1968). The only negative study is McDowell (1928). This threefold difference appears whether the child's speech is examined directly by a speech-language pathologist or whether one merely relies on parental report. The articulation defect usually antedates the stutter and is independent of age of onset of stuttering. In only one study (Andrews & Harris, 1964) have intelligence, speech development, and articulation proficiency been measured on

the same children; they were found to be independent of one another.

A recent survey of practicing speech-language pathologists supports these research findings. They reported that in elementary school stutterers in treatment, emotional disturbance was rare (2%), reading (6%) and learning (7%) difficulties were evident, but the most frequent concomitant problems were articulation (16%) and language disorder (10%) (Blood & Seider, 1981).

Electroencephalography

If stutterers have abnormalities in their speech system independent of intelligence, then it is important to decide where these hypothesized abnormalities reside. Electroencephalographic (EEG) studies have a long pedigree in stuttering research and an excess of abnormal findings should be evident, if only because stuttering is more common in persons with brain damage; yet the evidence remains equivocal. Andrews and Harris (1964), and Okasha, Moneim, Bishry, Kamel, & Moustafa (1974) conducted examinations of population samples of nonstutterers and stutterers; the first found no excess of abnormalities among the stutterers, while the second did. Sayles (1971) and Graham (1966) conducted blind controlled trials on samples of convenience which are unlikely to be representative. The findings of these studies were conflicting.

Laterality

An excess of EEG abnormalities would tell us nothing about the nature of stuttering, so more specific investigations are necessary. Speech centers reside in the left hemisphere in most persons. Is there any evidence that idiopathic stutterers have poorly lateralized speech centers? There are no facts in regard to handedness, and none in regard to laterality and EEG, evoked cortical potentials, brain-stem evoked responses, contingent negative variation, or tests of central auditory function. Actually, the most reliable index of speech laterality, the Wada intracarotid sodium amytal test, has generated a fact: *All six idiopathic stutterers who were tested had unilateral speech centers; all five stutterers with organic brain lesions showed bilateral representation* (A) (Andrews, Quinn, & Sorby, 1972; Jones, 1966; Luessenhop, Boggs, Laborwit, & Walle, 1973).

Moore and his group (Moore, Craven, & Faber, 1982; Moore & Haynes, 1980; Moore & Lang, 1977; Moore & Lorendo, 1980) have replicated evidence that *stutterers show more right hemispheric alpha suppression during speech-related tasks than do nonstutterers* (D); but Pinsky and McAdam (1980) are in disagreement, although their sample was small. Moore and his colleagues (Moore, 1976; Hand & Haynes, Note 3) used the half field visual reaction time paradigm to demonstrate that *stutterers are more inclined than normals to process linguistic material in the right hemisphere* (C). This work is interesting and there is an

---

*Notes refer to unpublished sources. See end of article for full documentation.

urgent need for an independent group to replicate these findings.

The dichotic listening test has also been proposed as a test related to cerebral dominance for speech. Differences in speech lateralization between groups of stutterers and nonstutterers have been sought in 22 studies. In nine studies (Brady & Berson, 1975; Curry & Gregory, 1969; Sommers, Brady, & Moore, 1975; Davenport, Note 4; Mattingly, Note 5; Perrin & Eisenson, Note 6; Ponsford, Note 7; Prins & Walton, Note 8; Strong, Note 9) only three of which have been published, a significant difference has been found; but in 13 studies (Dorman & Porter, 1975; Gruber & Powell, 1974; Liebetrau & Daly, 1981; Pinsky & McAdam, 1980; Quinn, 1972, 1976; Rosenfield & Goodglass, 1980; Slorach & Noehr, 1973; Sussman & MacNeilage, 1975; Barrett, Keith, Agnello, & Weiler, Note 10; Cerf & Prins, Note 11; McNeil & Athen, Note 12; Phelps, Note 13), of which nine have been published and whose methodology was superior to the three published positive studies, no significant group differences were found. There is, therefore, no fact. Yet, in many of the negative studies there has been a tendency for some individual stutterers to produce reduced laterality scores. This could well be due to a small proportion of acquired stutterers masquerading as idiopathic stutterers.

Central Auditory Functioning

Tests of central auditory function show that *stutterers are poorer at recognition/recall of competing messages but do not show differences concerning the hemispheric laterality of this deficit* (B). Statistically significant group differences have been reported with the *Synthetic Sentence Identification of an Ipsilateral Competing Message* by Toscher and Rupp (1978) and Molt and Guilford (1979); Hall and Jerger (1978) reported likewise, but without statistical test. Hannley and Dorman (1982) did not find this difference in treated stutterers. Barrett et al. (Note 10) found stutterers to be significantly poorer at word/syllable identification when the competition was dichotic (*Staggered Spondaic Word Test* and dichotic consonant vowel syllable). The latter finding was confirmed by Rosenfield and Goodglass (1980). Because dichotic studies have focused on the laterality issue, differences in the percent of stimuli recognized have typically not been examined; but in seven out of eight studies where methodology and data report allowed us to ascertain mean identification rates, there was a trend, sometimes substantial (Pinsky & McAdam, 1980; Sussman & MacNeilage, 1975) for stutterers to be less successful at recognizing and recalling the stimulus words. Moreover, Stocker and Parker (1977) in a related paradigm found stutterers to have difficulties in auditory recall of linguistic material. Quite independent of this, but related to hearing, MacCulloch and Eaton (1971) and Brown, Sambrooks, and MacCulloch (1975) found that *stutterers had reduced pain thresholds for intense auditory stimulation* (C).

Sensory-Motor Performance

In recent years, however, it is tests of sensory-motor performance that have been of most interest. Adams and Hayden (1976), exploring parameters of vocalization control, found stutterers to be slower in the onset and offset of voice in response to a tone. Since then there have been many examinations of auditory voice reaction time (Adams & Hayden, 1976; Cross & Luper, 1979, three findings; Cross, Shadden, & Luper, 1979; Cullinan & Springer, 1980; McFarlane & Shipley, 1981; Murphy & Baumgartner, 1981; Prosek, Montgomery, Walden, & Schwartz, 1979; Reich, Till, Goldsmith, & Prins, 1981; Venkatagiri, 1981, 1982; Cross & Cooke, Note 14; Lewis, Ingham, & Gervens, Note 15; Starkweather, Franklin, & Smigo, Note 16; Watson & Alfonso, Note 17). *Ten of these showed differences in auditory voice reaction time and six did not* (B). There have been seven examinations of voice reaction time to visual stimuli (McFarlane & Shipley, 1981; Prosek et al., 1979; Starkweather, Hirschman, & Tannenbaum, 1976; Cross & Cooke, Note 14; Lewis et al., Note 15; Watson & Alfonso, Note 17; Adler & Starkweather, Note 18); *in five of these stutterers were slower* (B). Similarly, in the case of auditory-manual reaction time, there are *six reports of slower performance in stutterers* (B) (Cross & Cooke, Note 14; Starkweather et al., Note 16; Cross, Note 19; Cross, Note 20) and two studies which find no difference (Prosek et al., 1979; Reich et al., 1981). There is, as yet, insufficient evidence regarding visual-manual reaction time. In each of the three reaction time paradigms for which data do exist, a consistent pattern emerges: About two-thirds of studies report stutterer-nonstutterer differences. Some of the negative reports are explicable in terms of inadequate power due to small sample sizes. Power issues may also account for the lack of resolution of the questions of stutterer-nonstutterer differences in variability of reaction times, and about the point in the test sequence at which optimal performance is reached.

However, consistently negative results obtained in reaction time research in our laboratory led us to approach this area with caution. We are at present preparing for publication reports of three studies using a variety of reaction time paradigms and comparing adult stutterers with controls matched for age, sex, and occupational status. In the first study we compared nine stutterers and nine controls on an auditory discrimination reaction time task using pure tones varying in frequency, and including both finger press and voice (/ ə /) conditions. The second study, which compared 13 stutterers and 13 controls, replicated the previous discrimination reaction time task and added simple finger and voice reaction time tasks to pure-tone stimuli, as well as comparing short and long stimulus durations. The third study replicated the auditory voice onset/offset paradigms used by Adams and Hayden (1976) and Lewis et al. (Note 15) with 20 stutterers and 20 controls. In none of these studies have we been able to demonstrate a significant reaction time deficit in our stutterers. All three studies employed computer methods of generating stimuli, randomizing interstimulus interval durations and target-nontarget ratios, and measuring reaction time latencies, and we are satisfied that power was adequate in at least the latter two studies. The extent of conflict in the reaction time results presently available suggests to us that the relationships involved are complex. Since this is currently an active research area, the facts detailed above may well change.

Reaction times are crude analogs of the constraints underlying the control of speech production, which is inherently a dynamic task. So it is of interest that *in a pursuit auditory-motor tracking task stutterers lag behind nonstutterers in generating a coherent response* (C). This difference in response times, based on the tracking performance of 12 stutterers and 12 controls (Neilson & Neilson, Note 21; Neilson, in press) was demonstrated using two different forms of tracking stimuli—short stimuli modeled on those used by Sussman and MacNeilage (1975) and a longer stimulus designed to give more precise tracking response characteristics. A replication study of similar size has recently been completed in these laboratories using only the longer stimulus. Methodology was precisely as before, with the exception that the subjects were allowed only minimal practice and did not have to reach a performance criterion before doing the test proper. Again, the mean response time of the stuttering group was significantly slower, but, contrary to expectation, the effect size of this difference was diminished rather than enhanced by the lack of practice.

To summarize the essential stutterer-nonstutterer differences: There is robust evidence that stutterers as a group differ in IQ distribution, are late and poor talkers, have difficulties in stimulus recognition/recall in complex auditory tasks, and lag in tests of sensory-motor response. It should be remembered, however, that an individual stutterer may show none of these differences.

PART 3. VARIABILITY OF STUTTERING

As in Part 2 all the data presented concern the behaviors of groups of stutterers.

Variation by Time

Stuttering is supposed to be variable; but in six studies with adults, *when frequency was measured 3 to 17 months apart prior to treatment, no significant difference was found between initial and repeated measurements* (B) (see Andrews & Harvey, 1981). Of course, for each individual fluency varies as does proficiency with any skilled act, but it seems that most mild stutterers will be mild tomorrow and next year, and most severe stutterers will be likewise.

Variation by Situation

For individuals, stuttering may vary from situation to situation; but in groups of adults *stuttering frequency does not vary significantly when speaking or reading to one person, speaking with a number of persons, and speaking on the telephone* (B) (Andrews & Harvey, 1981; Blood & Hood, 1978; Boberg, 1976; Boberg & Sawyer, 1977; Resick, Wendiggensen, Ames, & Meyer, 1978). It is important to realize that these situations are representative of everyday speech situations. *In an analog experiment the frequency of stuttering has been shown to increase when reading to an audience of increasing size* (A) (Porter, 1939; Siegel & Haugen, 1964), but this is not a situation encountered in real life.

Variation by Language Factors

More than 90 percent of stuttering occurs on the initial syllable of the utterance (Hahn, 1942; Johnson & Brown, 1935). *Words starting with consonants, words early in a sentence, and longer words are all more likely to be stuttered* (A) (Brown, 1937, 1945; St. Louis, 1979; Taylor, 1966). All these conditions have been claimed to describe words of more, rather than less uncertainty, uncertainty being defined as the predictability of the occurrence of a particular word, given the context. This situation appears similar to the conditions which determine the locus of hesitations in normal speech (see Soderberg, 1967, 1971).

Special Conditions Which Immediately Eliminate the Stutter

There has always been interest in conditions under which stuttering is reduced or absent. *In seven conditions, chorus reading* (A) (Adams & Ramig, 1980; Andrews, Howie, Dozsa, & Guitar, 1982; Ingham & Packman, 1979; Johnson & Rosen, 1937), *lipped speech* (A) (Commodore & Cooper, 1978; Perkins, Rudas, Johnson, & Bell, 1976), *prolonged speech and DAF* (A) (Andrews et al., 1982; Goldiamond, 1965), *rhythmic speech* (A) (Andrews et al., 1982; Johnson & Rosen, 1937; Martin & Haroldson, 1979; Perkins, Bell, Johnson, & Stocks, 1979), *shadowing* (A) (Andrews et al., 1982; Cherry & Sayers, 1956), *singing* (A) (Andrews et al., 1982; Witt, 1925), *and slowed speech* (B) Andrews et al., 1982; Johnson & Rosen, 1937), *the frequency of stuttering is reduced by 90 to 100 percent*.

In four of these conditions, facts concerning associated changes in other speech parameters have been established. *In chorus reading the reading rate can increase* (C) (Ingham & Carroll, 1977; Ingham & Packman, 1979), in part because of the nature of the task and in part as a secondary effect of the absence of stuttering. *In rhythmic speech there is an increase in segment duration* (A) (Andrews et al., 1982; Klich & May, 1982; Perkins et al., 1979), *but the reduction in frequency is not dependent on changed vocal level* (C) (Brayton & Conture, 1978; Conture & Metz, Note 22), *or modality of stimulation* (A) (Brady, 1969; Conture & Metz, Note 22), *or slowed overall speech rate* (A) (Brady, 1969; Fransella & Beech, 1965; Hanna & Morris, 1977). *In singing there is an increase in duration of voiced segments* (C)

(Colcord & Adams, 1979; Healey, Mallard, & Adams, 1976). *In slowed speech there is an increase in pause time* (A) (Andrews et al., 1982; Healey & Adams, 1981a), and *in prolonged speech/DAF there is an increase in fundamental frequency* (A) (Lechner, 1979; Soderberg, Note 23) *and an increase in segment duration* (A) (Andrews et al., 1982; Perkins et al., 1979; Wingate, 1969; Soderberg, Note 23).

Special Conditions Which Gradually Eliminate the Stutter

In the seven previous conditions the reduction in stuttering is immediate. *In response-contingent stimulation of stuttering, regardless of the motivational system subserving the stimulation, the frequency of stuttering is progressively reduced and can reach zero* (A) (Andrews, 1974; Andrews et al., 1982; Ingham & Andrews, 1973; James, 1981; Martin & Haroldson, 1982; Siegel, 1970). The reduction can occur without alteration in the fluent speech rate (syllables per minute of fluent speech) although the usual measure of speech rate (syllables per minute of speech) will show an increase because of the reduction of stuttering. *Identical noncontingent stimulation in experimentally naive subjects produces no change in the frequency of stuttering* (A) (Ingham & Andrews, 1973; Lanyon & Barocas, 1975). Biggs and Sheehan (1969) also explored this issue but their findings may have been confounded by the masking properties of their stimulus.

Special Conditions Which Immediately Reduce the Stutter

In six conditions the frequency of stuttering is reduced by 50 to 80 percent: speaking alone (A) (Hood, 1975; Porter, 1939; Quinn, 1971), *speaking in time to rhythmic movement* (A) (Andrews et al., 1982; Barber, 1939; Johnson & Rosen, 1937), *delayed auditory feedback of 50–150 msec* (A) (Burke, 1975; Soderberg, Note 23), *masking* (B) (Cherry & Sayers, 1956; Garber & Martin, 1977), *change in pitch* (A) (Johnson & Rosen, 1937; Ramig & Adams, 1980), *whispering* (A) (Bruce & Adams, 1978; Cherry & Sayers, 1956; Commodore & Cooper, 1978; May & Hackwood, 1968; Perkins et al., 1976). *The change in masking is independent of vocal level* (B) (Anthony, 1968; Cherry & Sayers, 1956; Garber & Martin, 1977), *although this normally increases* (A) (Adams & Moore, 1972; Brayton & Conture, 1978; Garber & Martin, 1977), *as does the fundamental frequency* (A) (Brayton & Conture, 1978; Lechner, 1979).

Special Conditions Which Gradually Reduce the Stutter

In two conditions, haloperidol (Burns, Brady, & Kuruvilla, 1978; Quinn & Peachey, 1973) *and EMG feedback from speech muscles* (Craig & Cleary, 1982; Guitar, 1975; Lanyon, 1977), *the frequency of stuttering decreases progressively but is not eliminated* (A). There are no data on other changes in speech associated with these reductions. *In the adaptation condition a temporary reduction of up to 50 percent of the baseline frequency of stuttering occurs when the same material is read aloud repeatedly* (A) (Bruce & Adams, 1978; Johnson & Knott, 1937). *Some reduction in stuttering is evident in repeated episodes of self-formulated speech* (B) (Bloom & Silverman, 1973; Kroll & Hood, 1974; Rousey, 1958). *The percent reduction is less in severe stutterers than mild stutterers* (A) (Bloom & Silverman, 1973; Siegel & Haugen, 1964; Shulman, 1955). *The full adaptation effect does not carry across whispered reading trials to audible reading* (A) (Brenner, Perkins, & Soderberg, 1972; Bruce & Adams, 1978), *and also does not continue when there is uncertainty about the task* (A) (Kroll & Hood, 1976; Wingate, 1972).

PART 4. TREATMENT

We recently used the empirical meta-analytic technique to review studies of the treatment of stuttering (Andrews, Guitar, & Howie, 1980). These were mainly in adults, but did include some children. We concluded that five treatments (prolonged speech, precision fluency shaping, rhythmic speech, airflow therapy, and attitude change) had been demonstrated to produce significant benefits. For reasons discussed therein, rhythmic speech was not a treatment to be preferred. More recent data have also made it less likely that the airflow techniques on their own, taught over a short term, can confer a long-lasting benefit (Andrews & Tanner, 1982a, 1982b; Ladouceur, Cote, Leblond, & Bouchard, 1982).

When treatments do not result in demonstrable benefit, researchers often lose interest in completing the study, or if completed, editors become reluctant to publish. If treatment is genuinely of no benefit, then the published reports of benefit may only represent the few false positive findings, the mass of true negative findings remaining unpublished. Rosenthal (1979) has suggested a means for examining this problem and estimating the number of unpublished null results which would be required to gainsay the published studies. When Rosenthal's formula is applied to the attitude studies, it is clear that only six null results would overthrow the tentative meta-analytic finding that attitude therapy is of benefit. Bearing in mind the wide range of clinicians who have over the years attempted to benefit stutterers by the use of attitude therapy, it does seem likely that at least six unpublished null results exist; therefore, we conclude that attitude therapy is unlikely to be of benefit. One problem implicit in the meta-analysis was that only studies which reported outcome data in terms that allowed calculation or estimation of mean and standard deviation could be coded. Hence studies using either response-contingent time-out techniques or language retraining strategies could not be included (Costello, 1975; Martin, Kuhl, & Haroldson, 1972; Ryan, 1974; Stocker & Upsrich, 1976).

For the present review an additional strategy seemed to be required to examine the apparently successful therapies. Bloodstein (1981, p. 386) listed 11 tests that he and others had felt ought to be satisfied before a treatment could be considered successful. In brief, these tests required a treatment to be successful with a wide range of stutterers when measured objectively, repeatedly, and unexpectedly across nonclinic situations over a period of 1 to 2 years. In addition, speech should sound natural, abnormal speech attitudes should be normalized, and the results should not be invalidated by either excessive dropouts from treatment or the effects of spontaneous remission. Finally, treatments should continue to be effective when used in different clinics and when conducted by different therapists as part of their routine service role.

Using these criteria only *the prolonged speech and precision fluency shaping strategies have reported sufficient data to meet the majority of these requirements*. If we rely on the reports of these procedures analyzed by Andrews et al. (1980) the following profile emerges. Data on more than 150 subjects have been reported for both treatments. These subjects, both adolescents and adults, have had their speech assessed by reliable and objective techniques on a number of occasions from the end of treatment to 18 months or more later. In addition, evidence has been presented that speech attitudes change towards normality. Further, it is unlikely that either regression to the mean or an excessive drop-out rate could invalidate these claims. As comparable reports on both treatments have come from a number of clinics, and it is clear that both treatments are in routine service use, it is unlikely that the later reports of benefit are due to the halo that surrounds a new treatment, or the charisma associated with a particular clinician (see Andrews et al., 1980, for relevant references).

What, then, are the problems? In both treatments a long period of time is spent in training subjects to speak in a different way—controlled rate, gentle onset of utterance, and continuous phonation with correct juncturing. The amount of training in this new speech technique seems important, for Andrews et al. (1980) showed hours of therapy to be the single best predictor of outcome. When these targets have been achieved within the clinic, each subject undertakes a series of planned speech assignments outside the clinic. In these assignments and initially in most everyday situations, subjects are required to consciously speak in the desired fashion. They will thus be fluent by design rather than automatically. This raises an assessment problem, for if they can be fluent by design, surely posttreatment assessments could be contaminated by this problem and relapse might well be evident especially when their speech is assessed unexpectedly or without their knowledge. However, proponents of the prolonged speech technique have produced evidence that *immediately after treatment overt/covert differences are evident, but 6 to 27 months after treatment the frequency of residual stuttering is not significantly different whether subjects are assessed overtly or covertly* (A) (An-

drews & Craig, 1982; Howie, Woods, & Andrews, 1982; Ingham, 1975). No such data have been produced concerning the posttreatment assessment of subjects treated by the precision fluency shaping technique.

Both techniques appear to produce considerable reduction in stuttering. The average subject, who originally stuttered on some 14 percent of his or her syllables, stutters on only 1 to 2 percent 18 months to 2 years after treatment. This is the average result, and while some subjects are never heard to stutter, most still regard themselves as stutterers who are now able to speak fluently. However, by 2 years some subjects will have relapsed and again be in need of treatment (Howie, Tanner, & Andrews, 1981). *Both programs can produce subjects whose treated speech is sufficiently natural that they can pass as normal speakers* (A) (Frayne, Coates, & Marriner, 1977; Hames & Runyan, Note 24), although *in the more rigorous paired-choice paradigm both naive and trained listeners can detect, more often than would be predicted by chance, which person is the treated stutterer and which the always normal speaker* (A) (Runyan & Adams, 1978, 1979), so residual differences obviously persist in the speech of some subjects.

There is one further, and to us, very disturbing fact. *The speech-language pathology profession entertains negative views about stutterers as persons and holds pessimistic views about the benefits of therapy* (A) (Ragsdale & Ashby, 1982; St. Louis & Lass, 1981; Woods & Williams, 1976; Yairi & Williams, 1970). This research refers to the U.S. speech-language pathology profession, but it is our impression that speech-language pathologists in England, Canada, and Australia have similar views. For 20 years there has been good evidence that stutterers, as people, are no different from anybody else. For 10 years there has been good evidence that a planned and disciplined approach to therapy is effective. Yet these negative stereotypes persist, unsupported by empirical evidence. The authors of this review are neither stutterers nor speech-language pathologists and are at a loss to understand how such negative stereotypes can continue to be believed. We can only surmise that some academics who teach speech-language pathologists have not assimilated the new knowledge and have continued to teach the diagnosogenic/mental health approach to stuttering that was current 30 years ago.

PART 5. THEORIES

The previous sections were based on empirical evidence. The reader should be warned that this section contains opinions, for it represents an explicit statement as to how we view the data. It might be helpful if we briefly recapitulate the findings which theoretical explanations should encompass.

In Part 1 we established that idiopathic stuttering begins sometime between the onset of speech and puberty, median age 4 years. It usually begins with the occurrence of repetitions which, together with prolongations, are necessary and sufficient for the disorder to be diagnosed. Other speech symptoms and associated movements and avoidance behaviors appear later in some children. In severe stutterers even the speech between stutters is judged to be abnormal.

The prevalence is about 1 percent until puberty but it then falls to about .8 percent at the age of 16. Estimates of the risk of ever stuttering vary around a median of 4.9 percent. About three quarters of children recover by the age of 16. Three times as many boys as girls stutter and this proportion increases with age. In children and adults, stuttering can be acquired after brain damage, hence the increased prevalence in persons with cerebral palsy, epilepsy, and other neurological conditions. Stutterers come from families in which there is an increased risk of first degree relatives themselves being stutterers. The risk to these relatives varies by sex of relative and sex of proband, and as an indication of the magnitude of the genetic effect the risk of stuttering in a monozygotic co-twin is nearly 80 percent. These data are consistent with the inheritance of stuttering in the majority of cases although severity of stuttering itself does not appear to be inherited. As discordant monozygotic twins exist, environmental factors must play some part. Acquired brain damage is the only environmental factor that has so far been conclusively demonstrated.

In Part 2 a number of differences between groups of stutterers and nonstutterers were described. Stutterers score half a standard deviation lower on tests of intelligence. There are two corollaries to this finding: They show half a year school grade disadvantage and the prevalence in educationally subnormal children is tripled. Stutterers and their parents are just as, and no more, neurotic than nonstutterers. Stutterers are more likely to be delayed in speech development, perform less well on language tests, and show articulation disorders independent of their stuttering.

Many comparisons of neurological function have been performed. There are no established differences concerning laterality when measured by handedness, dichotic word test, or intracarotid sodium amytal although there is increased right-hemisphere alpha suppression during speech-related tasks. Stutterers perform less well on tests of central auditory function and show reduced auditory pain thresholds. Stutterers are slower in auditory and visual voice reaction times and in auditory-motor pursuit tracking tasks.

Some of these differences, like late and poor talking, may be primarily associated with stuttering; others such as the intelligence deficit may be associated with factors inhibiting recovery; and others like the reaction-time deficits could even be associated, not with stuttering per se, but with the articulation and learning difficulties which are themselves directly associated with being a persistent stutterer (see Cullinan & Springer, 1980). If 75 percent of stutterers recover, then many of these differences may be attributes which cause stuttering to persist, unless they have been shown to be evident in preschool stutterers, in which case a primary association with stuttering would seem likely. Apart from the evidence concerning late and poor talking, most of

these data are derived from comparisons of stutterers older than 5. Obviously there are problems in testing younger children in these complex ways, but it does need to be done.

Part 3 focused on factors which vary the frequency of stuttering. There are no systematic variations by time or by ordinary situations. Stuttering is more likely to occur when reading to an audience of increasing size and is more likely on the initial sound of a word and on words of greater uncertainty. It can be immediately eliminated in seven conditions: chorus reading, lipped speech, prolonged speech, rhythmic speech, shadowing, singing, and instructions to slow. It can be progressively eliminated by response-contingent stimulation. It can be immediately reduced in six conditions: speaking alone, speaking with rhythmic movement, delayed auditory feedback, masking, change in pitch, and whispering. Lastly there are three conditions—adaptation, speech muscle EMG feedback, and haloperidol—which progressively reduce the stutter. Many of these factors cause changes which appear dramatic and the reason behind the change might seem important for ideas about stuttering. However, there is growing evidence that many of these conditions also vary the frequency of nonfluencies evident in the speech of normal speakers. That is, these conditions must be accounted for by conceptualizations which fit models of normal speech control as well as models of stuttering.

In Part 4 we noted that although there are many accounts of the successful treatment of stuttering, only two techniques, the prolonged speech and precision fluency shaping techniques, have been sufficiently documented to satisfy Bloodstein's (1981) criteria for successful treatment. The single most important ingredient in these programs appears to be the length of time spent in these particular forms of speech retraining. The resulting improved speech is stable across situations and over time so that at 2 years the average subject only stutters on 1 to 2 percent of his syllables. Many subjects pass as normal speakers, although, in a paired-choice situation, residual differences in the fluent speech can be detected.

This compilation of research findings assumes that stutterers basically share characteristics in common and that one subgroup of stutterers will not be different from other subgroups of stutterers in meaningful ways. Van Riper (1971) divided his subjects into four tracks and Daly (1981) used the Van Riper tracks to subdivide his subjects. Unfortunately, neither of these subject groups was representative of the population of stutterers. In this laboratory we took the Andrews and Harris (1964) population sample of young stutterers and used the Van Riper track criteria to subdivide them into groups: 44 percent were allocated to Track 1, 18 percent to Track 2, 4 percent to Track 3, and 16 percent to Track 4. The remaining 19 percent were unclassifiable.

If division in this way is to be of value, group membership should be associated with other antecedent or consequent variables. We did a regression analysis and could find no significant association between the Andrews and Harris variables and track membership. Furthermore, when the scores of this sample of stutterers were analyzed by Q technique factor analysis which associates subjects rather than variables, we could find no correspondence between this factor structure and the groupings proposed by Van Riper. Thus, we are not impressed that there are valid subgroupings of stutterers and hence find no justification in this theoretical section for considering stuttering as other than a homogeneous syndrome.

Good theories should be able to account for the established facts. Ideally they should also be parsimonious and be stated in a few general constructs, yet be sufficiently precise to allow predictions amenable to further experimental test. As is traditional, Bloodstein divides theories into three groups: stuttering as a neurotic response, stuttering as learned behavior, and stuttering as a physiological defect.

Stuttering as a Neurotic Response

Psychoanalytic explanations for stuttering were prevalent 40 years ago (viz., Fenichel, 1945, chap. 15). Stuttering was variously viewed as satisfying oral or anal erotic needs and/or as an expression of repressed hostility. Thus, the moment of stuttering represented the unconscious need to suppress speech. Implicit in these and later formulations (Glauber, 1958; Travis, 1957) is that stuttering is but one symptom of a neurotic conflict which would also be evident both in other neurotic symptoms and in disturbed interpersonal relationships, particularly those with parents. Each of these elements has been examined and found not to be true. First, stuttering is nonsyndromic, that is, it does not cluster with any other behavior problems (Glow & Glow, 1980) and in this it differs from emotional disorders in children. Second, both stutterers and their parents show no greater evidence of neurotic symptoms than do nonstuttering children or their parents.

This information has been known for 20 years, yet many still believe there is some abnormality in the stutterer's parent-child relationship. The parent bonding instrument is a recent technique (Parker, 1979) which has proven to be both a reliable and valid measure to assess the proposition that parents may be neglecting and/or overprotective in regard to their child. In this laboratory we compared a series of 50 stutterers and 50 matched controls on the instrument. There were no significant differences in the reports of parenting behaviors between the groups. Specifically, 33 percent of stutterers and 29 percent of controls reported their mothers as providing low care/high protection, and 32 percent of stutterers and 27 percent of controls reported that their fathers behaved in this fashion. (These results will be the subject of a separate report.)

When support cannot be obtained for the corollaries of the basic constructs on which a theory rests, then it is pointless to ask whether other predictions derived from the theory are consistent with the data. Stuttering is not a neurotic disorder.

Stuttering as Learned Behavior

In the late 1930s, Kelly, working in Iowa, formulated a personal construct theory which held that behavior was a product of one's attitudes. Johnson (1955, 1959), also in Iowa at that time, applied this to stuttering and formulated a theory that children became stutterers because others (usually parents) wrongly labeled normal nonfluencies as stuttering. The children, believing they were stuttering, began to react to and avoid these nonfluencies so that their speech behavior did become abnormal.

The evidence is not on Johnson's side. First, investigations of the speech of very young children show that those regarded as stutterers display three times as many part-word repetitions and prolongations as do nonstutterers, but the excess is not so pronounced for other classes of nonfluency. Whether they showed these repetitions on the day their parents first thought of them as stuttering is unknown and probably unknowable. Certainly, if the evidence from the parental bonding instrument on there being no evidence of overprotectiveness in the parents of stutterers is borne out, then the original construct seems even more unlikely. Nevertheless, the theory has been sufficiently influential to ask which of the facts established in Parts 1–4 could have been predicted.

In Part 1 the genetic information is inconsistent with Johnson's hypothesis. Even the celebrated family tree (Gray, 1940) used in support of his position has been reanalyzed and found to be consistent with the genetic position (Howie, 1976). The stutterer-nonstutterer differences (Part 2) are consistent with the proposition that genetic influences are important in the onset of stuttering; that is, stutterers are constitutionally different. Similarly, the facts described in Part 3 would not have been predicted by Johnson's original position; but the results of treatment (Part 4) could have been, for these techniques give a stutterer extensive experience of speaking without stuttering so that his deviant attitudes should normalize (Andrews & Cutler, 1974). Relapse should be more frequent in those who retained abnormal attitudes, but research in this laboratory does not yet provide strong support for this position. In a study of 62 stutterers the correlation between the immediate posttreatment S24 scores (Andrews & Cutler, 1974) and the frequency of stuttering 10 months after treatment was .36, and, in other words, explained only 13 percent of the outcome variance. It is of interest that an extensive attempt to change attitudes which deliberately followed the Kelly/Johnson position (Fransella, 1972) produced only modest benefits in speech when compared to the result of the speech retraining programs, a result inconsistent with the Johnson hypothesis.

Several attempts have been made to formulate concepts about stuttering within the framework of learning theory (e.g., Brutten & Shoemaker, 1967; Shames & Sherrick, 1963; Sheehan, 1953; Wischner, Note 25). These formulations fall into two basic categories. First, there are those theories which view stuttering primarily as an avoidance response; second, there are those theories which view stuttering not as a unitary phenomenon but as the interaction of at least two distinct behavioral phenomena. The most comprehensive form of the first category is that proposed by Sheehan (1953, 1975). He considered stuttering to be the result of conflict between the opposing drives to speak and to hold back from speaking. Consequently, an approach-avoidance conflict (cf. Miller, 1944) arises, in which the motivational drives subserving both approach and avoidance are simultaneously aroused. When the approach drive is dominant, fluent speech ensues, while when the avoidance drive is dominant, nonspeech or silence ensues. However, when the two drives are in equilibrium, such that the gradient for avoidance crosses the gradient for approach, stuttering results. The occurrence of the stutter reduces the fear presumed to underlie the avoidance drive, thereby reducing the avoidance drive and allowing the approach motivational system to dominate. Sheehan has extended this role theory formulation to include the conflict resulting from the choice between remaining silent or not remaining silent, thereby describing a "double approach-avoidance conflict" (Miller, 1944). While the source of the original avoidance is not clearly delineated, Sheehan postulated possible origins in learned speech anxieties and/or unconscious personality factors but did not cite supporting evidence for these constructs; indeed there appears to be none.

Unspecified classical conditioning of hypothetical central motivational states such as fear and anxiety were proposed by Sheehan (1975, p. 126) in his avoidance model. Lack of specification of these hypothetical states excludes the possibility that empirical evidence could have been provided in support of his theory. In contrast, Shames and Sherrick (1963) specified completely operant models of stuttering. They proposed that punishment for normal nonfluency in childhood results in an altered form of nonfluency, namely struggle and silence, which is reinforced by the termination of some of the aversive consequences of the original forms of nonfluency. The altered nonfluency occasions punishment, thereby instituting a constant shifting of reinforcement schedules for avoidance of the negative consequences of stuttering.

The major example of the second category of theories is that proposed by Brutten and Shoemaker (1967). They suggested that the core characteristics of stuttering, namely part-word and word repetitions and sound prolongations, belong to one response class while the secondary stutterings belong to another class. Specifically, they argue that stress may produce autonomic reactions capable of disrupting speech in some individuals. The negative emotion so aroused becomes classically conditioned with concurrent stimuli, such that these stimuli become eliciting stimuli. Thus, the core characteristics of stuttering represent a behavioral failure or disintegration created by negative emotion, while the secondary symptoms are instrumentally acquired adjustive

responses. These authors argue that the particular pattern of the disruption, namely speech disruption, is probably not a learned characteristic but that the relationship between eliciting stimuli and the arousal or emotionality that induces the behavioral/motor disruption is learned via classical conditioning.

Thus, while the above theorists agree that stuttering involves learned modifications of speech behavior, they differ in the mechanisms hypothesized to underlie the learning. Sheehan proposes a conflict-based instrumental model of approach-avoidance while Brutten and Shoemaker propose a two-factor model whereby two distinct processes operate to occasion and maintain the various aspects of stuttering. While the Sheehan model appears to provide an adequate description of how stuttering may be maintained, the predictive power of the model is not clear, since it is largely concerned with hypothetical motivational states. In addition, the source of the conflict responsible for the original stuttering is not supported by the empirical evidence concerning the psychosocial background of stutterers.

The purely operant model of stuttering also, by implication, involves some qualitative differences in the child-rearing practices of stutterers' parents in that it attributes the origins of stuttering to punishment for childhood nonfluency, a parental behavior that has been looked for and not found. The model does, however, predict that stuttering behaves as a lawful operant. Even the evidence for this last proposition is somewhat equivocal. Many of the investigations conducted to investigate the amenability of stuttering to instrumental contingencies have produced ambiguous results by virtue of the stimuli employed as punishing agents. Specifically, known fluency-inducing agents such as loud noise have been employed as putative aversive consequences for stuttering (e.g., Biggs & Sheehan, 1969; Flanagan, Goldiamond, & Azrin, 1958), and further, hedonically ambiguous stimuli such as verbal stimuli have also been employed (e.g., Cooper, Cady, & Robbins, 1970). Clearly, the data on the effect of punishment are unsatisfactory and further demonstration of the effect of unambiguously negative consequences for stuttering is required.

The most parsimonious learning model appears to be that proposed by Brutten and Shoemaker, although the predictions generated by these authors are not the only logically possible set of predictions. These authors argue that core stuttering behaviors, being elicited by stress, are idiosyncratic and unlearned and that the secondary behaviors are instrumentally learned coping behaviors. On this basis they argue that only the secondary symptoms should be amenable to instrumental contingencies. The evidence suggests that, in fact, all stuttering behaviors can be reduced by instrumental contingencies (Andrews, 1974; Costello & Hurst, 1981; Ingham & Andrews, 1973). While this finding presents an apparent contradiction, Andrews et al. (1982) have put forward an interpretation which suggests that there is mobilization of additional central cortical capacity under instrumental contingencies so that speech motor control improves. This proposition allows for improvement in both the central core behaviors and the instrumentally acquired behaviors because of the influence of the response-contingent reinforcement.

Stuttering as a Physiological Deficit

These models refer to a momentary failure of the complicated coordinations involved in fluent speech, the failure being identifiable as a moment of stuttering. Many stutterers are quite certain that emotional stress can precipitate such a breakdown and despite the lack of supporting research for this premise, it does form the basis for Brutten and Shoemaker's (1967) elegant theory of stuttering. Most breakdown theories, however, stem from the proposition that stutterers have a reduced physiological capacity to coordinate speech. Some workers have posited a perceptual deficit, some a motor defect, and others a central deficit. The evidence concerning motor models of stuttering was recently reviewed by St. Louis (1979).

An early breakdown theory was proposed by Orton and Travis (see Travis, 1978). This theory of incomplete cerebral dominance languished because available indicators of speech lateralization showed no stutterer-nonstutterer differences. Out of all the more modern indicators of speech lateralization only the recent work by Moore and his group has shown stable differences; stuttering males appear to use their right hemisphere for processing verbal stimuli more than nonstuttering males. According to Moore and Haynes (1980) stuttering occurs because right-hemisphere processing, which is claimed not to be a segmental processor, has a reduced capacity to handle the temporal-segmental relationships necessary to the production of individual phrases or utterances. The viability of this proposal depends on two lines of evidence being supported by further research. First, the stutterer-nonstutterer difference measure needs refinement, for the size of the present effect is small, less than half a standard deviation; and the distribution of stutterers' scores appears to lie completely within the distribution of the normal males, which is poor support for a qualitative difference in cortical processing style. The second issue concerns the importance of the underlying concept—does the right hemisphere process verbal material independent of the time dimension and is this important for fluent speech? These authors make no attempt to relate their findings to the facts established in Parts 1 to 4 of this article.

West (1958) and Eisenson (1958) had speculated about a physiological difference in speech competence called dysphemia, the presence of which would predispose a person to stuttering. More recently Adams (1974, 1978) and Perkins et al. (1976, 1979) independently held that stuttering might represent a failure of coordination of respiration, phonation, and articulation. Adams and his coworkers held some hope that the vocal difficulties might be primary, but a recent and thorough review of this difficult area by Starkweather (1982) has found little support for this idea as yet and his review should be read by those wishing to familiarize themselves with this area. Nevertheless, both the Adams and the Perkins positions on systems discoordination are supported by the data on fluency-inducing conditions which Perkins et al. (1979) suggested provide more effective planning time for voice onset coordinations, a position which places the postulated abnormality within the cerebrum.

Zimmermann (1980b; Zimmermann, Smith, & Hanley, 1981), on the basis of cineradiographic studies, suggested that stuttering involves changes in reflex interactions among respiratory, laryngeal, and supralaryngeal structures, a proposal which places the site of the abnormality within the brain stem. His preliminary model was developed from the motor control literature, especially that concerned with coordinative structures, but apart from hypothesizing that the stutterer can remain fluent by taking more time and keeping his velocity of movement down, Zimmermann has been properly cautious about relating his theory to many of the established facts about stuttering.

In contrast to Zimmermann, who sees stuttering as a purely motor disorder, our present theoretical position, now to be outlined, focuses on the central processing subserving speech production. Specifically, it focuses on the putative processes of integration within the central nervous system which establish and adaptively maintain the relationship between motor events and the sensory consequences generated by those events. This approach to stuttering as a disorder of sensory-motor processing has been developed in detail by Neilson (in press). Its origins were in the once popular conceptualization of stuttering as a sensory feedback disorder.

In 1953 Fairbanks (1954) presented a closed-loop model of the speech mechanism as a servosystem controlled by continuous auditory feedback of preprogrammed units of intent. The work of Lee (1951) on delayed auditory feedback and of Cherry and Sayers (1956) on masking led to much enthusiasm for stuttering as an analog of servomechanism instability with auditory feedback providing continuous error correction. This whole idea fell into disrepute following the persuasive arguments of Wingate (1969, 1970) and Lane and Tranel (1971).

Like others interested in speech production (Borden & Harris, 1980; Laver, 1980; Abbs & Kennedy, Note 26), Neilson realized that the once apparently contradictory positions of the centralists, who advocated open-loop preprogrammed control, and the peripheralists, who advocated closed-loop feedback control, could be subsumed in a hybrid conceptualization that allows both to be operative. Moreover, such conceptualizations can be hierarchical, allowing multiple levels of open- and closed-loop control. For instance, at one level of closed-loop control the feedback may be virtually continuous and corrective, ensuring that a selected response is executed according to its planned, preprogrammed formulation (e.g., reflex compensation for load fluctuation). At another level of closed-loop control the feedback may be evaluative and only able to influence movement at a minimum of a reaction time delay (e.g., picking up a pebble from the bottom of a pool). It is with the processes which involve this latter type of feedback operating at the level of response selection rather than response execution that our hypothesis regarding stuttering is particularly concerned.

As proposed by Neilson (in press), based on more general theorizing on motor control mechanisms (Neilson, Neilson, & O'Dwyer, Note 27) this feedback is used to establish and maintain an internal neuronal "model" of the relationship between self-generated sensory input (or reafference) and the motor output (or efference) which gives rise to that input. Such internal models are conceived as representing a general mathematical operator or "mapping" between motor and sensory events. They are postulated as being stored in the inverse sensory-to-motor form in order to subserve the generation of desired movement by providing the neural "translation" between the desired sensory input and the requisite motor output. Note that this allows novel movements to be performed, the appropriate commands being generated from the desired sensory image, even though that particular sensory event may not have previously occurred. This makes understandable why skilled motor performance can continue under conditions of feedback deprivation as in, to take a well-known example, the maintenance of intelligible speech in those who become deaf. Nevertheless, this efference-reafference model relating sensory input to motor output and vice versa continues to be updated in terms of whatever current feedback is available. In normal circumstances updating of a well-entrenched model may be minimal, but this ability to monitor and, when necessary, amend, provides the motor control system with its adaptive capability to deal with both external and internal changes.

In the terms of this conceptualization of hybrid, adaptive control of speech and on the basis of her auditory-motor tracking experiments, Neilson (in press) has hypothesized that, due to inadequate central capacity, stutterers have a diminished ability to deal with the relationship between motor activity and the associated sensory or reafferent activity produced during speech. As a consequence the stutterer, in order to speak fluently, must either spend additional time occupied with this relationship or must utilize additional capacity at the expense of other functions.

To us, this hypothesis appears to provide the best fit with the available data about stuttering (Andrews, 1981). The postulated inadequacy in central processing capacity might well be inherited in terms of a particular pattern of cortical organization. (For example, the right-hemisphere preponderance postulated by Moore could be genetically determined and obviously a similar consequence could result from the global or focal reduction in cortex that follows head injury or cerebrovascular accident.) Slower voice onset times, poorer performance on tests of central auditory function, delayed speech development, prevalence of articulation errors, and the slower auditory-motor response times for

discrete and continuous stimuli could all be expressions of this deficit in central processing capacity. Conversely, higher intelligence might well allow some predisposed children to compensate for this deficit and either never stutter or recover quickly. The deficit may be inherited with sex limitation, thereby explaining the preponderance of boys from the beginning. In addition, the female tendency to process linguistic material in both hemispheres (McGlone, 1980) may be protective and account for the more rapid recovery rate in girls.

This view would suggest that whether one will become a stutterer depends on one's neurological capacity for these sensory-to-motor and motor-to-sensory transformations and the demand posed by the speech act. Thus, stuttering should, as it does, have a maximal frequency of onset at a time when an explosive growth in language ability outstrips a still-immature speech motor apparatus, that is, between the ages of 3 and 7. Recovery should, therefore, occur when the motor capacity for coordinated speech catches up with a language development that has plateaued, and again that is probably so. Of course in both cases the imbalance could be further affected by an unusual speech environment such as especially fast-talking or slow-talking parents.

Our position would predict that conditions under which stuttering worsens are conditions in which the speech motor control task is more difficult, for example, the first word in an utterance. Fluency-inducing conditions are those in which the control task is simplified. Chorus reading, shadowing, singing, and prolonged speech may involve reduced control demands at either the linguistic or prosodic levels (Andrews et al., 1982). In lipped speech, whispering, and masking, the external feedback element is restricted, thus simplifying the information input for the model update task. In rhythmic speech, speaking with rhythmic movement, slowed speech, and probably speaking alone either the fluent speech rate and/or the articulation rate is reduced, thereby giving more time for the update of the underlying sensory-motor model. The adaptation effect might well depend on the repeated rehearsal of the same task performed without distraction so that the model requires minimal modification and hence the control task is progressively simplified. Response-contingent stimulation is associated with none of these changes and we have hypothesized elsewhere (Andrews et al., 1982) that stutterers must utilize additional capacity at the expense of other functions.

What, then, are the problems? The major problem concerns severity of stuttering. It is independent of the family history of stuttering and therefore not likely to be inherited; thus it should not be associated with the postulated deficit in central capacity for efferent-reafferent modeling. It is not yet clear what determines the frequency of the primary symptoms of stuttering. A partial solution, at least for secondary symptoms, is to accept the Brutten and Shoemaker (1967) position on the instrumental behaviors and regard them as learned. Certainly we can see no better way of accounting for the more complex speech symptoms and associated body movements. Indeed, there is nothing new in such a combined theoretical approach (cf. Yates, 1963).

What could determine the frequency of the primary symptoms of repetitions and prolongations? If the sensory-motor model is constantly updated in terms of prevailing sensory feedback, then the frequent occurrence of stuttering may lead to a model being updated on the basis of distorted information. When this model is reused, stuttering may become more likely. Thus, in effect, severe stutterers could continually practice their stuttering.

Why, then, do speech retraining treatments benefit stutterers? First, by requiring slowed and prolonged or stretched speech, the task is simplified and produces nonstuttered but abnormal speech. Then, as this is gradually approximated to normal speech, these treatment programs give subjects extensive practice in controlling their speech in terms of its sensory consequences, this time with a progressively normalized sensory-motor model. Likewise a recurrence of stuttering can be controlled by practice of fluent speech under controlled conditions so that once again correct models are used.

As a last issue we would like to note that many but not all of the above statements could be made in regard to Zimmermann's reflex position, so it is helpful to look for a critical experiment that might help to decide between the two. If the sensory-motor modeling theory is valid, then a distractor, because it occupies central cortical capacity, should cause stuttering to worsen and not, as is fondly believed, to reduce. Presumably if the distractor was a competing activity like mental arithmetic, the brain stem would not be involved, and so in Zimmermann's view stuttering would not alter. Some support for this trade-off between frequency of stuttering and a competing mental activity has been produced recently by Kamhi and McOsker (1982).

We have three concluding remarks. First, it must be clear that a considerable amount is known about stuttering. Persons who describe it as "a mysterious and ill-understood disorder" are merely confessing that they have not read the recent literature. Second, the information in this review is already somewhat dated, for work published in 1982 was probably done in 1979 or 1980, and by the time this review is published it will, in some respects, be out of date. Last, this review is an interim statement of how we view stuttering, for our view will change with the advent of new information. Science only issues interim reports.

ACKNOWLEDGMENTS

This review was written with support from the National Health and Medical Research Council of Australia and from the Clearview Foundation. The principal author would like to express his gratitude for the hospitality and advice received during his recent visit to the United States from Drs. Starkweather and Borden at Temple University, Drs. Guitar and Daniloff at the University of Vermont, Dr. Shipp at the University of California at San Francisco, and Drs. Curlee and Hixon at the University of Arizona at Tucson. We would also like to thank our reviewers and editors for the interest and care they have taken with this article.

NOTES

1. Zenner, A.A., & Shepherd, W.P. (1980). *Trait anxiety of stutterers and nonstutterers*. Paper presented to the annual convention of the American Speech-Language-Hearing Association, Detroit, 1980. *Asha, 22,712.* (Abstract)

2. Kline, M.L., & Starkweather, C.W. (1979). *Receptive and expressive language performance in young stutterers*. Paper presented to the annual convention of the American Speech-Language-Hearing Association, Atlanta, 1979. *Asha, 21, 797.* (Abstract)

3. Hand, C.R., & Haynes, W.R. (1981). *Hemispheric and reaction time differences in stutterers and nonstutterers*. Paper presented to the annual convention of the American Speech-Language-Hearing Association, Los Angeles.

4. Davenport, R.W. (1979). *Dichotic listening in four severity levels of stuttering*. Paper presented to the annual convention of the American Speech-Language-Hearing Association, Atlanta, 1979. *Asha, 21, 769.* (Abstract)

5. Mattingly, S.C. (1970). *The performance of stutterers and nonstutterers on two tasks of dichotic listening*. Paper presented to the annual convention of the American Speech-Language-Hearing Association, New York.

6. Perrin, K.L., & Eisenson, J. (1970). *An examination of ear preference for speech and nonspeech stimuli in a stuttering poupulation*. Paper presented to the annual convention of the American Speech-Language-Hearing Association, New York.

7. Ponsford, R.E. (1975). *Correlates of cerebral dominance for speech perception in stutterers*. Doctoral Dissertation, Fuller Theological Seminary, Pasadena, California.

8. Prins, D., & Walton, W. (1971). *Effects of monaural and binaural DAF upon the speech of stutterers in relation to response in a dichotic listening task*. Paper presented to the annual convention of the American Speech and Hearing Association, Chicago.

9. Strong, J.C. (1978). *Dichotic speech perception: A comparison between stutterers and nonstutterers*. Paper presented to the annual convention of the American Speech-Language-Hearing Association, San Francisco, 1978. *Asha, 20, 728.* (Abstract)

10. Barrett, K.H., Keith, R.W., Agnello, J.G., & Weiler, E.M. (1979). *Central auditory processing of stutterers and nonstutterers*. Paper presented to the annual convention of the American Speech-Language-Hearing Association, Atlanta, 1979. *Asha, 21, 769.* (Abstract)

11. Cerf, A., & Prins, D. (1974). *Stutterers' ear preference for dichotic syllables*. Paper presented to the annual convention of the American Speech and Hearing Association, Las Vegas.

12. McNeil, M., & Athen, J. (1977). *Stutterers' reliability on a dichotic listening task*. Paper presented to the annual convention of the American Speech and Hearing Association, Chicago.

13. Phelps, J.B. (1977). *The performance of stutterers and nonstutterers on selected dichotic listening tasks.* Paper presented to the annual convention of the American Speech-Language-Hearing Association, Chicago.

14. Cross, J., & Cooke, P.A. (1979). *Vocal and manual reaction times of adult stutterers and nonstutterers.* Paper presented to the annual convention of the American Speech-Language-Hearing Association, Atlanta, 1979. *Asha, 21,* 693. (Abstract)

15. Lewis, J.I., Ingham, R.J., & Gervens, A. (1979). *Voice initiation and termination times in stutterers and normal speakers.* Paper presented to the annual convention of the American Speech-Language-Hearing Association, Atlanta, 1979. *Asha, 21,* 693. (Abstract)

16. Starkweather, C.W., Franklin, S., & Smigo, T. (1981). *Voice and finger reaction times of stutterers and nonstutterers.* Paper presented to the annual convention of the American Speech-Language-Hearing Association, Los Angeles.

17. Watson, B.C., & Alfonso, P.J. (1980). *Comparison of LRT and VOT values between stutterers and nonstutterers.* Paper presented to the annual convention of the American Speech-Language-Hearing Association, Detroit, 1980. *Asha, 22,* 683. (Abstract)

18. Adler, J.B., & Starkweather, C.W. (1979). *Hemispheric differences in vocal and articulatory reaction times to linguistic and nonlinguistic visual stimuli in stutterers and nonstutterers.* Paper presented to the annual convention of the American Speech-Language-Hearing Association, Atlanta, 1979. *Asha, 21,* 769. (Abstract)

19. Cross, D.E. (1978). *Finger reaction times of stuttering and nonstuttering children and adults.* Poster session presented to the annual convention of the American Speech-Language-Hearing Association, San Francisco, 1978. *Asha, 20,* 730. (Abstract)

20. Cross, D.E. (1980). *Hemispheric asymmetries and stuttering: Evidence from choice reaction time.* Paper presented to the annual convention of the American Speech-Language-Hearing Association, Detroit, 1980. *Asha, 22,* 746. (Abstract)

21. Neilson, M.D., & Neilson, P.D. (1979). *Systems analysis of tracking performance in stutterers and normals.* Paper presented to the annual convention of the American Speech-Language-Hearing Association, Atlanta, 1979. *Asha, 21,* 770. (Abstract)

22. Conture, E.G., & Metz, D.E. (1974). *Some effects of rhythmic stimulation on the speaking behavior of stutterers.* Unpublished manuscript.

23. Soderberg, G.A. (1959). *A study of the effects of delayed auditory side-tone on four aspects of stutterers' speech during oral reading and spontaneous speaking.* Doctoral Dissertation, Ohio State University. (University Microfilms No. 60-796)

24. Hames, P.E., & Runyan, C.M. (1978). *Comparison of perceptual analyses of stutterers' fluency: Paired/single stimuli.* Paper presented to the annual convention of the American Speech-Language-Hearing Association, San Francisco, 1978. *Asha, 20,* 728. (Abstract)

25. Wischner, G.J. (1947). *Stuttering behavior and learning: A program of research.* Doctoral Dissertation, University of Iowa.

26. Abbs, J.H., & Kennedy, J.G. (1980, Spring-Summer). Neurophysiological processes of speech movement control. *SMCL Preprints,* Speech Motor Control Laboratories, Waisman Center, University of Wisconsin, Madison.

27. Neilson, P.D., Neilson, M.D., & O'Dwyer, N.J. (1982, September). *Acquisition of motor skill in tracking tasks: Learning internal models.* Paper presented to the Otago Symposium on Motor Memory and Control, University of Otago, Department of Physical Education, New Zealand.

REFERENCES

Adams, M.R. (1974). A physiologic and aerodynamic interpretation of fluent and stuttered speech. *Journal of Fluency Disorders, 1,* 35–67.

Adams, M.R. (1978). Stuttering theory, research, and therapy: The present and future. *Journal of Fluency Disorders, 3,* 139–147.

Adams, M.R., & Hayden, P. (1976). The ability of stutterers and nonstutterers to initiate and terminate phonation during production of an isolated vowel. *Journal of Speech and Hearing Research, 19,* 290–296.

Adams, M.R., & Moore, W.H., Jr. (1972). The effects of auditory masking on the anxiety level, frequency of dysfluency, and selected vocal characteristics of stutterers. *Journal of Speech and Hearing Research, 15,* 572–578.

Adams, M.R., & Ramig, P. (1980). Vocal characteristics of normal speakers and stutterers during choral reading. *Journal of Speech and Hearing Research, 23,* 457–469.

Agnello, J.G. (1975). Voice onset and voice termination features of stutterers. In L.M. Furst & L.C. Furst (Eds.), *Vocal tract dynamics and dysfluency.* New York: Speech and Hearing Institute.

Andrews, G. (1974). The etiology of stuttering. *Australian Journal of Human Communication Disorders, 2,* 8–12.

Andrews, G. (1981). Stuttering: A tutorial. *Australian and New Zealand Journal of Psychiatry, 15,* 105–109.

Andrews, G., & Craig, A. (1982). Stuttering: Overt and covert measurement of the speech of treated stutterers. *Journal of Speech and Hearing Disorders, 47,* 96–99.

Andrews, G., & Cutler, J. (1974). Stuttering therapy: The relation between changes in symptom level and attitudes. *Journal of Speech and Hearing Disorders, 39,* 312–319.

Andrews, G., Guitar, B., & Howie, P. (1980). Meta-analysis of the effects of stuttering treatment. *Journal of Speech and Hearing Disorders, 45,* 287–307.

Andrews, G., & Harris, M. (1964). *The syndrome of stuttering.* Clinics in Developmental Medicine (No. 17). London: Heinemann.

Andrews, G., & Harvey, R. (1981). Regression to the mean in pretreatment measures of stuttering. *Journal of Speech and Hearing Disorders, 46,* 204–207.

Andrews, G., Howie, P.M., Dozsa, M., & Guitar, B.E. (1982). Stuttering: Speech pattern characteristics under fluency-inducing conditions. *Journal of Speech and Hearing Research, 25,* 208–216.

Andrews, G., Quinn, P.T., & Sorby, W.A. (1972). Stuttering: An investigation into cerebral dominance for speech. *Journal of Neurology, Neurosurgery and Psychiatry, 35,* 414–418.

Andrews, G., & Tanner, S. (1982a). Stuttering treatment: Replication of the regulated breathing method. *Journal of Speech and Hearing Disorders, 47,* 138–140.

Andrews, G., & Tanner, S. (1982b). Stuttering: The results of 5 days treatment with an airflow technique. *Journal of Speech and Hearing Disorders, 47*, 427–429.

Anthony, J. (1968). The relationship between masking noise and severity of stuttering. *Ohio Journal of Speech and Hearing, 3*, 39–46.

Backus, O. (1938). Incidence of stuttering among the deaf. *Annals of Otolaryngology, Rhinology and Laryngology, 47*, 632–635.

Barber, V. (1939). Studies in the psychology of stuttering: XV. Chorus reading as a distraction in stuttering. *Journal of Speech Disorders, 4*, 371–383.

Berry, M.F. (1938). Developmental history of stuttering children. *Journal of Pediatrics, 12*, 209–217.

Biggs, B., & Sheehan, J. (1969). Punishment or distraction? Operant stuttering revisited. *Journal of Abnormal Psychology, 74*, 256–262.

Bjerkan, B. (1980). Word fragmentations and repetitions in the spontaneous speech of 2–6-year-old children. *Journal of Fluency Disorders, 5*, 137–148.

Blood, G.W., & Hood, S.B. (1978). Elementary school-aged stutterers' disfluencies during oral reading and spontaneous speech. *Journal of Fluency Disorders, 3*, 155–165.

Blood, G.W., & Seider, R. (1981). The concomitant problems of young stutterers. *Journal of Speech and Hearing Disorders, 46*, 31–33.

Bloodstein, O. (1960a). The development of stuttering: I. Changes in nine basic features. *Journal of Speech and Hearing Disorders, 25*, 219–237.

Bloodstein, O. (1960b). The development of stuttering: II. Development phases. *Journal of Speech and Hearing Disorders, 25*, 366–376.

Bloodstein, O. (1981). *A handbook on stuttering* (3rd ed.). Chicago: National Easter Seal Society.

Bloom, C.M., & Silverman, F.H. (1973). Do all stutterers adapt? *Journal of Speech and Hearing Research, 16*, 518–521.

Boberg, E. (1976). Intensive group therapy program for stutterers. *Human Communication, 1*, 29–42.

Boberg, E., & Sawyer, L. (1977). The maintenance of fluency following intensive therapy. *Human Communication, 2*, 21–28.

Bohme, G. (1968). Stammering and cerebral lesions in early childhood. Examinations of 802 children and adults with cerebral lesions. *Folia Phoniatrica, 20*, 239–249.

Borden, G.J., & Harris, K.S. (1980). *Speech science primer*. Baltimore: Williams & Wilkins.

Brady, J.P. (1969). Studies on the metronome effect on stuttering. *Behavior Research and Therapy, 7*, 197–204.

Brady, J.P., & Berson, J. (1975). Stuttering, dichotic listening and cerebral dominance. *Archives of General Psychiatry, 32*, 1449–1452.

Brayton, E.R., & Conture, E.G. (1978). Effects of noise and rhythmic stimulation on the speech of stutterers. *Journal of Speech and Hearing Research, 21*, 285–294.

Brenner, N.C., Perkins, W.H., & Soderberg, G.A. (1972). The effect of rehearsal on frequency of stuttering. *Journal of Speech and Hearing Research, 15*, 483–486.

Brown, S.F. (1937). The influence of grammatical function on the incidence of stuttering. *Journal of Speech Disorders, 2*, 207–215.

Brown, S.F. (1945). The loci of stuttering in the speech sequence. *Journal of Speech Disorders, 10*, 181–192.

Brown, S.F., & Hull, H.C. (1942). A study of some social attitudes of a group of 59 stutterers. *Journal of Speech Disorders, 7*, 323–324.

Brown, T., Sambrooks, J.E., & MacCulloch, M.J. (1975). Auditory thresholds and the effect of reduced auditory feedback on stuttering. *Acta Psychiatrica Scandinavica, 51*, 297–311.

Bruce, M.C., & Adams, M.R. (1978). Effects of two types of motor practice on stuttering adaptation. *Journal of Speech and Hearing Research, 21*, 421–428.

Brutten, E.J., & Shoemaker, D.J. (1967). *The modification of stuttering*. Englewood Cliffs, NJ: Prentice-Hall.

Burke, B.D. (1975). Variables affecting stutterers' initial reactions to delayed auditory feedback. *Journal of Communication Disorders, 8*, 141–155.

Burns, D., Brady, J.P., & Kuruvilla, K. (1978). The acute effect of haloperidol and apomorphine on the severity of stuttering. *Biological Psychiatry, 13*, 255–264.

Byrne, M.E. (1931). A follow-up study of 1000 cases of stutterers from the Minneapolis public schools. *Proceedings of the American Society for the Study of Disorders of Speech*.

Cherry, C., & Sayers, B. McA. (1956). Experiments upon the total inhibition of stammering by external control and some clinical results. *Journal of Psychosomatic Research, 1*, 233–246.

Colcord, R.D., & Adams, M.R. (1979). Voicing duration and vocal SPL changes associated with stuttering reduction during singing. *Journal of Speech and Hearing Research, 22*, 468–479.

Commodore, R.W., & Cooper, E.B. (1978). Communicative stress and stuttering frequency during normal, whispered, and articulation-without-phonation speech modes. *Journal of Fluency Disorders, 3*, 1–12.

Conradi, E. (1912). Speech defects and intellectual progress. *Journal of Educational Psychology, 3*, 35–38.

Cook, T.D., & Leviton, L.C. (1980). Reviewing the literature: A comparison of traditional methods with meta-analysis. *Journal of Personality, 48*, 499–572.

Cooper, E.B., Cady, B.B., & Robbins, C.J. (1970). The effect of the verbal stimulus words *wrong, right*, and *tree* on the disfluency rates of stutterers and nonstutterers. *Journal of Speech and Hearing Research, 13*, 239–244.

Costello, J.M. (1975). The establishment of fluency with time-out procedures: Three case studies. *Journal of Speech and Hearing Disorders, 40*, 216–231.

Costello, J.M., & Hurst, M.R. (1981). An analysis of the relationship among stuttering behaviors. *Journal of Speech and Hearing Research, 24*, 247–256.

Cox, M.D. (1982). The stutterer and stuttering: Neuropsychological correlates. *Journal of Fluency Disorders, 7*, 129–140.

Craig, A.R., & Cleary, P.J. (1982). Reduction of stuttering of young male stutterers by electromyographic feedback. *Biofeedback and Self Regulation, 7*, 241–255.

Cross, D.E., & Luper, H.L. (1979). Voice reaction time of stuttering and nonstuttering children and adults. *Journal of Fluency Disorders, 4*, 59–77.

Cross, D.E., Shadden, B.B., & Luper, H.L. (1979). Effects of stimulus ear presentation on the voice reaction time of adult stutterers and nonstutterers. *Journal of Fluency Disorders, 4*, 45–58.

Cullinan, W.L., & Springer, M.T. (1980). Voice initiation times in stuttering and nonstuttering children. *Journal of Speech and Hearing Research, 23*, 344–360.

Curlee, R.F. (1981). Observer agreement on disfluency and stuttering. *Journal of Speech and Hearing Research, 24*, 595–600.

Curran, M.F., & Hood, S.B. (1977). Listener ratings of severity for specific disfluency types in children. *Journal of Fluency Disorders, 2*, 87–97.

Curry, F.K.W., & Gregory, H.H. (1969). The performance of stutterers on dichotic listening tasks thought to reflect cerebral dominance. *Journal of Speech and Hearing Research, 12*, 72–82.

Daly, D.A. (1981). Differentiation of stuttering subgroups with Van Riper's developmental tracks: A preliminary study. *Journal of the National Student Speech Language Hearing Association*, 89–101.

Darley, F.L. (1955). The relationship of parental attitudes and adjustments to the development of stuttering. In W. Johnson & R.R. Leutenegger (Eds.), *Stuttering in children and adults*. Minneapolis: University of Minnesota Press.

Donnan, G.A. (1979). Stuttering as a manifestation of stroke. *Medical Journal of Australia, 1*, 44–45.

Dorman, M.F., & Porter, R.J. (1975). Hemispheric lateralization for speech perception in stutterers. *Cortex, 11*, 181–185.

Eisenson, J. (1958). A perseverative theory of stuttering. In J. Eisenson (Ed.), *Stuttering: A symposium*. New York: Harper & Row.

Fairbanks, G. (1954). Systematic research in experimental phonetics: 1. A theory of the speech mechanism as a servosystem. *Journal of Speech and Hearing Disorders, 19*, 133–139.

Fenichel, O. (1945). *The psychoanalytic theory of neurosis*. New York: W.W. Norton.

Few, L.R., & Lingwall, J.B. (1972). A further analysis of fluency within stuttered speech. *Journal of Speech and Hearing Research, 15*, 356–363.

Flanagan, B., Goldiamond, I., & Azrin, N. (1958). Operant stuttering: The control of stuttering behavior through response-contingent consequences. *Journal of the Experimental Analysis of Behavior, 1*, 173–177.

Floyd, S., & Perkins, W.H. (1974). Early syllable dysfluency in stutterers and nonstutterers: A preliminary report. *Journal of Communication Disorders, 7*, 279–282.

Fransella, F. (1972). *Personal change and reconstruction*. London: Academic Press.

Fransella, F., & Beech, H.R. (1965). An experimental analysis of the effect of rhythm on the speech of stutterers. *Behaviour Research and Therapy, 3*, 195–201.

Frayne, H., Coates, S., & Marriner, N. (1977). Evaluation of post treatment fluency by naive subjects. *Australian Journal of Human Communication Disorders, 5*, 48–54.

Fritzell, B. (1976). The prognosis of stuttering in school children: A 10-year longitudinal study. In *Proceedings of the XVI Congress of the International Society of Logopedics and Phoniatrics*, Basel: Karger.

Garber, S.F., & Martin, R.R. (1977). Effects of noise and increased vocal intensity on stuttering. *Journal of Speech and Hearing Research, 20*, 233–240.

Gens, G.W. (1950). Correlation of neurological findings, psychological analyses and speech disorders among institutionalized epileptics. *Training School Bulletin, 47*, 3–18.

Glauber, I.P. (1958). The psychoanalysis of stuttering. In J. Eisenson (Ed.), *Stuttering: A symposium*. New York: Harper & Row.

Glow, R.A., & Glow, P.H. (1980). Non-syndromic behavior problems in children. In J.W.G. Tiller & P.R. Martin (Eds.), *Behavioral Medicine*. Proceedings of the Geigy Psychiatric Symposium. Melbourne: Geigy.

Godai, U., Tatarelli, R., & Bonanni, G. (1976). Stuttering and tics in twins. *Acta Geneticae Medicae et Gemellologiae, 25*, 369–375.

Goldiamond, I. (1965). Stuttering and fluency as manipulatable operant response classes. In L. Krasner & L.P. Ullman (Eds.), *Research in behavior modification*. New York: Holt, Rinehart, & Winston.

Graham, J.K. (1966). A neurologic and electroencephalographic study of adult stutterers and matched normal speakers. *Speech Monographs, 33*, 290. (Abstract)

Gray, M. (1940). The X family: A clinical and laboratory study of a "stuttering" family. *Journal of Speech Disorders, 5*, 343–348.

Gruber, L., & Powell, R.L. (1974). Responses of stuttering and nonstuttering children to a dichotic listening task. *Perceptual and Motor Skills, 38*, 263–264.

Guitar, B. (1975). Reduction of stuttering frequency using analog electromyographic feedback. *Journal of Speech and Hearing Research, 18*, 672–685.

Hahn, E.F. (1942). A study of the relationship between stuttering occurrence and phonetic factors in oral reading. *Journal of Speech Disorders, 7*, 143–151.

Hall, J.W., & Jerger, J. (1978). Central auditory function in stutterers. *Journal of Speech and Hearing Research, 21*, 324–337.

Hanna, R., & Morris. S. (1977). Stuttering, speech rate, and the metronome effect. *Perceptual and Motor Skills, 44*, 452–454.

Hannley, M., & Dorman, M.F. (1982). Some observations on auditory functioning and stuttering. *Journal of Fluency Disorders, 7*, 93–108.

Harms, M.A., & Malone, J.Y. (1939). The relationship of hearing acuity to stammering. *Journal of Speech Disorders, 4*, 363–370.

Healey, E.C. (1982). Speaking fundamental frequency characteristics of stutterers and nonstutterers. *Journal of Communication Disorders, 15*, 21–29.

Healey, E.C., & Adams, M.R. (1981a). Rate reduction strategies used by normally fluent and stuttering children and adults. *Journal of Fluency Disorders, 6*, 1–14.

Healey, E .C., & Adams, M.R. (1981b). Speech timing skills of normally fluent and stuttering children and adults. *Journal of Fluency Disorders, 6*, 233–246.

Healey, E.C., Mallard, A.R., & Adams, M.R. (1976). Factors contributing to the reduction of stuttering during singing. *Journal of Speech and Hearing Research, 19*, 475–480.

Hegde, M.N. (1972). Stuttering, neurotocism and extraversion. *Behaviour Research and Therapy, 10*, 395–397.

Helm, N.A., Butler, R.B., & Benson, D.F. (1978). Acquired stuttering. *Neurology, 28*, 1159–1165.

Heltman, H.J., & Peacher, G.M. (1943). Misarticulation and diadokokinesis in the spastic paralytic. *Journal of Speech Disorders, 8*, 137–145.

Hillman, R.E., & Gilbert, H.R. (1977). Voice onset time for voiceless stop consonants in the fluent reading of stutterers and nonstutterers. *Journal of the Acoustical Society of America, 61*, 610–611.

Hood, S.B. (1975). Effect of communicative stress on the frequency and form-types of disfluent behavior in adult stutterers. *Journal of Fluency Disorders, 1*, 36–47.

Horlick, R.S., & Miller, M.H. (1960). A comparative personality study of a group of stutterers and hard of hearing patients. *Journal of General Psychology, 63,* 259–266.

Howie, P.M. (1976). The identification of genetic components in speech disorders. *Australian Journal of Human Communication Disorders, 4,* 155–163.

Howie, P.M. (1981a). Concordance for stuttering in monozygotic and dizygotic twin pairs. *Journal of Speech and Hearing Research, 24,* 317–321.

Howie, P.M. (1981b). Intra pair similarity in frequency of disfluency in monozygotic and dizygotic twin pairs containing stutterers. *Behavior Genetics, 11,* 227–237.

Howie, P.M., Tanner, S., & Andrews, G. (1981). Short- and long-term outcome in an intensive treatment program for adult stutterers. *Journal of Speeach and Hearing Disorders, 46,* 104–109.

Howie, P.M., Woods, C.L., & Andrews, G. (1982). Relationship between covert and overt speech measures immediately before and immediately after stuttering treatment. *Journal of Speech and Hearing Disorders, 47,* 419–422.

Huffman, E.S., & Perkins, W.H. (1974). Dysfluency characteristics identified by listeners as "stuttering" and "stutterer." *Journal of Communication Disorders, 7,* 89–96.

Ingham, R.J. (1975). A comparison of covert and overt assessment procedures in stuttering therapy outcome evaluation. *Journal of Speech and Hearing Research, 18,* 346–354.

Ingham, R.J., & Andrews, G. (1973). An analysis of a token economy in stuttering therapy. *Journal of Applied Behavior Analysis, 6,* 219–229.

Ingham, R.J., & Carroll, P.J. (1977). Listener judgment of differences in stutterers' nonstuttered speech during chorus- and nonchorus-reading conditions. *Journal of Speech and Hearing Research, 20,* 293–302.

Ingham, R.J., & Packman, A. (1979). A further evaluation of the speech of stutterers during chorus- and nonchorus-reading conditions. *Journal of Speech and Hearing Research, 22,* 784–793.

Ingram, R.S. (1963). Late and poor talkers. In M. Bax (Ed.), *The child who does not talk.* London: Heinemann/Spastic Society.

James, J.E. (1981). Punishment of stuttering: Contingency and stimulus parameters. *Journal of Communication Disorders, 14,* 375–386.

Jameson, A.M. (1955). Stammering in children: Some factors in the prognosis. *Speech, 19,* 60–67.

Johnson, W. (1955). A study of the onset and development of stuttering. In W. Johnson & R.R. Leutenegger (Eds.), *Stuttering in children and adults.* Minneapolis: University of Minnesota Press.

Johnson, W. (1959). *The onset of stuttering.* Minneapolis: University of Minnesota Press.

Johnson, W., & Brown, S.F. (1935). Stuttering in relation to various speech sounds. *Quarterly Journal of Speech, 21,* 481–496.

Johnson, W., & Knott, J.R. (1937). Studies in the psychology of stuttering: I. The distribution of moments of stuttering in successive readings of the same material. *Journal of Speech Disorders, 2,* 17–19.

Johnson, W., & Rosen, B. (1937). Studies in the psychology of stuttering: VII. Effect of certain changes in speech pattern upon frequency of stuttering. *Journal of Speech Disorders, 2,* 105–109.

Jones, R.K. (1966). Observations on stammering after localized cerebral injury. *Journal of Neurology, Neurosurgery and Psychiatry, 29,* 192–195.

Kamhi, A.G., & McOsker, T.G. (1982). Attention and stuttering: Do stutterers think too much about speech? *Journal of Fluency Disorders, 7,* 309–321.

Kidd, K.K. (1980). Genetic models of stuttering. *Journal of Fluency Disorders, 5,* 187–201.

Kidd, K.K., Heimbuch, R.C., Records, M.A., Oehlert, G., & Webster, R.L. (1980). Familial stuttering patterns are not related to one measure of severity. *Journal of Speech and Hearing Research, 23,* 539–545.

Klich, R.J., & May, G.M. (1982). Spectrographic study of vowels in stutterers' fluent speech. *Journal of Speech and Hearing Research, 25,* 364–370.

Kroll, R.M., & Hood, S.B. (1974). Differences in stuttering adaptation between oral reading and spontaneous speech. *Journal of Communication Disorders, 7,* 227–237.

Kroll, R.M., & Hood, S.B. (1976). The influence of task presentation and information load on the adaptation effect in stutterers and normal speakers. *Journal of Communication Disorders, 9,* 95–110.

Ladouceur, R., Cote, C., Leblond, G., & Bouchard, L. (1982). Evaluation of regulated-breathing method and awareness training in the treatment of stuttering. *Journal of Speech and Hearing Disorders, 47,* 422–426.

Lane, H., & Tranel, B. (1971). The Lombard sign and the role of hearing in speech. *Journal of Speech and Hearing Research, 14,* 677–709.

Lanyon, R.I. (1977). Effect of biofeedback-based relaxation on stuttering during reading and spontaneous speech. *Journal of Consulting and Clinical Psychology, 45,* 860–866.

Lanyon, R.I., & Barocas, V.S. (1975). Effects of contingent events on stuttering and fluency. *Journal of Consulting and Clinical Psychology, 43,* 786–793.

Lanyon, R.I., Goldsworthy, R.J., & Lanyon, B.P. (1978). Dimensions of stuttering and relationship to psychopathology. *Journal of Fluency Disorders, 3,* 103–113.

Laver, J. (1980). Monitoring systems in the neurolinguistic control of speech production. In V.A. Fromkin (Ed.), *Errors in linguistic performance: Slips of the tongue, ear, pen and hand.* New York: Academic Press.

Lechner, B.K. (1979). The effects of delayed auditory feedback and masking on the fundamental frequency of stutterers and nonstutterers. *Journal of Speech and Hearing Research, 22,* 343–353.

Lee, B.S. (1951). Artificial stutter. *Journal of Speech and Hearing Disorders, 16,* 53–55.

Liebetrau, R.M., & Daly, D.A. (1981). Auditory processing and perceptual abilities of organic and functional stutterers. *Journal of Fluency Disorders, 6,* 219–231.

Louttit, C.M., & Halls, E.C. (1936). Survey of speech defects among public school children of Indiana. *Journal of Speech Disorders, 1,* 73–80.

Luessenhop, A.J., Boggs, J.S., Laborwit, L.J., & Walle, E.L. (1973). Cerebral dominance in stutterers determined by Wada testing. *Neurology, 23,* 1190–1192.

MacCulloch, M.J., & Eaton, R. (1971). A note on reduced auditory pain threshold in 44 stuttering children. *British Journal of Disorders of Communication, 6,* 148–153.

Mann, M.B. (1955). Nonfluencies in the oral reading of stutterers and nonstutterers of elementary school age. In W. Johnson &

R.R. Leutenegger (Eds.), *Stuttering in children and adults.* Minneapolis: University of Minnesota Press.

Martin, R.R., & Haroldson, S.K. (1979). Effects of five experimental treatments on stuttering. *Journal of Speech and Hearing Research, 22,* 132–146.

Martin, R.R., & Haroldson, S.K. (1982). Contingent self-stimulation for stuttering. *Journal of Speech and Hearing Disorders, 47,* 407–413.

Martin, R.R., Kuhl, P., & Haroldson, S. (1972). An experimental treatment with two preschool stuttering children. *Journal of Speech and Hearing Research, 15,* 743–752.

May, A.E., & Hackwood, A. (1968). Some effects of masking and eliminating low frequency feedback on the speech of stammerers. *Behavior Research and Therapy, 6,* 219–223.

McAllister, A.H. (1937). *Clinical studies in speech therapy.* London: University of London Press.

McDowell, E.D. (1928). *The educational and emotional adjustments of stuttering children.* New York: Columbia University Teachers College.

McFarlane, S.C., & Shipley, K.G. (1981). Latency of vocalization onset for stutterers and nonstutterers under conditions of auditory and visual cueing. *Journal of Speech and Hearing Disorders, 46,* 307–312.

McGlone, J. (1980). Sex differences in human brain asymmetry: A critical survey. *The Behavioral and Brain Sciences, 3,* 215–263.

Meltzer, H. (1935). Talkativeness in stuttering and non-stuttering children. *Journal of Genetic Psychology, 46,* 371–390.

Metz, D.E., Conture, E.G., & Caruso, A. (1979). Voice onset time, frication, and aspiration during stutterers' fluent speech. *Journal of Speech and Hearing Research, 22,* 649–656.

Miller, N.E. (1944). Experimental studies of conflict. In J. McV. Hunt (Ed.), *Personality and the behavior disorders.* New York: Ronald Press.

Molt, L.F., & Guilford, A.M. (1979). Auditory processing and anxiety in stutterers. *Journal of Fluency Disorders, 4,* 255–267.

Moore, W.H., Jr. (1976). Bilateral tachistoscopic word perception of stutterers and normal subjects. *Brain and Language, 3,* 434–442.

Moore, W.H., Jr., Craven, D.C., & Faber, M.M. (1982). Hemispheric alpha asymmetries of words with positive, negative, and neutral arousal values preceding tasks of recall and recognition: Electrophysiological and behavioral results from stuttering males and nonstuttering males and females: *Brain and Language, 17,* 211–224.

Moore, W.H., Jr., & Haynes, W.O. (1980). Alpha hemispheric asymmetry and stuttering: Some support for a segmentation dysfunction hypothesis. *Journal of Speech and Hearing Research, 23,* 229–247.

Moore, W.H., Jr., & Lang, M.K. (1977). Alpha asymmetry over the right and left hemispheres of stutterers and control subjects preceding massed oral readings: A preliminary investigation. *Perceptual and Motor Skills, 44,* 223–230.

Moore, W.H., Jr., & Lorendo, L.C. (1980). Hemispheric alpha asymmetries of stuttering males and nonstuttering males and females for words of high and low imagery. *Journal of Fluency Disorders, 5,* 11–26.

Morley, M.E. (1957). *The development and disorders of speech in childhood.* Edinburgh: Livingstone.

Murphy, M., & Baumgartner, J.M. (1981). Voice initiation and termination time in stuttering and nonstuttering children. *Journal of Fluency Disorders, 6,* 257–264.

Murray, H.L., & Reed, C.G. (1977). Language abilities of preschool stuttering children. *Journal of Fluency Disorders, 2,* 171–176.

Neilson, M.D. *Stuttering and the control of speech: A systems analysis approach.* Cambridge, England: Cambridge University Press (in press).

Nelson, S.E., Hunter, N., & Walter, M. (1945). Stuttering in twin types. *Journal of Speech Disorders, 10,* 335–343.

Okasha, A., Bishry, Z., Kamel, M., & Hassan, A.H. (1974). Psychosocial study of stammering in Egyptian children. *British Journal of Psychiatry, 124,* 531–533.

Okasha, A., Moneim, S.A., Bishry, Z., Kamel, M., & Moustafa, M. (1974). Electroencephalographic study of stammering. *British Journal of Psychiatry, 124,* 534–535.

Panelli, C.A., McFarlane, S.C., & Shipley, K.G. (1978). Implications of evaluating and intervening with incipient stutterers. *Journal of Fluency Disorders, 3,* 41–50.

Parker, G. (1979). Parental characteristics in relation to depressive disorders. *British Journal of Psychiatry, 134,* 138–147.

Perkins, W.H., Bell, J., Johnson, L., & Stocks, J. (1979). Phone rate and the effective planning time hypothesis of stuttering. *Journal of Speech and Hearing Research, 22,* 747–755.

Perkins, W., Rudas, J., Johnson, L., & Bell, J. (1976). Stuttering: Discoordination of phonation with articulation and respiration. *Journal of Speech and Hearing Research, 19,* 509–522.

Perozzi, J.A., & Kunze, L.H. (1969). Language abilities of stuttering children. *Folia Phoniatrica, 21,* 386–392.

Pinsky, S.D., & McAdam, D.W. (1980). Electroencephalographic and dichotic indices of cerebral laterality in stutterers. *Brain and Language, 11,* 374–397.

Pizzat, F.J. (1951). A personality study of college stutterers. *Speech Monographs, 18,* 240–241. (Abstract)

Porter, H.K. (1939). Studies in the psychology of stuttering: XIV. Stuttering phenomena in relation to size and personnel of audience. *Journal of Speech Disorders, 4,* 323–333.

Prins, D. (1972). Personality, stuttering severity, and age. *Journal of Speech and Hearing Research, 15,* 148–154.

Prosek, R.A., Montgomery, A.A., Walden, B.E., & Schwartz, D.M. (1979). Reaction-time measures of stutterers and nonstutterers. *Journal of Fluency Disorders, 4,* 269–278.

Prosek, R.A., & Runyan, C.M. (1982). Temporal characteristics related to the discrimination of stutterers' and nonstutterers' speech samples. *Journal of Speech and Hearing Research, 25,* 29–33.

Quinn, P.T. (1971). Stuttering: Some observations on speaking when alone. *Journal of the Australian College of Speech Therapists, 21,* 92–94.

Quinn, P.T. (1972). Stuttering: Cerebral dominance and the dichotic word test. *Medical Journal of Australia, 2,* 639–643.

Quinn, P.T. (1976). Cortical localization of speech in normals and stutterers. *Australian Journal of Human Communication Disorders, 4,* 118–120.

Quinn, P.T., & Andrews, G. (1977). Neurological stuttering—A clinical entity? *Journal of Neurology, Neurosurgery and Psychiatry, 40,* 699–701.

Quinn, P.T., & Peachey, E.C. (1973). Haloperidol in the treatment of stutterers. *British Journal of Psychiatry, 123,* 247–248.

Ragsdale, J.D., & Ashby, J.K. (1982). Speech-language pathologists connotations of stuttering. *Journal of Speech and Hearing Research, 25,* 75–80.

Ramig, P., & Adams, M.R. (1980). Rate reduction strategies used by stutterers and nonstutterers during high- and low-pitched speech. *Journal of Fluency Disorders, 5,* 27–41.

Reich, A., Till, J., Goldsmith, H., & Prins, D. (1981). Laryngeal and manual reaction times of stuttering and nonstuttering adults. *Journal of Speech and Hearing Research, 24,* 192–196.

Resick, P.A., Wendiggensen, P., Ames, S., & Meyer, V. (1978). Systematic slowed speech: A new treatment for stuttering. *Behavior Research and Therapy, 16,* 161–167.

Rosenbek, J., Messert, B., Collins, M., & Wertz, R.T. (1978). Stuttering following brain damage. *Brain and Language, 6,* 82–96.

Rosenfield, D.B. (1972). Stuttering and cerebral ischemia. *New England Journal of Medicine, 287,* 991.

Rosenfield, D.B., & Goodglass, H. (1980). Dichotic testing of cerebral dominance in stutterers. *Brain and Language, 11,* 170–180.

Rosenthal, R. (1979). The "file-drawer problem" and tolerance for null results. *Psychological Bulletin, 86,* 638–641.

Rousey, C.L. (1958). Stuttering severity during prolonged spontaneous speech. *Journal of Speech and Hearing Research, 1,* 40–47.

Runyan, C.M., & Adams, M.R. (1978). Perceptual study of the speech of "successfully therapeutized" stutterers. *Journal of Fluency Disorders, 3,* 25–39.

Runyan, C.M., & Adams, M.R. (1979). Unsophisticated judges' perceptual evaluations of the speech of "successfully treated" stutterers. *Journal of Fluency Disorders, 4,* 29–38.

Ryan, B.P. (1974). *Programmed therapy for stuttering in children and adults.* Springfield, IL: Charles C Thomas.

St. Louis, K.O. (1979). Linguistic and motor aspects of stuttering. In N.J. Lass (Ed.), *Speech and language: Advances in basic research* (Vol. 1). New York: Academic Press.

St. Louis, K.O., & Lass, N.J. (1981). A survey of communicative disorders students' attitudes toward stuttering. *Journal of Fluency Disorders, 6,* 49–79.

Sander, E.K. (1961). Reliability of the Iowa Speech Disfluency Test. *Journal of Speech and Hearing Disorders,* Monograph Supplement, *7,* 21–30.

Sayles, D.G. (1971). Cortical excitability, perseveration, and stuttering. *Journal of Speech and Hearing Research, 14,* 462–475.

Schindler, M.D. (1955). A study of educational adjustments of stuttering and non-stuttering children. In W. Johnson & R.R. Leutenegger (Eds.), *Stuttering in children and adults.* Minneapolis: University of Minnesota Press.

Seider, R.A., Gladstien, K.L., & Kidd, K.K. Recovery and persistence of stuttering among relatives of stutterers. *Journal of Speech and Hearing Disorders* (in press).

Shames, G.H., & Sherrick, C.E., Jr. (1963). A discussion of nonfluency and stuttering as operant behavior. *Journal of Speech and Hearing Disorders, 28,* 3–18.

Sheehan, J.G. (1953). Theory and treatment of stuttering as an approach-avoidance conflict. *Journal of Psychology, 36,* 27–49.

Sheehan, J.G. (1975). Conflict theory and avoidance reduction therapy. In J. Eisenson (Ed.), *Stuttering: A second symposium.* New York: Harper & Row.

Shulman, E. (1955). Factors influencing the variability of stuttering. In W. Johnson & R.R. Leutenegger (Eds.), *Stuttering in children and adults.* Minneapolis: University of Minnesota Press.

Siegel, G.M. (1970). Punishment, stuttering and disfluency. *Journal of Speech and Hearing Research, 13,* 677–714.

Siegel, G.M., & Haugen, D. (1964). Audience size and variations in stuttering behavior. *Journal of Speech and Hearing Research, 7,* 381–388.

Silverman, E-M., & Williams, D.E. (1967). A comparison of stuttering and nonstuttering children in terms of five measures of oral language development. *Journal of Communication Disorders, 1,* 305–309.

Slorach, N., & Noehr, B. (1973). Dichotic listening in stuttering and dyslalic children. *Cortex, 9,* 295–300.

Soderberg, G.A. (1967). Linguistic factors in stuttering. *Journal of Speech and Hearing Research, 10,* 801–810.

Soderberg, G.A. (1971). Relation of word information and word length to stuttering disfluencies. *Journal of Communication Disorders, 4,* 9–14.

Sommers, R.K., Brady, W.A., & Moore, W.H. (1975). Dichotic ear performances of stuttering children and adults. *Perceptual and Motor Skills, 41,* 931–938.

Starkweather, C.W. (1982). Stuttering and laryngeal behavior: A review. *ASHA Monographs, 21,* 1–45.

Starkweather, C.W., Hirschman, P., & Tannenbaum, R.S. (1976). Latency of vocalization onset: Stutterers versus nonstutterers. *Journal of Speech and Hearing Research, 19,* 481–492.

Stocker, B., & Parker, E. (1977). The relationship between auditory recall and dysfluency in young stutterers. *Journal of Fluency Disorders, 2,* 177–187.

Stocker, B., & Upsrich, C. (1976). Stuttering in children and level of demand. *Journal of Childhood Communication Disorders, 1,* 116–131.

Sussman, H.M., & MacNeilage, P.F. (1975). Studies of hemispheric specialization for speech production. *Brain and Language, 2,* 131–151.

Taylor, I.K. (1966). What words are stuttered? *Psychological Bulletin, 65,* 233–242.

Toscher, M.M., & Rupp, R.R. (1978). A study of the central auditory processes in stutterers using the Synthetic Sentence Identification (SSI) test battery. *Journal of Speech and Hearing Research, 21,* 779–792.

Travis, L.E. (1957). The unspeakable feelings of people, with special reference to stuttering. In L.E. Travis (Ed.), *Handbook of speech pathology.* New York: Appleton-Century-Crofts.

Travis, L.E. (1978). The cerebral dominance theory of stuttering: 1931–1978. *Journal of Speech and Hearing Disorders, 43,* 278–281.

Van Riper, C. (1971). *The nature of stuttering.* Englewood Cliffs, NJ: Prentice-Hall.

Venkatagiri, H.S. (1981). Reaction time for voiced and whispered /a/ in stutterers and nonstutterers. *Journal of Fluency Disorders, 6,* 265–271.

Venkatagiri, H.S. (1982). Reaction time for /s/ and /z/ in stutterers and nonstutterers. *Journal of Communication Disorders, 15,* 55–62.

Wall, M.J. (1980). A comparison of syntax in young stutterers and nonstutterers. *Journal of Fluency Disorders, 5,* 345–352.

Wendahl, R.W., & Cole, J. (1961). Identification of stuttering during relatively fluent speech. *Journal of Speech and Hearing Research, 4,* 281–286.

West, R. (1958). An agnostic's speculations about stuttering. In J. Eisenson (Ed.), *Stuttering: A symposium.* New York: Harper & Row.

Westby, C.E. (1979). Language performance of stuttering and nonstuttering children. *Journal of Communication Disorders, 12*, 133–145.

Williams, A.M., & Marks, C.J. (1972). A comparative analysis of the ITPA and PPVT performance of young stutterers. *Journal of Speech and Hearing Research, 15*, 323–329.

Williams, D.E., & Silverman, F.H. (1968). Note concerning articulation of school-age stutterers. *Perceptual and Motor Skills, 27*, 713–714.

Wingate, M.E. (1962). Personality needs of stutterers. *Logos, 5*, 35–37.

Wingate, M.E. (1964). A standard definition of stuttering. *Journal of Speech and Hearing Disorders, 29*, 484–489.

Wingate, M.E. (1969). Sound and pattern in "artificial" fluency. *Journal of Speech and Hearing Research, 12*, 677–686.

Wingate, M.E. (1970). Effect on stuttering of changes in audition. *Journal of Speech and Hearing Research, 13*, 861–873.

Wingate, M.E. (1972). Deferring the adaptation effect. *Journal of Speech and Hearing Research, 15*, 547–550.

Wingate, M.E. (1976). *Stuttering: Theory and treatment.* New York: Irvington.

Witt, M.H. (1925). Statistische Erhebungen uber den Einfluss des Singens und Flusterns auf das Stottern. *Vox, 11*, 41–43.

Woods, C.L., & Williams, D.E. (1976). Traits attributed to stuttering and normally fluent males. *Journal of Speech and Hearing Research, 19*, 267–278.

World Health Organization. (1977). *Manual of the International statistical classification of diseases, injuries, and causes of death* (Vol. 1). Geneva: World Health Organization.

Yairi, E., & Clifton, N.F., Jr. (1972). Disfluent speech behavior of preschool children, high school seniors, and geriatric persons. *Journal of Speech and Hearing Research, 15*, 714–719.

Yairi, E., & Williams, D.E. (1970). Speech clinicians' stereotypes of elementary-school boys who stutter. *Journal of Communication Disorders, 3*, 161–170.

Yates, A.J. (1963). Delayed auditory feedback. *Psychological Bulletin, 60*, 213–232.

Zimmermann, G. (1980a). Articulatory dynamics of fluent utterances of stutterers and nonstutterers. *Journal of Speech and Hearing Research, 23*, 95–107.

Zimmermann, G. (1980b). Stuttering: A disorder of movement. *Journal of Speech and Hearing Research, 23*, 122–136.

Zimmermann, G.N., Smith, A., & Hanley, J.M. (1981). Stuttering: In need of a unifying conceptual framework. *Journal of Speech and Hearing Research, 24*, 25–31.

Concordance for Stuttering in Monozygotic and Dizygotic Twin Pairs

Pauline M. Howie

Several lines of evidence converge to provide increasingly strong evidence that stuttering is under genetic control. At the simplest level, many studies show that stutterers more frequently report a family history of stuttering than nonstutterers (see, for example, a recent review by Sheehan & Costley, 1977). At a more complex level, the incidence of stuttering in various relatives of stutterers is higher than the population incidence (Andrews & Harris, 1964; Johnson, 1959; Kant & Ahuja, 1970; Kidd, Kidd, & Records, 1978), and it increases with increasingly close relationship to the stutterer (Andrews & Harris, 1964; Johnson, 1959). Although these family incidence studies have not always incorporated the appropriate age corrections (Andrews & Harris, 1964), the obtained incidence patterns are encouragingly consistent with one another. Furthermore, both Andrews and Harris (1964) and Kidd et al. (1978) reported a higher incidence of stuttering in the relatives of female stutterers than in the relatives of male stutterers, a finding difficult to explain in purely environmental terms.

Kidd (1977) statistically tested the fit of stuttering family incidence data to two contrasting genetic models—a single major locus model and a multifactorial model—and reported that both fit the data equally well, an encouraging finding for genetic theory though the question of exactly how the stuttering genotype is transmitted is left unanswered.

All family incidence research is hampered by the confounding of environmental similarity with genetic similarity, with the consequence that observed intrafamily similarity in stuttering could still conceivably reflect cultural rather than genetic transmission. Investigations of individuals raised apart from their biological families provide an effective means of separating environment and genes, although even here, prenatal environmental factors may be confounded with genetic factors. Twin studies also allow control for within-family environmental variables. The rationale of the twin method is that because identical or monozygotic (MZ) twins share all their genes and fraternal or dizygotic (DZ) twins share on average only half their genes, any greater intrapair similarity observed in MZ twins is attributable to inherited factors. This rationale requires the assumption that MZ twins share equally similar environments as do DZ twins, an assumption which has recently received some empirical support (Lytton, 1977; Matheny, Wilson, & Dolan, 1976; Plomin, Willerman, & Loehlin, 1976; Scarr, 1968).

Traditionally, twin studies of stuttering have compared MZ and DZ twins on *pair-wise* concordance rates (Allen, Harvald, & Shields, 1967), that is, the percentage of pairs concordant for stuttering in a sample of twins selected to contain at least one stutterer. The existing literature (Table 1) contains reports of 50 MZ pairs, 78 percent of which were concordant for stuttering, and 78 DZ pairs, 9 percent of which were concordant for stuttering. With only one exception (Graf, 1955), all studies confirm the genetic hypothesis of higher concordance in MZ than in DZ twins. However, even the more systematic of these studies (Graf, 1955; Nelson, Hunter, & Walter, 1945; Seeman, 1967) reveal serious methodological shortcomings. Stuttering diagnosis and zygosity classification were not independent and were based on unreliable or ill-defined criteria. Most studies combined same- and opposite-sex DZ twins, thus confounding sex with zygosity. Concordance rates were not corrected for age (necessary because some young discordant pairs may eventually become concordant) or for independence of ascertainment [necessary because concordant pairs may be twice as likely as discordant pairs to be identified in a search for affected pairs (Allen et al., 1967; Smith, 1974)]. Most of these shortcomings are likely to bias results in favor of a genetic hypothesis, and thus little confidence can be placed in the results of the early studies.

The aim of the present research was therefore to establish whether the previously reported concordance patterns for stuttering would be replicated when the twin method was applied with greater methodological stringency.

Reprinted from *Journal of Speech and Hearing Research*, 24, no. 3 (September 1984), 317–321. Copyright © 1984 American Speech-Language-Hearing Association.

TABLE 1. Summary of studies of concordance for stuttering in twins.

Researcher	Number of pairs			
	MZ twins		DZ twins	
	Discordant	Concordant	Discordant	Concordant
Nelson et al. (1945)	1	9	28	2
Graf (1955)	6	1	7	2
Seeman (1967)	0	14	32	1
Gedda, Branconi, & Bruno (1960)	1	1	3	1
Andrews & Harris (1964)	0	1	1	1
Brodnitz (1951)	0	1	0	—
Yoshimashu (1941)	0	1	0	—
Shields (1962)	1	1	0	—
Juel-Nielsen (1965)	2	0	0	—
Early reports collected by Seeman	0	10	0	—
Total	11	39 (78%)	71	7 (9%)

METHOD

Subjects

The subjects were 30 same-sex twin pairs, each pair containing at least one stutterer or former stutterer. Ages ranged from 6 to 27 years (mean, 13.52 years; standard deviation, 5.81). Seventeen pairs were ascertained by searching files in all public speech clinics in Sydney and Melbourne. Another 13 pairs volunteered in response to a newspaper request.

Diagnosis of Zygosity

Twin pairs were classified as either monozygotic (MZ) or dizygotic (DZ), based on the following four criteria: (a) blood grouping for nine systems: ABO, Rhesus, MNSs, P, Lutheran, Kell, Lewis, Duffy, Kidd (Race & Sanger, 1968). Permission for blood tests was granted by 22 pairs, six of whose HLA tissue typing was also available; (b) total ridge counts and maximal palmar ATD angle (Holt, 1968); (c) cephalic index (Weiner & Lourie, 1969); and (d) height.

In seven pairs, DZ classification was certain because of the presence of at least one blood type difference. For each remaining pair, the probability of dizygosity was calculated, given the observed intrapair differences and similarities on the four criteria (Maynard-Smith & Penrose, 1955; Race & Sanger, 1968). The calculated probability of dizygosity was less than .05 in all but three of the pairs classified as MZ and greater than .95 in all but four of the pairs classified as DZ. Final classification was based on the probabilities examined

in conjunction with intrapair differences in iris color, hair color and form, earlobe attachment, and finger ridge patterns. Zygosity was assessed by two judges, one of whom had direct contact with the twins, while the other made the diagnosis on the basis of profile and full-face photographs and all the relevant data. Thus, the second judge had no information about stuttering concordance. The zygosity classifications of the two judges agreed in every case.

Speech Samples and Diagnosis of Stuttering

For each subject, two 500-word speech samples were recorded: a monologue with standard instructions ("Tell the story of a book or film"); and a conversation with the experimenter on standardized topics. The recordings of the 60 subjects were arranged on audiotape in random order, and stuttering was diagnosed by a speech pathologist who had never met the twins and had no knowledge of twin pair membership or zygosity, thus ensuring independence of stuttering diagnosis and zygosity classification. The clinician had to categorize the subject as either a stutterer or a nonstutterer, according to a standard definition (*International Classification of Diseases*, WHO, 1977). In one MZ pair, the clinician diagnosed neither co-twin as a stutterer. This pair was eliminated from the calculation of concordance rates. The reliability of the clinician's stuttering diagnosis was assessed by comparison with the mothers' diagnoses of stuttering, based on the same standard definition. Table 2 shows the agreement between mothers and clinician. Diagnoses agreed in 50 of the 60 subjects and may be regarded as consistent in at least five other subjects. The individual diagnosed as a stutterer by the mother and as a nonstutterer by the clinician was an intermittent stutterer according to the mother, a diagnosis independently corroborated by a teacher. The five cases in which the clinician diagnosed stuttering when the mother did not were divided among MZ pairs (2 cases) and DZ pairs (3 cases), and therefore did not affect the MZ-DZ concordance difference estimated on the basis of clinician diagnoses.

As a measure of stuttering severity, the clinician counted the number of disfluencies in each sample. Disfluencies were defined according to Johnson's (1961) criteria, and the scores were expressed as the number of disfluencies per 100 words. The two speech samples were combined to

TABLE 2. Agreement between diagnoses of stuttering by mothers and by clinician. Frequency of classification into each diagnostic category.

Clinician diagnosis	Maternal diagnosis			
	Stutterer	Former stutterer	Non-stutterer	Total
Stutterer	33	4	5	42
Nonstutterer	1	4	13	18
Total	34	8	18	60

form one score for each subject because disfluency scores in the two samples proved to be highly correlated. Both intrarater and interrater reliability were high: the Pearson Product Moment correlation between the clinician's first rating and a second rating of 10 randomly selected subjects was .99. The correlation between two independent judges' ratings of another 10 subjects was .87.

Calculation of Concordance for Stuttering

The most appropriate concordance rate for genetic research is the *proband-wise* rate, which estimates the risk of stuttering in the co-twin of stutterer and thus may be interpreted in genetic terms more meaningfully than the *pair-wise* rate (Smith, 1974). However, pair-wise rates were also calculated for comparison with previous research. The respective formulae (Allen et al., 1967) are: pair-wise rate = $\frac{1}{2}(C + x)/[\frac{1}{2}(C + x) + D']$, and proband-wise rate = $(C + x)/(C + x + D')$, where C = number of concordant pairs, x = number of concordant pairs in which both co-twins were independently ascertained (see Allen et al., 1967), and D' = number of discordant pairs, corrected for age.

Discordant pairs were counted as full pairs if they were 12 years or older, and if not, they were given a weighting of between 0 and .9 depending on the proportion of risk of stuttering already passed. Andrews and Harris's (1964) empirically based estimates of proportion of risk passed were used.

RESULTS

Table 3 shows the frequencies of concordant and discordant MZ and DZ pairs and the derived pair-wise and proband-wise concordance rates, corrected for age and independence of ascertainment. Male and female data are presented separately, although the numbers are not large enough to justify separate statistical analysis. The ratio of males to females was very similar in the two groups (2.20:1 for MZ and 2.25:1 for DZ).

It is clear that whether pair-wise or proband-wise rates are used, concordance for stuttering is considerably higher in MZ twins than in DZ twins. Ten of the 16 MZ pairs were concordant for stuttering, producing a corrected pair-wise concordance rate of .63. By contrast, only three of the 13 DZ pairs were concordant, producing a corrected pair-wise concordance rate of .19. Chi-square analyses were performed using Yate's correction for continuity (Siegel, 1956), which has the effect of increasing the conservatism of the test. Because the direction of the relationship between concordance and zygosity was predicted, a one-tailed test was used. Analysis of the combined sexes sample showed a significant relationship between frequency of pair-wise concordance and zygosity, whether corrected frequencies ($\chi^2 = 3.27$, $p < .05$) or uncorrected frequencies ($\chi^2 =$

TABLE 3. Frequency of concordant and discordant pairs among MZ and DZ twins, and the derived pair-wise and proband-wise concordance rates, corrected for age and independence of ascertainment. Calculation formulae are given in the text.

Variable	All twins		Males		Females	
	MZ	DZ	MZ	DZ	MZ	DZ
Number of concordant pairs	10	3	7	3	3	0
Number of discordant pairs	6[a]	10	4[a]	6	2	4
Corrected pair wise concordance rate	.63	.19	.64	.29	.60	0
Corrected probandwise concordance rate	.77	.32	.78	.45	.75	0

[a]One of the 7 discordant MZ pairs was eliminated from concordance calculations because neither co-twin was identified as a stutterer by the clinician (see text).

3.05, $p < .05$) were used. Male and female subgroups followed a similar pattern. Analysis of concordance based on maternal diagnoses of stuttering produced essentially the same results. The genetic hypothesis of higher MZ than DZ concordance for stuttering was therefore confirmed. Examination of the proband-wise concordance rates in Table 3 indicates that the estimated risk of stuttering in the MZ co-twin of a stutterer is .77, and .32 in the DZ co-twin of a stutterer.

Comparison of Volunteer and Clinic Subjects

Because the twin sample was drawn from two different sources, it was important to establish whether the two subgroups differed in any way which might bias results. The clinic and volunteer groups were similar in age and MZ:DZ ratio, but not surprisingly, the average stuttering severity was significantly lower in stutterers of the volunteer group (mean disfluencies per 100 words = 6.35, standard deviation = 5.30) than in the stutterers of the clinic group (mean disfluencies = 13.63, standard deviation = 11.07, $t = 2.39$, $p < .05$). The volunteer group also contained a lower proportion of concordant twins (regardless of zygosity) than the clinic group, though the difference was not significant. Thus, the volunteer group was free of the most serious source of sampling bias in twin studies: over-reporting of concordant MZ pairs (Neel & Schull, 1954).

DISCUSSION

The findings of this study support the hypothesis that genetic factors are involved in the etiology of stuttering. Concordance for stuttering was significantly greater in identical twins than in fraternal twins, whether the diagnosis of clinician or mother was used, and thus the results of the early and methodologically dubious studies of twin concordance for stuttering (Table 1) were essentially replicated. This finding is consistent with the family incidence literature, which also strongly suggests a genetic contribution to stuttering. The small number of females in the present study precluded the possibility of testing the concordance hypothesis separately for males and females. A larger study would enable questions to be asked about male-female differences in the extent or nature of the genetic contribution to stuttering. It may also provide a test of the fit of different models of genetic transmission, as single major genes and multifactorial models of transmission such as those suggested by Kidd's (1977) "best fit" solutions to his family data may predict quite different patterns of male and female concordance.

Although the present results essentially confirm the earlier research, they suggest that the early studies exaggerated the extent of the MZ-DZ discrepancy in concordance. The presence of at least six discordant pairs among the 17 MZ pairs in this study suggests that MZ discordance for stuttering is not as rare as most of the earlier research implied. The demonstrated reliability of the classification of zygosity and stuttering makes it unlikely that misclassification could account for the observed MZ discordance in the present study.

One of the problems of concordance research is that because independence of stuttering diagnosis and zygosity classification is crucial, parental reports are not acceptable as a primary source of data. Thus, valuable information from parents about recovered or intermittent stuttering is not usable, whereas a professional's diagnosis of stuttering based on speech samples taken during a restricted time period is usable. In this study, the mothers reported recovered stuttering in several twins, and these individuals were classed as stutterers for the purpose of calculating concordance rates based on maternal diagnosis. However, the concordance rates calculated from maternal diagnoses were very similar to those based on clinician diagnosis. Thus, the inevitable exclusion of some former stutterers from the clinician concordance rates apparently did not depress the resulting rates, probably because in this study as in other research (Boehmler, 1958; Tuthill, 1946) the clinician was more likely than the parent to diagnose nonfluent speech as stuttering (Table 2).

While the evidence clearly supports a genetic hypothesis, the presence of MZ discordance is of theoretical significance, because if the genetically identical co-twin of a stutterer does not necessarily become a stutterer, genetic factors alone are clearly not sufficient to produce stuttering. This conclusion is supported by the fact that the estimated risk of .32 of stuttering in the DZ co-twins of stutterers (Table 3: proband-wise concordance rate) is higher than the generally reported risk of approximately .20 for siblings of stutterers (Andrews & Harris, 1964; Kidd et al., 1978). The

genetic similarity between DZ co-twins is the same as between siblings, but the environmental similarity is presumably greater in DZ co-twins, and therefore a finding of higher risk of stuttering in DZ co-twins of stutterers than in their siblings, if stable and significant, would again implicate nongenetic factors in the etiology of stuttering.

The isolation of environmental variables and understanding of their interaction with genetic factors is a task for future research. It may also be possible for future research to isolate specific symptoms or dimensions of stuttering which are and are not under genetic control. Quantitative measures of various dimensions of stuttering are required to answer this question. In another paper (Howie, in press), an examination of MZ and DZ co-twin similarity in the frequency of different disfluency types provides some evidence of genetic contribution to the overall frequency of disfluency and to the frequency of occurrence of blocks and prolongations but not to the frequency of disfluencies of the repetition or interjection type.

The presence of discordant MZ twins in the present study also has implications for the interpretation of genealogical studies of stuttering. If, as MZ discordance implies, genotypically predisposed individuals do not always display the phenotype of stuttering, incidence figures in family studies of stuttering will underestimate the frequency of occurrence of the genotype. This may explain why the obtained family incidence figures fall well below classical Mendelian single gene expectations. It may be that by broadening diagnostic criteria, or by identifying a marker of the genotype, classical transmission patterns will emerge. Alternatively, several genes may be involved in the stuttering genotype, as pointed out by Kay and Andrews (Andrews & Harris, 1964) and by Kidd (1977). The presence of discordant MZ pairs is equally compatible with a multifactorial model of the etiology of stuttering.

What implications do these findings have for the treatment of stuttering? It is of importance that a genetic view of the etiology of stuttering is in no way inconsistent with a symptom-oriented approach to its clinical management. Successful treatment of a condition does not necessarily depend on reversing the conditions of its cause. It is also possible to compensate in some way for the initial deficiency, as in the modification of diet in the treatment of phenylketonuria, which is an inherited condition. Thus, the treatment of stuttering may be seen as the training of new behaviors and attitudes to compete with and compensate for disordered behaviors, whether these behaviors are the result of environmental or genetic factors.

ACKNOWLEDGMENTS

This research was completed as part of the requirements of a doctoral degree at the University of New South Wales, Sydney, Australia, under the supervision of Dr. Gavin Andrews. The author wishes to acknowledge the support of

Gavin Andrews at all stages of the project, and the invaluable genetic guidance of Dr. David Hay, of Latrobe University, Melbourne, Australia.

REFERENCES

Allen, G., Harvald, B., & Shields, J. (1967). Measures of twin concordance. *Acta Genetica* (Basel), *17*, 475–481.

Andrews, G., & Harris, M. (1964). *The syndrome of stuttering.* London: Heinemann Books Ltd.

Boehmler, R.M. (1958). Listener responses to nonfluencies. *Journal of Speech and Hearing Research, 1,* 132–141.

Brodnitz, F.A. (1951). Stuttering of different types in identical twins. *Journal of Speech Disorders, 16,* 334–336.

Gedda, L., Branconi, L., & Bruno, G. (1960). Su alcuni casi di balbuzie in coppie gemellari mono- e dizigotiche. *Acta Geneticae Medicae et Gemellologiae, 9,* 407–426.

Graf, O. (1955). Incidence of stuttering among twins. In W.J. Johnson & R.R. Leutenegger (Eds.), *Stuttering in children and adults.* Minneapolis: University of Minnesota Press.

Holt, S.B. (1968). *The genetics of dermal ridges.* Springfield, IL: Charles C. Thomas.

Howie, P.M. Intrapair similarity in frequency of disfluency in MZ and DZ twin pairs containing stutterers. *Behavior Genetics,* in press.

Johnson, W.J. (1959). *The onset of stuttering.* Minneapolis: University of Minnesota Press.

Johnson, W.J. (1961). Measurements of oral reading and speaking rate and disfluency of adult male and female stutterers and nonstutterers. *Journal of Speech and Hearing Disorders Monograph Supplement, 7,* 1–20.

Juel-Nielsen, N. (1965). Individual and environment: A psychiatric-psychological investigation of monozygotic twins reared apart. *Acta Psychiatrica Scandinavica Supplement 183.*

Kant, K., & Ahuja, Y.R. (1970). Inheritance of stuttering. *Acta Medica Auxologica, 2,* 179–191.

Kidd, K.K. (1977). A genetic perspective on stuttering. *Journal of Fluency Disorders, 2,* 259–269.

Kidd, K.K., Kidd, J.R., & Records, M.A. (1978). The possible causes of the sex ratio in stuttering and its implications. *Journal of Fluency Disorders, 3,* 13–23.

Lytton, H. (1977). Do parents create, or respond to differences in twins? *Development Psychology, 13,* 456–459.

Matheny, A.P., Wilson, R.S., & Dolan, A.B. (1976). Relations between twins' similarity of appearance and behavioral similarity: Testing an assumption. *Behavior Genetics, 6,* 343–351.

Maynard-Smith, S.M., & Penrose, L.S. (1955) Monozygotic and dizygotic twin diagnosis. *Annals of Human Genetics, 19,* 273–289.

Neel, J.V., & Schull, W.J. (1954). *Human heredity.* Chicago: University of Chicago Press.

Nelson, S.E., Hunter, N., & Walter, M. (1945). Stuttering in twin types. *Journal of Speech Disorders, 10,* 335–343.

Plomin, R., Willerman, L., & Loehlin, J.C. (1976). Resemblance in appearance and the equal environments assumption in twin studies of personality traits. *Behavior Genetics, 6,* 43–52.

Race, R.R., & Sanger, R. (1968). *Blood groups in man.* London: Spottiswoode.

Scarr, S. (1968). Environmental bias in twin studies. In S. Vandenberg (Ed.), *Progress in human behavior genetics.* Baltimore: Johns Hopkins Press.

Seeman, M. (1967). *Les troubles du language chez l'enfant* (M. Musafia, Trans.). Brussels: Presses Académiques.

Sheehan, J.G., & Costley, M.S. (1977). A reexamination of the role of heredity in stuttering. *Journal of Speech and Hearing Disorders, 52,* 47–59.

Shields, J. (1962). *Monozygotic twins brought up apart and brought up together.* London: Oxford University Press.

Siegel, S. (1956). *Non parametric statistics for the behavioral sciences.* New York: McGraw-Hill.

Smith, C. (1974). Concordance in twins: Methods and interpretation. *American Journal of Human Genetics, 26,* 454–466.

Tuthill, C.A. (1946). A quantitative study of extensional meaning with special reference to stuttering. *Speech Monographs, 13,* 81–98.

Weiner, J.S., & Lourie, J.A. (Eds.). (1969). *Human biology: A guide to field methods.* Oxford: Blackwell Scientific Publications.

World Health Organization (WHO). (1977). *International classification of diseases. Manual of the international statistical classification of diseases, injuries, and causes of death* (9th rev.). Geneva: WHO.

Yoshimashu, S. (1941). Psychopathie und Kriminalität. *Psychiatria et Neurologia Japonica, 45,* 455–531.

Molecular Genetics: The Key to the Puzzle of Stuttering?

Nancy J. Cox

Phrases like gene cloning and recombinant DNA have moved from science fiction into mainstream biological science and, lately, back into popular nonfiction. Though it is now common to read about breakthroughs made with the new tools from moelcular biology, it may not be easy for scientists in other disciplines to see how useful these tools might be to them. This report will bring you up to date on these molecular genetic tools and speculate on what these tools might reveal about the nature of stuttering.

STUTTERING AS A GENETIC DISORDER

Stuttering has long been recognized as a familial disorder. Family studies have shown that the risk of stuttering in relatives of a person who stutters is increased over that for the general population (Andrews & Harris, 1964; Kidd, 1977) and that the pattern of transmission in families is consistent with predictions derived from genetic models (Kidd, Heimbuck, & Records, 1981; Cox, Kramer, & Kidd, 1984). In contrast, purely environmental models do not provide a good explanation for the observed transmission (Kidd et al., 1981; Cox, Seider, & Kidd, 1984).

There is little satisfaction, however, in saying that genetic models are compatible with the data on stuttering when a variety of quite different genetic models are all equally compatible with the data. It is clear that genes are not the entire story; monozygotic twins, who have identical genetic makeup, are not always concordant for stuttering (Howie, 1981). In fact, the genetic component to stuttering is unlikely to be simple. There may be many different genes involved, each of which individually has small effect but which in combination with each other and with some environmental predisposing factors can produce the pattern of stuttering observed in families. Alternatively, there may be only one or at most a few genes which are important for stuttering, again allowing for the interaction of environmental predisposing factors.

Even if we could precisely specify the genetic model for stuttering, it would give us little additional insight into the nature of the disorder. Knowing exactly how the primary defect is transmitted would still not tell us what that defect is. But consider the possibility that we could actually identify the gene or genes responsible for the transmission of stuttering. Would it be a gene or genes involved in the complex developmental process of hemispheric lateralization? Or perhaps the gene would code for a structural protein in the larynx which is abnormal in persons who stutter and prevents appropriately coordinated communication with speech centers in the brain. Imagine what insights this knowledge would provide on the nature of recovery from stuttering. Consider what implications the findings might have for our understanding of normal brain development.

Could the "new" genetics really do all this? Until we understand these tools and can evaluate their power and limitations, we can't really answer this question. The next section provides a schematic overview of the new developments in molecular genetics that are relevant for studies of disorders like stuttering.

THE "NEW" GENETICS (AS WELL AS THE OLD)

DNA (deoxyribonucleic acid) is the basic material of life. The twisted ladder configuration of DNA has a special significance. The deoxyribose sugar forms the backbone of the ladder, while the bases thymine (T), adenine (A), guanine (G), and cytosine (C) form the rungs of the ladder, thymine pairing with adenine and cytosine pairing with guanine. It is the sequence of these bases, read three at a time, which determines what amino acids are brought together to form the proteins which ultimately form us. The segment of DNA which contains the sequence coding for a particular protein is the "gene" for that protein.

Human DNA is organized into 23 pairs of chromosomes; a parent passes on one of each pair to a child. When we speak of the gene which codes for a particular protein, we are actually referring to a pair of genes, one on each chromosome, each of which can produce the protein. When there is DNA sequence variation in the gene that codes for a protein, the gene is said to be polymorphic and the alternative forms of the gene are called polymorphisms or alleles. Since

Reprinted from *ASHA, 30*, no. 4, 36–37. Copyright © 1988 American Speech-Language-Hearing Association.

genes come in pairs, it is possible for one individual to have two different forms (alleles) of the same gene. The two alleles have an equal probability (i.e., 50%) of being passed on to any child. But it is obvious that the genes on a single chromosome would tend to be inherited together. Consider two genes found on the same pair of chromosomes, gene A with alleles designated A1 and A2 and gene B with alleles designated B1 and B2 (Figure 1). When a parent passes on the chromosome with the A1 allele, the child should also inherit the B1 allele. This would always be the case if not for the phenomenon of genetic recombination. In this process, a pair of homologous chromosomes may exchange genetic material. In our example, if a recombination occurs at a point between the A and B genes then the A1 allele would be passed on with the B2 allele instead of the B1 allele. The probability of recombination is proportional to the distance between two genes. The farther apart two genes on the same chromosome are, the more likely is a recombination between them. In fact, genes far apart on the same chromosome are no more likely to be transmitted together than genes on different chromosomes. Recombination is not an unnatural or unusual occurrence, it is just nature's way of shuffling the DNA variation into different combinations.

Variation in the DNA sequence can lead to variation in the proteins produced; such genetic variation is responsible for many of the visible differences between individuals. A genetic disease is caused by variation in DNA, but we may not know what abnormal protein produces the disease. In order to identify the gene that gives rise to the abnormal disease-producing protein, we could undertake genetic studies of families in which the disease occurs. Imagine that we could place uniquely marked tags at regular intervals on each of the chromosome pairs in the parents of such families. We could then watch how the tags were transmitted to the

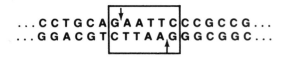

Figure 2. The recognition sequence of the restriction enzyme EcoRI is denoted by the box and the cutting sites are denoted by arrows. Adenine is represented by A, thymine by T, cytosine by C, and guanine by G.

children in the family, paying special attention to what tags seem to be transmitted along with illness in the family. Recent breakthroughs in molecular biology have provided us with just such marker tags.

The key to developing these markers was the isolation of a group of enzymes from bacteria. These enzymes are called restriction enzymes and they have the ability to cut DNA at specific sites. Figure 2 shows the recognition and cutting sites for one such enzyme, EcoRI; different enzymes have different recognition sites. The important feature is that an enzyme will cut the DNA at its recognition site, and *only* at its recognition site, so that the resulting set of fragments is completely reproducible.

Figure 3 illustrates schematically the process of applying these marker tags. Briefly, DNA can be extracted from a small sample of whole blood and digested with a restriction enzyme. The resulting collection of fragments can be size-fractionated by electrophoresing the digested DNA in an agarose gel. The DNA is then transferred from the gel to a membrane in a blotting procedure that preserves the size-fractionation achieved by electrophoresis. A piece of DNA may then be labeled, radioactively for example, and then hybridized to the complementary DNA trapped on the membrane. The labeled piece of DNA is called a probe; it may be a random, nonfunctional piece of DNA, or it may contain sequences which code for a protein or part of a protein.

Figure 4 illustrates schematically the application of the process described above to DNA that has a polymorphic restriction enzyme recognition site. This means that the set of bases which form the recognition and cutting site for some enzyme has been altered, perhaps by just one base, on some chromosomes, so that the DNA is no longer cleaved at that site. As shown in the figure, the DNA that would hybridize with the probe has two invariant restriction enzyme recognition sites and one site which may be present or absent. When the variable site is present, the marker DNA would hybridize to a fragment of DNA 3000 bases (or 3 kilobases 3Kb) in length. When the variable site is absent, the probe would hybridize to a fragment of DNA 5 Kb in length, since the next invariant cut site is 2 Kb further from the variable site. Variation in DNA sequences detected by variation in the length of the DNA fragments after digestion with restriction enzymes is called restriction fragment length polymorphisms or RFLPs.

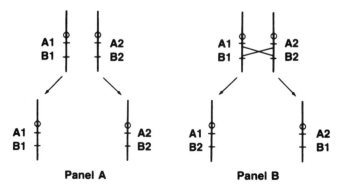

Figure 1. Schematic representation of a pair of chromosomes going into separate gametes. In panel A, on the left, the chromosome pair has not undergone a recombination, and so the markers A1 and B1 will be passed on together, as will the markers A2 and B2. In panel B, on the right, a recombination has occurred between the A and B genes. Therefore A1 will be passed on with B2, and A2 will be passed on with B1.

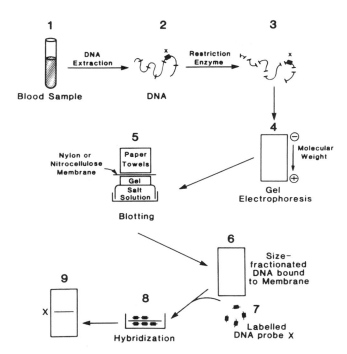

Figure 3. (1) A small sample of whole blood is collected and (2) DNA is extracted. (3) The DNA is digested with a restriction enzyme which cuts the DNA at specific sites. (4) These pieces of DNA are size-fractionated in a process called electrophoresis. The digested DNA is placed in a small hole at one end of an agarose gel and an electric current is applied; the DNA migrates toward the positive (+) pole, but the smaller fragments (low molecular weight) migrate through the gel faster than the larger fragments. After the current has been applied some length of time, there is a size gradient in the gel. (5) The DNA in the gel is then transferred to a special kind of membrane in a blotting procedure. A salt solution is drawn up through the gel, carrying the DNA with it. The salt solution passes through the membrane and is absorbed by the paper towels, but the DNA is trapped by the membrane. (6) The DNA is "bound" to the membrane in a perfect reflection of the size fractionation achieved by the electrophoresis. (7) A piece of DNA, X, is labeled, either radioactively or by some other technique. The labeled DNA is called a probe. (8) The X probe is hybridized to the DNA on the membrane. The base sequence of the probe seeks its complementary sequence in the DNA on the membrane—A pairs with T and C pairs with G. Only sequences perfectly complementary to the probe will hybridize with it. (9) The labeled membrane is then processed to show where the probe hybridized. The position of the "band" of hybridization depends on the size of the DNA fragment which contained the sequence complementary to the X probe.

Probes which detect RFLPs are the marker tags that we can use to follow pieces of DNA through families. Geneticists are working hard to provide enough of these markers to saturate each of the chromosomes. Depending on how closely spaced we require the markers to be, the human genome may be saturated with reasonably polymorphic

markers in 2 to 3 years. There are already several chromosomes that have many areas of full saturation.

This method of following pieces of DNA in families with a disease is referred to as a linkage study; the disease is said to be "mapped" when a particular marker or set of markers have been identified that clearly cosegregate with the disease. This, of course, is only the first step in characterizing the gene or genes responsible for the disease. Once the general site of the gene has been identified by its proximity to one of the markers, then a variety of molecular strategies are used to identify the actual gene involved and determine how it causes the disease.

The first diseases to which these markers were successfully applied were those which had clear, well understood patterns of transmission. Cystic fibrosis, for example, is a genetic disease with a recessive pattern of inheritance. This means that each person born with cystic fibrosis has abnormal "cystic" alleles at the cystic fibrosis gene on both of their chromosomes. Both parents of a child with cystic fibrosis have a normal allele at the cystic fibrosis gene on one of their chromosomes and a "cystic" allele at this gene on the other chromosome. Although they have one copy of the "cystic"

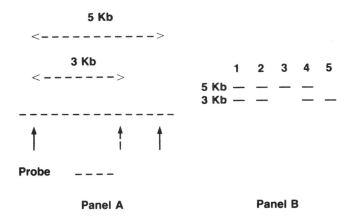

Figure 4. Panel A illustrates the invariant restriction enzyme cutting sites with solid arrows and the variable cutting site with a dashed arrow. When the variable site is absent, the probe would hybridize to a piece of DNA 5000 bases (or 5 kilobases = 5 Kb) in length. When the variable site is present, the probe would hybridize to a piece of DNA 3 Kb in length. Panel B illustrates schematically how this restriction fragment length polymorphism would be visualized in a hybridization of labeled probe to a membrane with DNA from members of a family. The father's DNA is shown in track 1; he has one chromosome with the variable site and one chromosome without. The mother's DNA is shown in track 2, and she has the same type as the father. The first child's DNA in track 3 indicates that this child inherited the chromosome without the variable site from each of his parents. The second child's DNA in track 4 shows the same type as the parents, indicating this child inherited a chromosome with the variable site from one parent and a chromosome without the variable site from the other parent. Track 5 shows that the third child has inherited the chromosome with the variable site from each of her parents.

allele, they appear normal and have none of the symptoms of the disease themselves—the "cystic" allele is recessive to the normal allele. Huntington disease is a genetic disease with a dominant pattern of inheritance. Thus, the Huntington's allele is dominant to the normal allele at this gene, and the presence of only one Huntington's allele will cause a person to be affected with the disease.

Although the inheritance patterns for cystic fibrosis and Huntington disease had long been known, the chromosomal location of the genes and the gene products which ultimately cause the diseases were not known. Both genes have recently been mapped using the RFLP marker methods just described (Gusella et al., 1983; Knowlton et al., 1985; Wainwright et al., 1985; White et al., 1985). Studies are well underway to isolate the actual genes and determine the gene products.

Of course, as we have already noted, stuttering does *not* have a simple, well characterized pattern of transmission. Of what use are the molecular methods for a trait with such a complex pattern of transmission? Recent reports of genetic studies in the psychiatric disorder of manic-depressive illness should lead us to be optimistic.

Like stuttering, manic-depressive illness is a behavioral disorder which has a significant but complex pattern of familial transmission. Unlike stuttering, manic-depressive illness is characterized by a variety of additional complications for genetic studies, such as late age-of-onset, diagnostic overlap with other disorders, and cohort effects in the prevalence of illness. Nevertheless, a recent linkage study of manic-depression in a large Amish family found evidence that susceptibility to illness was transmitted through the family along with markers on the short arm of chromosome 11 (Egeland et al., 1987). While the gene increasing susceptibility to manic-depression in this family has not yet been identified, an enzyme thought to be a good candidate for involvement in psychiatric illness had previously been mapped to this area of chromosome 11 and may turn out to be the guilty gene. However, studies in other pedigrees in which manic-depression is being transmitted indicate that the disease is likely to be heterogeneous; the same gene is not responsible for illness in all families transmitting manic-depression. The candidate enzyme mapped to chromosome 11 may be but one step in a long series; some families may have heritable defects at other enzymes in this pathway which lead to the same ultimate increased susceptibility to manic-depressive illness.

This mapping was the first demonstration that the new DNA markers will be useful in the study of diseases with complex inheritance patterns as well as with those showing simple patterns. Indeed, many geneticists now believe that linkage studies with DNA markers will be the only way to be certain whether there is a gene (or genes) involved in the transmission of such complex traits, since the patterns of transmission are compatible with so many different hypotheses.

APPLICATION OF MOLECULAR GENETIC TECHNIQUES TO STUTTERING— PITFALLS AND PAYBACKS

A good strategy for applying molecular genetics to stuttering would be to collect data on nuclear families with at least two affected children. Such families should not be difficult to find, since stuttering is relatively common and has onset in childhood. A modest blood sample (10 to 30 ml of blood is commonly collected, far less than donors to the Red Cross contribute) is all that is required from family members, although a more complete study would be desirable. The process illustrated in Figure 3 requires some specialized equipment and scientific expertise, but the overall cost is not prohibitive. What is the worst that could happen if such a study were to be undertaken? If several hundred probes were tested and none found to be linked to susceptibility to stuttering, the expense of collecting and analyzing the data would have yielded only "negative" information. Such an outcome might be expected if susceptibility to stuttering was a truly polygenic trait; in this situation, each individual gene contributes such a small amount to susceptibility that its effect cannot be detected against the background of the other genes and environmental fators which also contribute to susceptibility. Even so, we would still have more information on the etiology of stuttering than we have now.

It seems likely, however, that a single gene would be responsible for the major portion of susceptibility in at least some families, even if susceptibility to stuttering is transmitted as a polygenic trait in most families. A gene implicated in even a few families could provide a wealth of information on what factors might be involved in other families. Identification of the genetic component to susceptibility also provides one of the best ways to identify those elusive environmental factors which may increase susceptibility to stuttering. In a family showing linkage of stuttering to a particular gene, we would expect most, but not all, of the members of the family with the at-risk genetic constitution to express the trait of stuttering since even monozygotic twins with identical gene makeup will not always be concordant. By carefully comparing the birth and early developmental histories of those with the at-risk genetic constitutions who do not express their susceptibility to stuttering to their family members who expressed this same risk as stuttering, we might be able to identify environmental factors which predispose to stuttering. This same principle could, of course, be applied in studies of monozygotic twins. However, monozygotic twin pairs which include only one stutterer will occur much less frequently than sibling pairs. In addition, twins have a much more similar environment than siblings, since they share the same prenatal environment and history and grow up at the same time; thus, it is more difficult to identify differences.

The real payoff, of course, would be gaining an understanding of the basic defect in stuttering. My own belief is that susceptibility to stuttering is due to a developmental defect—key periods in normal brain development seem to coincide with the peak years of stuttering development and spontaneous recovery in children. Presumably, any genetic or environmental factor which could disrupt or delay this developmental process is a candidate for increasing susceptibility to stuttering. Because we know so little about how this development normally proceeds, any knowledge we could gain on developmental defects which can lead to stuttering could provide the foundation for an understanding of normal developmental processes. It is also possible that a better understanding of the primary defect would enable us to devise more effective treatments for stuttering or even prevention in susceptible individuals.

The new molecular genetic tools are powerful, with proven utility even for complex disorders. I believe there is a reasonable probability of success; these tools could provide us with a key piece in the puzzle of stuttering. And as with any puzzle, if you fill in one piece, it is often easier to recognize how the others fit together.

REFERENCES

Andrews, G., & Harris, M. (1964). *The syndrome of stuttering.* (Clinics in Develop. Med., No. 17). London: Spastics Society Medical Education and Information Unit in association with Wm. Heinemann Medical Books.

Cox, N.J., Kramer, P.L., & Kidd, K.K. (1984). Segregation analyses of stuttering. *Genetic Epidemiology, 1,* 245–253.

Cox, N.J., Seider, R.A., & Kidd, K.K. (1984). Some environmental factors and hypotheses for stuttering in families with several stutterers. *Journal of Speech and Hearing Research, 27,* 543–548.

Detera-Wadleigh, S.D., Berrettini, W.H., Goldin, L.R., Boorman, D., Anderson, S., & Gershon, E.S. (1987). Close linkage of c-Harvey-ras-1 and the insulin gene to affective disorders is ruled out in three North American pedigrees. *Nature, 325,* 806–808.

Egeland, J.A., Gerhard, D.S., Pauls, D.L., Sussex, J.N., Kidd, K.K., Allen, C.R., Hostetter, A.M., & Housman, D.E. (1987). Bipolar affective disorders linked to DNA markers on chromosome 11. *Nature, 325,* 783–787.

Gusella, J.F., Wexler, N.S., Conneally, P.M., Naylor, S.L., Anderson, M.A., Tanzi, R.E., Watkins, P.C., Ottina, K., Wallace, M.R., Sakaguchi, A.Y., et al. (1983). A polymorphic DNA marker genetically linked to Huntington's disease. *Nature, 306,* 234–238.

Hodgkinson, S., Sherrington, R., Gurling, H., Marchbanks, R., Reeders, S., Mallet, J., McInnis, M., Petursson, H., & Brynjolfsson, J. (1987). Molecular genetic evidence for heterogeneity in manic depression. *Nature, 325,* 805–806.

Howie, P.M. (1981). Concordance for stuttering in monozygotic and dizygotic twin pairs. *Journal of Speech and Hearing Research, 24,* 317–321.

Joffe, R.T., Harvath, Z., & Tarvybas, I. (1986). Bipolar affective disorder and thalassemia minor. *American Journal of Psychiatry, 143,* 933.

Kidd, K.K. (1977). A genetic perspective on stuttering. *Journal of Fluency Disorders, 2,* 259–269.

Kidd, K.K., Heimbuch, R.C., & Records, M.A. (1981). Vertical transmission of susceptibility to stuttering with sex-modified expression. *Proceedings of the National Academy of Science (USA), 78,* 606–610.

Knowlton, R.G., Cohen-Haguenaer, O., VanCong, N., Frezal, J., Brown, V.A., Barker, D., Braman, J.C., Schumm, J.W., Tsui, L.C., Buchwald, M., et al. (1985). A polymorphic DNA marker linked to cystic fibrosis is located on chromosome 7. *Nature, 318,* 380–382.

Wainwright, B.J., Scambler, P.J., Schmidtke, J., Watson, E.A., Law, H.Y., Farrall, M., Cooke, H.F., Eiberg, H., & Williamson, R. (1985). Localization of cystic fibrosis locus to human chromosome 7cen-q22. *Nature, 318,* 384–385.

White, R., Woodward, S., Leppert, M., O'Connell, P., Hoff, M., Herbst, J., Lalouel, J.M., & VandeWoude, G. (1985). A closely linked genetic marker for cystic fibrosis. *Nature, 318,* 382–384.

Stuttering: Speech Pattern Characteristics under Fluency-inducing Conditions

Gavin Andrews
Pauline M. Howie
Melinda Dozsa
Barry E. Guitar

There are three antecedents to this report. The first is the clinical observation that both syllable-timed speech and the prolonged speech induced by delayed auditory feedback seemed to derive their ability to inhibit stuttering from the nature of the particular speech patterns associated with each technique. In syllable-timed speech the duration of each syllable, the inverse of articulation rate, was of interest, whereas in prolonged speech the length of continuous phonation between pauses seemed an additional important variable. Furthermore, the inhibiting effect of each technique appeared to be potentiated when slow rates of speech were used. Indeed, Wingate (1969, 1970) had drawn attention to the possibility of some change in the manner of phonation associated with conditions which could inhibit stuttering. The second antecedent is Bloodstein's (1950) report of conditions under which stuttering was markedly reduced or absent, conditions which in the early 1970s were devoid of a unifying explanation. The third antecedent is experience with Goldman-Eisler's (1968) speech pause analyzer which allowed the measurement of phonation time and pause time, and thus the calculation of fluent speech rate, articulation rate, and phonation duration.

Preliminary work (Andrews, 1974) appeared promising, particularly as the results were consistent with an association between reduced stuttering and any condition in which the cortical load of speech formulation and execution could have been simplified. The ensuing years have seen considerable development in this area, but at no time has any research group investigated a variety of speech characteristics across a wide range of fluency-inducing conditions. Various attempts have been made to identify some characteristic common to all fluency-inducing conditions. Blood-

stein's questionnaire study of 204 stutterers reported reduced or absent stuttering in at least 95 percent of the respondents under the following conditions: speaking or reading alone, speaking in unison or when relaxed, speaking to an animal or infant, singing, speaking in time to a rhythmic stimulus (pacing), imitating a regional dialect, speaking and writing simultaneously, and swearing. Bloodstein suggested that fluency under these conditions could be explained either by reduced communicative responsibility, changes in speech pattern, or strong or unusual stimulation. Martin and Haroldson (1979) noted the need for studies of stutterers exposed to a range of fluency conditions. They measured the speech of 20 adult stutterers under four conditions: response contingent stimulation, masking, DAF, and rhythmic pacing. Stuttering frequency decreased significantly in all conditions, but the speech rate did not change in any of the conditions.

Wingate (1969, 1970) posited his hypothesis of changed phonation after reviewing evidence for reduced stuttering and changed speech patterns during pacing, singing, chorus reading, shadowing, masking, and delayed auditory feedback (DAF). Supporting this hypothesis, Adams, Lewis, and Besozzi (1973) suggested that improved fluency during slow, word-by-word speech might be explained in terms of simplification of transitions from phoneme to phoneme, and Adams and Reis (1971) interpreted their finding of reduced stuttering in totally voiced reading as due to the reduced need for phonatory adjustments. Bruce and Adams (1978) argued that their finding of absence of carry-over of adaptation effects from whispered to voiced reading indicated the importance of efficient laryngeal valving for voicing in determining the frequency of stuttering. Perkins, Rudas, Johnson, and Bell (1976) similarly posited simplification of phonatory-respiratory-articulatory coordinations to explain reduced stuttering from voiced to whispered and then to lipped speech. In a later paper, Perkins, Bell, Johnson, and Stocks (1979) reported greater stuttering

Reprinted from *Journal of Speech and Hearing Research*, 25, no. 2, 208–216. (June 1982). Copyright © 1982 American Speech-Language-Hearing Association.

reduction under conditions of reduced "phone rate" (speech rate excluding time spent pausing and stuttering) than under reduced syllable or word rate. They explained this in terms of increased speech planning time for voice onset coordinations available when phone rate is reduced. Other workers have explained decreased stuttering under certain conditions in terms of reduced linguistic complexity and the resulting decreased demands on speech planning (Haynes & Hood, 1978; Tornick & Bloodstein, 1976).

Clearly, before these various explanations of induced fluency in stutterers can be disentangled, the exact nature of any changes in speech characteristics occurring under these conditions requires further description. There is a gradually growing research literature in this area. In particular, changes in vocal intensity, fundamental frequency, and intraoral air pressure and flow have been examined. The speech characteristics with which our study is concerned are temporal variables associated with various aspects of speech rate, as well as the duration of phonation between pausing. To date, reports of changes in temporal characteristics of speech under fluency-inducing conditions have largely been restricted to investigations of vowel and consonant durations under a limited range of conditions. Increased duration of vowels have been reported during DAF (Wingate, 1970), and of vowels and consonants during pacing (Brayton & Conture, 1978). Perkins et al.'s (1979) report of decreased phone rate (a synonym for articulation rate) under DAF and slow syllable-timed speech also reflects lengthened syllables under these conditions. Brayton and Conture reported that consonant duration increased very slightly during masking, and Adams, Runyan, and Mallard (1974) reported that peak-to-peak consonant duration was unchanged during whispering. Healey and Adams (1978) reported increased duration of pauses as well as of consonants and vowels during deliberately slowed speech, and increased voicing duration has been reported during singing (Colcord & Adams, 1979; Healey, Mallard, & Adams, 1976).

Surprisingly, the evidence on speech rate during reduced stuttering is unclear, because of the confounding of stuttering frequency and speech rate. If stuttered utterances are included in total speaking time when speech rate is calculated, any decrease in speech rate accompanying reduced stuttering may be cancelled by the decrease in time spent stuttering, thus producing unchanged or increased speech rate (Adams & Hutchinson, 1974; Ingham & Packman, 1979). The absence of speech rate change accompanying fluency in Martin and Haroldson's study may reflect this cancellation. Measures of fluent speech rate (excluding stuttering time), or articulation rate, may be more appropriate in this context (Perkins et al., 1979). For example, by identifying fluent speech rate and holding it constant, Ingham and Packman were able to show that the ameliorative effects on stuttering of chorus reading did not depend on slowed speech.

The present study describes changes in some speech pattern characteristics in three stutterers speaking under 15

conditions believed to increase fluency using a simple technique in which tape recordings of speech were transformed into periods of speech sound and silence (Goldman-Eisler, 1968). This is the first time all these conditions have been explored within the same subjects using measures of phonation duration, speech rate, and sentence length. For both theoretical and clinical reasons we were concerned with describing the strategies that stutterers used to reduce their stuttering.

METHOD

General Procedure

The subjects were three adult male stutterers who had not undergone stuttering therapy. Each subject was measured on six baseline trials and 15 experimental trials, one for each of the 15 fluency-inducing conditions. Unless the particular requirements of the condition precluded it, the task for each baseline and experimental trial was to speak on one to five topics selected at random from a very large pack of topic cards copied from the subject index of *The Last Whole Earth Catalogue* (Portola Institute, 1971). The listener was a female experimenter who had no other contact or conversation with the subject. Each trial lasted 10 min. Between each experimental condition, repeated baseline trials were conducted until the frequency of stuttering returned to within the range established in the six original baseline trials. The design was therefore a repeated AB design. Subjects' speech was recorded with a Revox A77 recorder, in a sound protected room, with mouth-to-microphone distance held constant across all trials.

The Experimental Conditions

The conditions selected for investigation included 12 of those reviewed by Bloodstein (1950), as well as three further conditions which reflect techniques proven effective in stuttering therapy: response contingent stimulation, slowed speech rate, and prolonged or DAF-influenced speech. The order of the experimental conditions was chosen to facilitate the extinction of any effects of the previous conditions. Those conditions which might produce cognitive awareness of a fluency control technique (e.g., syllable-timed and prolonged/DAF speech) therefore were placed at the end of the series. Details of each condition follow in the order of their presentation. In conditions 9, 10, 12, 14, and 15 specific training was required and criteria were set for satisfactory performance before the experimental trial was begun. In the remaining conditions, the experimenter simply gave the necessary instructions and ensured that the subject understood by listening to a few phrases before beginning the trial.

The first 300 syllables of each 10-min recording were analyzed. Analysis of the durations of pauses and phonations was carried out using equipment based on Goldman-Eisler's

(1968, p. 143ff) specifications. Essentially, the analysis involved transforming speech signals derived from tape recordings into a train of pulses as long as the period of phonation between pauses of at least 250 msec. These pulses then were used to drive an event recorder to give a graphic representation of periods of speech and silence. The apparatus could detect pauses as short as 100 msec. The gain of the event recorder was set by the experimenter so that all audible speech sounds produced a corresponding marking in the visual record. After the visual record had been obtained, the text of the subject's speech was transcribed beneath it. This was done by fitting speech of a known time length between the cues written in real time on the visual records. "Cleaning up" of the text was not carried out; everything said was preserved regardless of grammatical accuracy. From the visual transcripts it was possible to measure the duration of each segment of speech sound (phonation) and silence (pause), and to locate and measure the duration of each stutter.

Stuttering frequency was measured as a percentage of syllables stuttered (%SS). Stutters were defined according to the World Health Organization criteria (1977). To determine the duration of stutters from the visual record, certain rules were established. Pauses and phonations that occurred between the first audible attempt at a phoneme and its final successful utterance were included as part of the duration of one stutter. Abnormal hesitations were included as stutters. As abnormal hesitations are for the most part silent, the judgment about whether to count these as stutters was based on whether the flow of speech was markedly interrupted and followed by a sound which seemed forced. If an abnormal hesitation was judged to be present, then the silent period contained therein and the terminal forced phoneme were included as one stutter. Filled pauses ("ah," "um") were counted as a separate entity unless they occurred during a stuttering period or preceded the onset of a stutter by a time interval of less than 250 msec, in which case they were included as part of a stutter.

Breaks in phonation of less than 250-msec duration were not counted as pauses and were included in the measurement of phonation. This minimum pause length was selected to minimize the likelihood of counting as pauses those breaks in phonation that were due to stop consonants, fricatives, and unvoiced sounds in general. Although single phonemes in these categories are generally briefer than 250 msec in running speech (Lisker & Abramson, 1967), the duration of sequences of three or four such phonemes (e.g., *textbook, asked politely*) could produce apparent breaks in phonation of this magnitude. Goldman-Eisler (1968) argued that a 250-msec minimum, although conservative, was desirable to ensure that speech discontinuities measured in her pause analysis were not due simply to such articulatory shifts. Since then, Love and Jeffress (1971) have reported stutterer/nonstutterer differences in the frequency of shorter pauses (150–250 msec), but this is another issue. Our study is concerned with the question of whether stutterers' speech under fluency-enhancing conditions differs from their speech under normal speaking conditions.

Counts were made of the length and frequency of all pauses, phonations, stutters, and filled pauses, plus the total number of syllables uttered. We deleted stutters and filled pauses from the analysis, then analyzed the resulting fluent speech segments to produce the following measures.

Mean Phonation Duration (in Sec).   Average length of all fluent speech between pauses greater than 250 msec. In simple terms this reflects utterance or phrase length. Phonations adjacent to a stutter were not used for this calculation because it could be difficult to determine whether or not the break in phonation was part of the stutter.

Pause Proportion.   Time spent in pauses, expressed as a proportion of total fluent speaking time (sum of fluent phonations and pauses).

Articulation Rate (Syllables per Sec).   Number of fluent syllables uttered, divided by total fluent phonation time. This measure is the reciprocal of syllable duration.

Fluent Speech Rate (Syllables per Sec).   Number of fluent syllables uttered divided by total fluent speaking time.

Mean Sentence Length.   Average number of words per "sentence." Sentences were determined by punctuating the written transcripts of speech into the shortest possible, grammatically correct sentences.

Reliability of Measures

Percentage of Syllables Stuttered.   To estimate intrajudge reliability for %SS, 35 conditions (including baselines) were randomly selected from across all subjects and rerated by the original judge. The correlation between first and second ratings was .96. For interjudge reliability, the correlations of %SS scores for two independent judges' ratings of speech samples from 40 randomly selected conditions was .93.

Speech Pattern Measures.   Assessment of reliability of these measures is time-consuming and therefore necessarily limited, each condition requiring approximately 100 hand measurements of duration from graphs of periods of sounds and silence. However, the following data demonstrate the replicability of the method.

To check the ability of the speech pause analyzer to reliably detect periods of sounds and silence, four randomly selected conditions from one subject were reanalyzed on the apparatus used by Goldman-Eisler at University College, London, and compared with the results from the speech pause analyzer used in our study. The resulting scores for mean phonation duration, fluent speech rate, and articulation rate are shown in Table 1. To assess intra- and interjudge reliability, six conditions were selected randomly from the

TABLE 1. Instrument comparability. Mean phonation duration (MPD), fluent speech rate (FSR), and articulation rate (AR) scores for four conditions derived from analyses using the present speech pause analyzer (column 1) and the Goldman-Eisler apparatus (column 2).

Condition number	MPD		FSR		AR	
	1	2	1	2	1	2
3	3.0	2.9	2.5	2.2	3.0	2.9
4	4.5	3.9	2.9	2.7	3.3	3.3
12	.3	.3	.7	.6	3.4	2.9
14	.5	.7	1.4	1.3	2.5	2.3
Mean	2.07	1.95	1.88	1.7	2.8	2.85

three subjects. Speech samples from five of these conditions were reanalyzed from the original tape recordings by the same experimenter as a check on intrajudge reliability (Table 2), and samples from four conditions were reanalyzed from the original tape recordings by a second experimenter as a check on interjudge reliability (Table 3). The similarity between the pairs of scores in these three tables is satisfactory.

RESULTS

Table 4 shows the percentage of syllables stuttered (%SS) for each subject under each original baseline and experimental condition, and the mean reduction in stuttering frequency as a percentage of the baseline mean. The speech pattern characteristic scores of each subject in each of the six initial

baseline and 15 experimental conditions are presented in the Appendix.

The data in Table 4 reveal that overall each subject's stuttering was reduced by some 70 percent, but there were some differences in individual response to the various conditions. In 38 of the 45 experimental trials (15 conditions by three subjects) stuttering was reduced to below the baseline range. In only one trial (Speak and write, Subject 2) did stuttering actually increase beyond the baseline range. In only three conditions was the mean percentage of reduction in stuttering less than 50 percent: Speak and write, Alone with cards, and Relaxed. Six conditions were associated with a greater than 90 percent reduction in stuttering. They were Prolonged/DAF speech, Singing, Chorus reading, Shadowing, Syllable-timed speech, and Response contingent. Descriptive statistics were used; inferential statistics would not have been appropriate in an exploratory study of three subjects. The magnitude of change in stuttering and other speech characteristics was computed using Cohen's effect size statistic (Cohen, 1977) to compare the changes in different measures. There were three subjects measured on six variables while speaking under 15 conditions. In Table 5 (see p. 45) an effect size for each measure in each condition is displayed. Each subject generated an effect size for each cell in the table; the median of these three effect sizes is shown. The two outlying values may be calculated from the data in the Appendix and Table 4 using the following formula:

$$ES = \frac{\text{Baseline mean} - \text{Experimental mean}}{\text{Baseline } SD}$$

TABLE 2. Intrajudge reliability. Mean phonation duration (MPD), pause proportion (PP), articulation rate (AR), and fluent speech rate (FSR) scores for five conditions on the first (1) and second (2) analyses by the same experimenter.

Condition	MPD		PP		AR		FSR	
	1	2	1	2	1	2	1	2
15	2.37	2.54	.3	.24	1.21	.95	.84	.72
3	2.98	3.20	.16	.13	3.00	2.90	2.50	2.50
Baseline 5	.74	.63	.41	.44	4.14	4.96	2.43	2.76
1	.59	.51	.69	.75	2.73	3.52	.94	.92
Baseline 1	1.42	1.44	.23	.20	4.27	4.00	3.29	3.18
Mean	1.62	1.66	.36	.35	3.07	3.27	2.00	2.02

TABLE 3. Interjudge reliability. Mean phonation duration (MPD), pause proportion (PP), articulation rate (AR), and fluent speech rate (FSR) scores for four conditions derived from the analyses of the first (1) and second (2) experimenters.

Condition	MPD		PP		AR		FSR	
	1	2	1	2	1	2	1	2
15	2.37	2.33	.30	.33	1.21	1.04	.84	.70
1	.59	.40	.69	.81	2.73	4.04	.94	.79
Baseline 1	1.42	1.52	.23	.20	4.27	3.96	3.29	3.15
Baseline 2	1.15	.68	.16	.31	3.45	4.54	2.87	3.13
Mean	1.38	1.23	.35	.41	2.92	3.40	1.99	1.94

TABLE 4. The frequency of stuttering in percentage of syllables stuttered for each subject under the first six baseline conditions and the 15 experimental conditions. The group mean stuttering reduction under each experimental condition is expressed in terms of percentage of decrease in stuttering frequency.

Experimental conditions		Stuttering frequency (%SS)			Group mean percentage decrease in stuttering
		Subject			
		1	2	3	
Baseline	1	22.0	19.0	6.3	
Baseline	2	18.7	12.1	2.8	
Baseline	3	14.0	15.1	6.6	
Baseline	4	15.1	19.6	9.6	
Baseline	5	16.0	17.6	7.2	
Baseline	6	13.3	9.0	6.0	
Mean baselines	1–6	16.5	15.4	6.4	
SD Baselines	1–6	3.2	4.2	2.2	
Speak and write		12.6	26.6	.0	18
Dialect		5.5	10.2	2.0	57
Singing		.0	.0	.4	98
Chorus reading		.0	.0	.0	100
Shadowing		1.2	1.3	.0	95
Animal		5.9	1.0	6.7	51
Alone		2.3	.8	4.1	72
Alone with cards		9.1	10.2	4.6	36
Relaxed		15.5	7.1	1.0	48
Response contingent		2.0	.0	.6	93
Slowing		.0	2.0	.0	96
Masking		11.6	7.9	1.4	52
Arm swing		7.1	2.4	.8	76
Syllable-timed		.0	4.1	.0	91
Prolonged/DAF		.8	.2	.0	98
Mean improvement over baseline					72

Thus an effect size of 1 reflects a change of 1 *SD* from the baseline mean.

In Table 5 the conditions are grouped according to the changes that occurred. Only effect sizes of greater than two standard deviation units are shown, because changes of this magnitude would likely be significant were a larger number of subjects tested. It is clear that lengthened mean phonation duration occurs consistently in four conditions: Chorus reading, Shadowing, Singing, and Prolonged/DAF. Slowed fluent speech rate occurs in six conditions: Prolonged/DAF, Syllable-timed speech, Speak and write, Slowing, Arm swing, and Relaxed. With the exception of Prolonged/DAF, increased phonation duration was never associated with slowed fluent speech rate. In the other conditions the two changes seem mutually exclusive; indeed in Syllable-timed speech, Speak and write, and Slowing, mean phonation

duration actually decreases in the presence of slowed fluent speech rate. Slowed fluent speech rates are apparently achieved by means of either decreased articulation rate (Prolonged/DAF, Syllable-timed speech) or increased pause proportion (Slowing), or by means of both of these slowing techniques (Speak and write). In the Arm swing and Relaxed conditions there was no clear evidence of changes in either articulation rate or pause proportion accompanying slowed fluent speech rate. Shortened sentence length, suggesting the possibility of reduced language complexity, was present in only two conditions: Animal and Slowing. In five conditions there were no consistent changes in any measured speech pattern characteristics among these subjects (Alone, Alone with cards, Dialect, Masking, and Response contingent).

To explore the extent to which the speech pattern measures can account for reductions in stuttering frequency, a multiple regression analysis was performed using the effect sizes for stuttering frequency change as the dependent variable and the effect sizes for change in the five speech pattern characteristics as the independent variables. Together, the five speech pattern variables accounted for 41 percent of the variance in stuttering frequency effect sizes.

DISCUSSION

Did Fluency Improve?

With the exception of Speak and write, Relaxed, and Alone with cards, all subjects showed some reduction in stuttering in all conditions, thus generally supporting previous reports of individual conditions believed to enhance fluency. It is clear that temporary fluency can be instated in stutterers with varying degrees of success.

The present results (see Table 5) do not identify any single strategy by which stuttering was always reduced and which may therefore be presumed necessary for fluency. In four speaking conditions, three of them associated with the elimination of independent language formulation, reduced stuttering appeared to be achieved via increased phonation duration. In others, it was achieved via decreased speech rate, often involving increased pausing or slower articulation.

The absence of change in fluent speech rate during Chorus reading in our study supports Ingham and Packman's (1979) finding that decreased fluent speech rate is not necessary for stuttering-reduction under this condition. Results in Table 5 suggest that the ameliorative effects of chorus reading are related to increased phonation duration, rather than to changed speech rate.

The evidence in this study of a decrease in articulation rate (and thus an increase in its inverse, syllable duration) associated with decreased stuttering under Prolonged/DAF, Singing, and Syllable-timed speech (Table 5) is consistent with findings in the literature reviewed earlier of increased vowel or consonant durations in the same conditions. It is

TABLE 5. Changes in stuttering frequency (SF), mean phonation duration (MPD), fluent speech rate (FSR), articulation rate (AR), pause proportion (PP), and sentence length (SL) under 15 fluency-inducing conditions. The change in each measure under each condition is expressed as the median effect size for the three subjects. A positive effect size indicates an increase over baseline mean. Blank entries for the speech pattern characteristics represent effect sizes of less than 2.

Experimental conditions	Effect sizes					
	SF	MPD	FSR	AR	PP	SL
Chorus reading	−3.7	8.5	—	—	—	—
Shadowing	−3.4	4.8	—	—	—	—
Singing	−3.7	9.3	—	−2.2	—	—
Prolonged/DAF	−3.7	2.5	−4.0	−4.7	—	—
Syllable-time	−2.9	−2.0	−3.3	−4.1	—	—
Speak and write	−1.2	−3.0	−4.3	−2.0	5.0	—
Slowing	−3.2	−3.0	−5.0	—	4.0	−2.7
Arm swing	−2.9	—	−3.4	—	—	—
Relaxed	−2.0	—	−2.0	—	—	—
Animal	−3.3	—	—	3.3	—	−3.9
Alone	−3.5	—	—	—	—	—
Alone with cards	−1.2	—	—	—	—	—
Dialect	−2.0	—	—	—	—	—
Masking	−1.8	—	—	—	—	—
Response contingent	−3.7	—	—	—	—	—

notable that in all five conditions in which slowed fluent speech rate accompanied reduced stuttering, subjects appeared to achieve this either by reducing articulation rate or by increasing pausing, but not both. Table 5 demonstrates this for Prolonged/DAF, Syllable-timed speech, and Slowing. Examination of the Appendix reveals that in Arm swing and Relaxed conditions, in which the mean effect sizes were not large enough to enter in Table 5, those subjects who did slow their fluent speech rate (Subjects 2 and 3) achieved this either by pausing or slowed articulation, but again not both. In the Slowing condition all three subjects increased pause proportion and only one (Subject 3, with the smallest pause proportion increase) slowed articulation rate markedly. This again suggests mutual exclusiveness of these two slowing strategies, a finding which is inconsistent with earlier reports of the combined use of both strategies, whether slowing occurs as a voluntary response to instruction (Healey & Adams, 1978) or as an "involuntary" by-product of pitch change (Ramig & Adams, 1980). It is interesting that in Syllable-timed speech, slowing was achieved via slowed articulation rather than increased pause proportion, at least in two of the three subjects. In this sense Prolongation and Syllable-timed speech are surprisingly similar to one another (see Appendix).

The design of this study ensured that the observed association between increased fluency and longer mean phonation duration or slower speech could not simply reflect the confounding effects of absence of stuttering in the speech sample analyzed. In both experimental and baseline conditions, only fluent speech segments were analyzed; therefore, speech rate variables were not contaminated by the act of stuttering. Furthermore, because phonations adjacent to stutters were not analyzed, the possibility of a spurious association between stuttering and shortened phonation duration could be excluded. Further weight to this conclusion was provided by the conditions in which stuttering lessened (notably, Response contingent stimulation), and no consequent increase in phonation duration was observed.

The reduced sentence length in Slowing and Animal conditions suggests that in some speech situations, simplified linguistic demands may account for some of the reduction in stuttering. Reduced demands for language formulation may also account for some of the reduced stuttering observed during Chorus reading, Shadowing, and Singing. This explanation is consistent with the Healey, Mallard, and Adams (1976) finding that a greater decrease in stuttering occurred when singing familiar, compared with unfamiliar, lyrics. The pair of conditions Alone and Alone with cards was included in this study to explore the possibility that any reduced stuttering when subjects were alone was not due to psychological variables associated with the absence of an audience (variables which were held constant in both conditions) but rather to linguistic variables, which were assumed to differ in the two conditions. However, because the reduction in sentence length in the Alone condition was minimal (effect size of less than 2 in all subjects), the preliminary assumption could not be made that any language simplification had occurred. These data are therefore not strong enough to resolve the issue conclusively. Replication is needed.

Implications for the Treatment of Stuttering

Because the majority of fluency-inducing conditions investigated in this study were accompanied either by increased phonation duration or by slowing, it might be assumed that those treatment techniques which are currently proving the most effective would incorporate a combination of these two speech pattern variables. Prolonged/DAF is the only condition which fits this description (Table 5). Andrews, Guitar, and Howie's (1980) recent analysis of the relative effectiveness of various stuttering treatments clearly indicates the superiority of prolonged speech treatment techniques; the present data provide some support for the effectiveness of this technique.

The results of the present study also suggest that treatment techniques which incorporate speech rate control should be effective. In the Andrews et al. (1980) review of treatment, only one study used slowed speech as the principal treatment (Peins, McGough, & Lee, 1972); thus, it was not possible to draw any conclusions about its effectiveness. Rhythmic speech techniques displayed a substantial treatment effect, secondary only to prolonged and gentle onset techniques, as might be predicted from the present results. Long-term maintenance of therapy gains was, however, less impressive for rhythmic speech techniques than for prolonged or gentle onset techniques.

Theoretical Implications

Funding limits for this research decreed small subject numbers, so the study must be regarded as exploratory. Replication with a larger group of subjects is essential if the roles of the individual speech pattern changes are to be defined more precisely. However, the opportunity for simultaneous investigation of a number of speech variables under a range of conditions provides a useful source of information about the nature of stuttering and its amelioration.

Armed with this information, it is instructive to reexamine the various theories outlined in the introduction. The present data provide empirical support for Bloodstein's hypothesis that speech pattern changes occur under some conditions; in 10 of the 15 conditions investigated here, some change in speech pattern occurred, whether in the form of phonation duration, articulation rate, or pause proportion (Table 1). We cannot draw conclusions about the viability of the other two explanations offered by Bloodstein. The data on the Alone conditions did not allow any resolution of the importance of variables associated with communicative responsibility, and the study was not designed to investigate the specific roles of strong or unusual stimulation. Wingate (1969, 1970) posited that changed phonation was operating in a number of conditions, and this was evident in Table 1. There were changes in phonation duration and speech rate variables in most of the conditions in which stuttering decreased. However, the Alone, Dialect, and Response contingent conditions showed no evidence of any change in the manner of phonation associated with decreased stuttering—it is difficult to visualize what kind of phonation change might be involved.

Two of the hypotheses outlined earlier (Andrews, 1974; Perkins et al., 1979) offer better prospects for a single explanation of all the conditions studied in the present investigation. The present results are consistent with the Perkins et al. (1979) hypothesis that fluency-facilitating conditions provide increased effective planning time, which may be achieved in a variety of ways. Some of these are (a) slowing of transitions (reflected in slowed articulation rate in the present study), (b) decreased frequency of coordinations or voice onsets required (reflected in increased mean phonation duration in this study), (c) increased predictability of voice onsets, and, finally, (d) reduced grammatical complexity (as reflected in shortened sentence length in the present study). Similarly, these results are consistent with the somewhat parallel hypothesis of Andrews (1974, 1981) that reduced stuttering is associated with conditions in which the neurophysiological demands of speech motor control and language formulation are reduced, which in the present study could have been simplified in a number of ways. Increased pausing or decreased articulation rate would allow increased time for planning, and the latter would also allow a slower rate of actual performance. Increased phonation duration could be associated with reduced control demand at both linguistic and prosodic levels. At the linguistic level longer phonation durations would reduce the frequency of decisions about what is to be said; at the prosodic level longer phonation durations would reduce the frequency of control decisions concerning intensity, intonation, and pausing. The demands of language formulation could be held to be reduced in conditions associated with no need for self-formulated language or with shortened, and hence simplified, sentence length.

However, both the effective planning time and the neurophysiological demand formulations leave some of the observations in this study unaccounted for. Three conditions in which stuttering was reduced (Alone, Dialect, Response contingent) were notable for the absence of change in any variables which might be associated with increased planning time or reduced neurophysiological demand. There may be variables responsible for reduced stuttering under these conditions which were not measured in the present study. Alternatively, it is still possible that the Alone and Dialect conditions may be explicable in terms of reduced linguistic complexity, and therefore may be consistent with these formulations, the sentence length measure used in the present study not being sufficiently sensitive to measure linguistic complexity. The Response contingent condition presents little threat to these ideas, for one implication of the demand model is that stuttering should not only improve when the linguistic or speech motor demands are reduced, but also when the functional capacity is temporarily increased and the demands held constant. Token reinforcement for fluency or time-out for stuttering were both effective, yet in neither condition was there evidence that the effect could be mediated in terms of reduced demand. Leaving aside learning theory explanations for the moment, both result in increased motivation and arousal consistent with a temporary increase in functional capacity.

The Masking condition in the present study produced only minimal decrease in stuttering. Nevertheless, there is sufficient evidence in the literature of the effectiveness of masking that this condition must be accounted for by any explanatory theory. In Masking the motor control task may be simplified by the absence of auditory feedback. In addition, Masking that reduces stuttering is usually associated with the Lombard effect of increased intensity and reduced rate, the latter change being consistent with reduced neurophysiological demand.

APPENDIX

Condition	Description
1. Speak and write	Speaking on stimulus card topics, while simultaneously writing down what was being said.
2. Dialect	Speaking in a regional dialect of the subject's choice.
3. Singing	Singing songs of subject's choice.
4. Chorus reading	Reading from newspaper in unison with two fluent speakers.
5. Shadowing	Subject presented (via monaural earphone), with recording of a fluent speaker reading a newspaper article and required to "shadow" the reader (see Cherry & Sayers, 1956, for criteria).
6. Animal	Speaking to a placid cat or dog. No topic cards used.
7. Alone	Speaking in the absence of a listener. Experimenter withdrew from laboratory. No topic cards used.
8. Alone with cards	As for condition 7, but with topic cards. This condition was run to determine whether reduced language complexity might account for any changes observed in conditions 6 and 7.
9. Relaxed	Speaking after undergoing Jacobsen's deep muscular relaxation. Trial began when subject was deeply relaxed (See Jacobsen, 1938, for criteria).
10. Response contingent	Response contingent stimulation (RCS) was administered until stuttering frequency stabilized over a 3-min period, after which the trial was begun with RCS still operating. For Subject 1, time out from positive reinforcement (Haroldson, Martin, & Starr, 1968) was used. After each stutter, a red light was displayed for 10 sec, during which time the subject was not permitted to speak. For Subjects 2 and 3, monetary reinforcement for increasing fluency was used (Ingham & Andrews, 1973).
11. Masking	See Cherry and Sayers. A recording of a wide-band 80-dB masking noise was played via binaural-occluding earphones during the entire trial.
12. Slowing	See Ingham, Martin, and Kuhl (1974). Subjects were required to speak at half their baseline speech rate. Feedback of the rate achieved was provided every 30 sec. When subjects had remained within the desired range for 5 minutes, the trial commenced.
13. Arm swing	Subjects were instructed to swing their arms in a rhythmic manner and to speak in time to these movements.
14. Syllable-timed	Syllable-timed rhythmic speech (Andrews & Harris, 1964) was instated using an earpiece metronome set at 90 beats per min. After 15-min practice the aid was withdrawn and the trial began.
15. Prolonged/DAF	Delayed auditory feedback (DAF) was administered at 250 msec delay (Goldiamond, 1965). Subjects were instructed to prolong each vowel and to keep the sound flowing continuously at whatever rate was comfortable. Training was continued until stuttering frequency stabilized over a 3-min period.

ACKNOWLEDGMENTS

This work was supported by a grant from the National Health and Medical Research Council, Canberra, Australia, for the years 1974–76.

REFERENCES

Adams, M., & Hutchinson, J. (1974). The effects of three levels of auditory masking on selected vocal characteristics and the frequency of disfluency of adult stutterers. *Journal of Speech and Hearing Research, 17,* 682–688.

Adams, M.R., Lewis, J.I., & Besozzi, T.E. (1973). The effect of reduced reading rate on stuttering frequency. *Journal of Speech and Hearing Research, 16,* 671–675.

Adams, M.R., & Reis, R. (1971). The influence of onset of phonation on the frequency of stuttering. *Journal of Speech and Hearing Research, 14,* 639–644.

Adams, M.R., Runyan, C., & Mallard, A.R. (1974). Airflow characteristics of the speech of stutterers and nonstutterers. *Journal of Fluency Disorders, 1,* 4–12.

Andrews, G. (1974). The etiology of stuttering. *Australian Journal of Human Communication Disorders, 2,* 8–12.

Andrews, G. (1981). Stuttering: A tutorial. *Australian and New Zealand Journal of Psychiatry, 15,* 105–109.

Andrews, G., Guitar, B., & Howie, P. (1980). Meta-analysis of the effects of stuttering treatment. *Journal of Speech and Hearing Disorders, 45,* 287–307.

Andrews, G., & Harris, M. (1964). The syndrome of stuttering. *Clinics in Developmental Medicine, No. 17.* London: Heinemann.

Bloodstein, O. (1950). A rating scale study of conditions under which stuttering is reduced or absent. *Journal of Speech and Hearing Disorders, 15*, 29–36.

Brayton, E.R., & Conture, E.G. (1978). Effects of noise and rhythmic stimulation on the speech of stutterers. *Journal o, Speech and Hearing Research, 21*, 285–294.

Bruce, M., & Adams, M.R. (1978). Effects of two types of motor practice on stuttering adaptation. *Journal of Speech and Hearing Research, 21*, 421–428.

Cherry, C., & Sayers, B. (1956). Experiments upon the total inhibition of stammering by external control, and some clinical results. *Journal of Psychosomatic Research, 1*, 233–246.

Cohen, J. (1977). *Statistical power analysis for the behavioral sciences.* New York: Academic Press.

Colcord, R.D., & Adams, M.R. (1979). Voicing duration and vocal sound pressure level changes associated with stuttering reduction during singing. *Journal of Speech and Hearing Research, 22*, 468–479.

Goldiamond, I. (1965). Stuttering and fluency as manipulatable operant response classes. In L. Krasner & L.P. Ullman (Eds.), *Research in behavior modification.* New York: Holt, Rinehart, & Winston.

Goldman-Eisler, F. (1968). *Psycholinguistics: Experiments in spontaneous speech.* London: Academic Press.

Haroldson, S.K., Martin, R.R., & Starr, C.D. (1968). Time-out as a punishment for stuttering. *Journal of Speech and Hearing Research, 11*, 560–566.

Haynes, W.O., & Hood, S.B. (1978). Disfluency changes in children as a function of the systematic modification of linguistic complexity. *Journal of Communicative Disorders, 11*, 79–93.

Healey, E.C., & Adams, M.R. (1978). *Rate reduction strategies used by normals and stutterers.* Paper presented at the Annual Convention of the American Speech and Hearing Association, San Francisco.

Healey, C., Mallard, A.R., & Adams, M.R. (1976). Factors contributing to the reduction of stuttering during singing. *Journal of Speech and Hearing Research, 19*, 475–480.

Ingham, R.J., & Andrews, G. (1973). An analysis of a token economy in stuttering therapy. *Journal of Applied Behavioral Analysis, 6*, 219–229.

Ingham, R.J., Martin, R.R., & Kuhl, P. (1974). Modification and control of rate of speaking by stutterers. *Journal of Speech and Hearing Research, 17*, 489–496.

Ingham, R.J., & Packman, A. (1979). A further evaluation of the speech of stutterers under chorus- and nonchorus-reading conditions. *Journal of Speech and Hearing Research, 22*, 784–793.

Jacobsen, E. (1938). *Progressive relaxation.* Chicago: University of Chicago Press.

Lisker, L., & Abramson, A.S. (1967). Some effects of context on voice onset time in English stops. *Language and Speech, 10*, 1–28.

Love, L.R., & Jeffress, L.A. (1971). Identification of brief pauses in the fluent speech of stutterers and nonstutterers. *Journal of Speech and Hearing Research, 14*, 229–240.

Martin, R., & Haroldson, S.K. (1979). Effects of five experimental treatments on stuttering. *Journal of Speech and Hearing Research, 22*, 132–146.

Peins, M., McGough, W.E., & Lee, B.S. (1972). Evaluation of a tape-recorded method of stuttering therapy: Improvement in a speaking task. *Journal of Speech and Hearing Research, 15*, 364–371.

Perkins, W.H., Bell, J., Johnson, L., & Stocks, J. (1979). Phone rate and the effective planning time hypothesis of stuttering. *Journal of Speech and Hearing Research, 22*, 747–755.

Perkins, W., Rudas, J., Johnson, L., & Bell, L. (1976). Stuttering: Discoordination of phonation with articulation and respiration. *Journal of Speech and Hearing Research, 19*, 509–522.

Portola Institute (1971). *The last whole earth catalogue.* Menlo Park, CA: Author/Random House.

Ramig, P., & Adams, M.R. (1980). Rate reduction strategies used by stutterers and nonstutterers during high- and low-pitched speech. *Journal of Fluency Disorders, 5*, 27–41.

Tornick, G.B., & Bloodstein, O. (1976). Stuttering and sentence length. *Journal of Speech and Hearing Research, 19*, 651–654.

Wingate, M.E. (1969). Sound and pattern in "artificial" fluency. *Journal of Speech and Hearing Research, 12*, 677–686.

Wingate, M.E. (1970). Effect on stuttering of changes in audition. *Journal of Speech and Hearing Research, 13*, 861–873.

World Health Organization. (1977). International Classification of Diseases. *Manual of the International Statistical Classification of Diseases, Injuries and Causes of Death* (9th rev.). Geneva: WHO.

CHAPTER 1 ADDITIONAL READINGS

Adams, M.R. (1984). Stuttering theory, research, and therapy: A five-year retrospective and look ahead. *Journal of Fluency Disorders, 9*, 103–113.

Adams, M.R. (1988). Five-year retrospective on stuttering theory, research, and therapy: 1982–1987. *Journal of Fluency Disorders, 13*, 399–406.

Adams, M.R., & Ramig, P. (1980). Vocal characteristics of normal speakers and stutterers during choral reading. *Journal of Speech and Hearing Research, 23*, 457–469.

Adams, M.R., Sears, R.L., & Ramig, P.R. (1982). Changes in stutterers and nonstutterers during monotoned speech. *Journal of Fluency Disorders, 7*, 21–35.

Attanasio, J.S. (1987). A case of late-onset or acquired stuttering in adult life. *Journal of Fluency Disorders, 12*, 287–290.

Colcord, R.D., & Adams, M.R. (1979). Voicing duration and vocal SPL changes associated with stuttering reduction during singing. *Journal of Speech and Hearing Research, 22*, 468–479.

Cox, M.D. (1982). The stutterer and stuttering: Neuropsychological correlates. *Journal of Fluency Disorders, 7*, 129–140.

Culler, M.H., & Freeman, F.J. (1984). Stuttering: The six blind men revisited. *Journal of Fluency Disorders, 9*, 89–92.

Deal, J.L. (1982). Sudden onset of stuttering: A case report. *Journal of Speech and Hearing Disorders, 47,* 301–304.

Fukawa, T., Yoshioka, H., Ozawa, E., & Yoshida, S. (1988). Difference of susceptibility to delayed auditory feedback between stutterers and nonstutterers. *Journal of Speech and Hearing Research, 31,* 475–479.

Gladstien, K.L., Seider, R.A., & Kidd, K.K. (1981). Analysis of the sidship patterns of stutterers. *Journal of Speech and Hearing Research, 24,* 460–462.

Gregory, H.H. (1986). Stuttering: A contemporary perspective. *Folia Phoniatrica, 38,* 89–120.

Ham, R., Fuccie, D., Cantrell, J., & Harris, D. (1984). Residual effect of delayed auditory feedback on normal speaking rate and fluency. *Perceptual and Motor Skills, 59,* 61–62.

Hayden, P.A., Adams, M.R., & Jordahl, N. (1982). The effects of pacing and masking on stutterers' and nonstutterers' speech initiation times. *Journal of Fluency Disorders, 7,* 9–19.

Healey, E.C., & Adams, M.R. (1981). Rate reduction strategies used by normally fluent and stuttering children and adults. *Journal of Fluency Disorders, 6,* 1–14.

Healey, E.C., & Howe, S.W. (1987). Speech shadowing characteristics of stutterers under diotic and dichotic conditions. *Journal of Communication Disorders, 20,* 493–506.

Homzie, M.J., Lindsay, J.S., Simpson, J., & Hasenstab, S. (1988). Concomitant speech, language and learning problems in adult stutterers and in members of their families. *Journal of Fluency Disorders, 13,* 261–277.

Howie, P.M. (1981). Intrapair similarity in frequency of disfluency in monozygotic and dizygotic twin pairs containing stutterers. *Behavior Genetics, 11,* 227–238.

Ingham, R.J., & Packman, A. (1979). A further evaluation of the speech of stutterers during chorus- and nonchorus-reading conditions. *Journal of Speech and Hearing Research, 22,* 784–793.

Kidd, K.K., Heimbuch, R.C., Records, M.A., Oehlert, G., & Webster, R.L. (1980). Familial stuttering patterns are not related to one measure of severity. *Journal of Speech and Hearing Research, 23,* 539–545.

Klouda, G.V., & Cooper, W.E. (1987). Syntactic clause boundaries, speech timing, and stuttering frequency in adult stutterers. *Language and Speech, 30,* 263–276.

Lebrun, Y., Leleux, C., Rousseau, J., & Devreux, F. (1982). Acquired stuttering. *Journal of Fluency Disorders, 8,* 323–330.

Lebrun, Y., Leleux, C., & Retif, J. (1987). Neurogenic stuttering. *Acta Neurochirurgica, 85,* 103–109.

Ludlow, C.L., Rosenberg, J., Salazar, A., Grafman, J., & Smutok, M. (1987). Site of penetrating brain lesions causing chronic acquired stuttering. *Annals of Neurology, 22,* 60–66.

Manning, W.H., Dailey, D., & Wallace, S. (1984). Attitude and personality characteristics of older stutterers. *Journal of Fluency Disorders, 9,* 207–215.

Perkins, W.H. (1983). The problem of definition: Commentary on "stuttering." *Journal of Speech and Hearing Disorders, 48,* 246–249.

Perkins, W.H., Bell, J., Johnson, L., & Stocks, J. (1979). Phone rate and the effective planning hypothesis of stuttering. *Journal of Speech and Hearing Research, 22,* 747–755.

Prins, D., & Beaudet, R. (1980). Defense preference and stutterers' speech disfluencies: Implications for the nature of the disorder. *Journal of Speech and Hearing Research, 23,* 757–768.

Prins, D., & Hubbard, C.P. (1988). Response contingent stimuli and stuttering: Issues and implications. *Journal of Speech and Hearing Research, 31,* 696–709.

Ramig, P.R., & Adams, M.R. (1980). Rate reduction strategies used by stutterers and nonstutterers during high- and low-pitched speech. *Journal of Fluency Disorders, 5,* 27–41.

Ramig, P.R., & Adams, M.R. (1981). Vocal changes in stutterers and nonstutterers in high- and low-pitched speech. *Journal of Fluency Disorders, 6,* 15–33.

Rosenfield, D.B., & Freeman, F.J. (1983). Stuttering onset after laryngectomy. *Journal of Fluency Disorders, 8,* 265–268.

Ryan, B.P., & Ryan, B.V. (1984). Additions to Andrews, Craig, Feyer, Hoddinott, Howie, and Neilson (1983) and to Andrews, Guitar, and Howie (1980). *Journal of Speech and Hearing Disorders, 49,* 429.

Seider, R.A., Gladstein, K.L., & Kidd, K.K. (1982). Language onset and concomitant speech and language problems in subgroups of stutterers and their siblings. *Journal of Speech and Hearing Research, 25,* 482–486.

Sermas, C.E., & Cox, M.D. (1982). The stutterer and stuttering: Personality correlates. *Journal of Fluency Disorders, 7,* 141–158.

Silverman, E.M., & Zimmer, C.H. (1979). Women who stutter: Personality and speech characteristics. *Journal of Speech and Hearing Research, 22,* 553–564.

Stephen, S.C., & Haggard, M.P. (1980). Acoustic properties of masking/delayed feedback in the fluency of stutterers and controls. *Journal of Speech and Hearing Research, 23,* 527–538.

Turnbaugh, K., Guitar, B., & Hoffman, P. (1981). The attribution of personality traits: The stutterer and nonstutterer. *Journal of Speech and Hearing Research, 24,* 288–291.

Venkatagiri, H.S. (1980). The relevance of DAF-induced speech disruption to the understanding of stuttering. *Journal of Fluency Disorders, 5,* 87–98.

Wingate, M.E. (1979). The first three words. *Journal of Speech and Hearing Research, 22,* 604–612.

Wingate, M.E. (1984a). Pause loci in stuttered and normal speech. *Journal of Fluency Disorders, 9,* 227–235.

Wingate, M.E. (1984b). Stutter events and linguistic stress. *Journal of Fluency Disorders, 9,* 285–300.

Young, M.A. (1985). Increasing the frequency of stuttering. *Journal of Speech and Hearing Research, 28,* 282–293.

Zimmermann, G.N. (1980). Stuttering: A disorder of movement. *Journal of Speech and Hearing Research, 23,* 122–136.

Zimmermann, G.N., Smith, A., & Hanley, J.M. (1981). Stuttering: In need of a unifying conceptual framework. *Journal of Speech and Hearing Research, 24,* 25–31.

CHAPTER TWO

Characteristics of Children Who Stutter

If we take a look at the literature prior to 1970, a majority of the research devoted to children who stutter focused on specific descriptions of their stuttering behavior in the early stages of the disorder, the establishment of differences between the speech and language development of stutterers and nonstutterers as well as the collection of data related to sex-ratios, prevalance statistics, and numbers of children who appeared to recover from stuttering (Andrews, Craig, Feyer, Hoddinott, Howie, and Neilson, 1983). For many years, too, there was a concerted effort made to construct theories of stuttering that would account for the onset, development, and maintenance of stuttering. Most of the research devoted to the early stages of stuttering was inspired by theories about the relationship between stuttering and nonfluent speech behavior commonly found in the speech of very young children (Bloodstein, 1987). However, after 1970, researchers abandoned theory development because of a lack of testable hypotheses that would support a given theory. Rather, researchers turned to other empirical issues related to systematic observations of stuttering behavior in children.

As stated in the Introduction of Chapter 1 of this book, the onset of stuttering typically occurs between the ages of 2 and 5, and if the stuttering persists, a child's disfluencies will continue to undergo a number of changes as the child gets older. At the onset of the disfluent behavior, the literature would suggest that the disfluencies of children identified as stuttering are similar in nature to the disfluencies of nonstutterers. However, there is no general consensus that early stuttering and normal nonfluencies are categorically different. Whether or not early stuttering is categorically or dimensionally different from normal nonfluencies is open to debate and in need of further research.

During the last decade considerable interest has been shown in developing clinically useful guidelines for the differentiation between incipient stutterers and normally nonfluent children. In 1977, Adams published a set of speech-related criteria that would help clinicians determine whether or not a child was in danger of becoming a stutterer. Adams' guidelines for identifying the frequency, type, and form of disfluencies exhibited by a disfluent child have been supplemented and refined through the research of Yairi and Lewis (1984) and Pindzola and White (1986). The Yairi and Lewis article can be found in this chapter while the Pindzola and White article can be found in Chapter 4.

A recent study and an article in this chapter by Hubbard and Yairi (1988) showed that preschool-age stutterers produced a significantly greater number of disfluencies on single words and/or adjacent words than did nonstutterers. The size of these clusters of disfluencies was also longer in the group of stutterers than in the matched, normally fluent subjects. Together, the above studies indicate that there is both an empirical and a clinical interest in determining the speech behaviors exhibited by children in the early stages of the disorder.

In 1982, Myers and Wall suggested several physiological, psycholinguistic, and psychosocial factors that appear to influence the onset and development of early childhood stuttering. The extent to which each of these factors interacts to account for the onset and development of the stuttering is still unknown. Nevertheless, it is probably necessary to consider the interrelationship or interaction of these variables as the best explanation for why stuttering occurs in some children and not in others. Thus, we appear to be on the threshold of an increased understanding of both the qualitative and quantitative differences that exist between incipient stutterers and normally nonfluent children.

In addition to discovering differences between the speech and nonspeech behaviors of young stutterers and nonstutterers, there is some evidence that there are minor differences in the way mothers of stuttering children and those of nonstuttering children communicate. Research by Langlois, Hanrahan, and Inouye (1986) has shown that mothers of stuttering children made significantly more demands of their children and asked a greater number of questions than did mothers of nonstutterers. Meyers and Freeman (1985) found that mothers interrupted children's disfluent speech more often than they interrupted a child's fluent speech moments. These investigators also found that mothers of stutterers talked significantly faster to both fluent and nonfluent children than did mothers of normally fluent children. Furthermore, when a child talked slowly during a fluent moment, the mother interacting with that child would increase her speech rate. These data indicate that there is a complex relationship between the interactions of mothers of stutterers and their children and the development and maintenance of stuttering.

A number of factors may explain this phenomenon, but this line of research holds some promise for providing clinically useful information for the diagnosis and management of stuttering in early childhood. In the article by Meyers in this chapter, it is reported that when young stutterers spoke with their mothers, fathers, and peers, there was no significant difference in the number of nonfluencies associated with the three conversational partners. These data suggest that familiar listeners do not affect the level of stuttering in young stutterers. Perhaps we need to investigate how other family members and peers respond and react to a child's disfluent speech.

Another potentially important issue that has surfaced recently in the literature is an attempt by Schwartz and Conture to subgroup young stutterers according to certain speech and nonspeech behaviors. The concept that stutterers are not homogeneous groups of people has been discussed for decades. We have thought for a long time that it might be more appropriate to regard stutterers as a heterogeneous population of individuals rather than a homogeneous one. Despite the recognition that the majority of research on adult stutterers implies a homogeneous model of stuttering, no one has attempted to explain conflicting research results from the standpoint of subgroups of stutterers. For this reason, the research of Schwartz and Conture represents an important contribution to the literature on stuttering in young children.

In addition to these recent trends in the behavioral research area, there has been increased attention given to the analysis of young stutterers' acoustic and physiological behaviors during their fluent and disfluent moments. Beginning in the mid to late 1970s and continuing to the present, there was a great deal of interest in comparing acoustical and physiological measures of adult stutterers' and nonstutterers' perceptually fluent speech. Both direct and indirect evidence shows that adult stutterers' fluency is characterized by heightened respiratory, laryngeal, and articulatory activity. A number of studies also have shown that certain instances of stutterers' fluent speech are associated with slower voice initiation and onset times, and longer vowel and consonant durations than nonstutterers' (see Adams, Freeman, & Conture, 1984; Adams, 1985 for a complete review).

As noted earlier, almost all of the research on stutterers' acoustical and physiological behaviors has been reported with adults. Although these findings are important in their own right, they say nothing about the behaviors of young stutterers. In reviewing the stuttering literature, one finds a paucity of research studies in these areas that have been published on children who stutter. In his review of research between 1970 and 1984 concerning the speech production abilities of stutterers, Adams (1987) was unable to find one published article dealing with an analysis of young stutterers' speech physiology. This is not surprising given that an analysis of children's stuttering using acoustic measures is a lot easier and less threatening to a child than taking direct measures of speech behavior from devices such as surface EMG or intra-oral air pressure and air flow sensors. However, it seems that we have spent the last 5 to 10 years figuring out why we have equivocal findings from measures of adult stutterers' fluency.

It is interesting to note that the results from the studies devoted to acoustic measures of young stutterers' fluency do not seem to show the extent of equivocal findings that we tend to see from studies dealing with adult stutterers. With the exception of the study by Adams (1987) who found that a small group of stutterers at the onset of stuttering possessed slower Voice Onset Time (VOT) and longer segment durations than matched normals, most of the findings indicate that there are no gross temporal differences between young stutterers' and nonstutterers' fluent speech (Winkler & Ramig, 1986; Zebrowski, Conture, & Cudahy, 1985). However, I do not believe that we have exhausted this line of research since many methodological and sampling issues have not been resolved. Continued research in this area with child stutterers will also allow us to address the question of whether the differences that we find for the adult stutterers are due to : (1) the result of being a stutterer for a long period of time, (2) the result of an inherited slowness or mistiming in a child's speech physiology that continues into adulthood, (3) a combination of both learned and inherited deficits in both speech and nonspeech activities, or (4) the result of some compensatory movement that stutterers adopt in order to control their stuttering. It is hoped that future research with young stutterers will provide some answers to these questions.

Even though an acoustical analysis of stutterers speech behavior is relatively simple and nonthreatening to a child, there is a concern that these measures are not refined enough to discover subtle difficulties that stutterers might show in their speech physiology. One of the first published studies of children's speech physiology was the study by Conture, Rothenberg, and Molitor (1986). They analyzed electroglottographic recordings from the fluent speech responses of 3- to 7-year-old stutterers and found that some stutterers had difficulty stabilizing and controlling laryngeal gestures during fluency. Conture, Colton, and Gleason (1988) explored the issue of simultaneous measurements of certain respiratory, laryngeal, and supralaryngeal events of young stutterers' fluent speech productions. Another similar study was conducted by Caruso, Conture, and Colton (1988). Perhaps Conture (1987) summed it up best when he said, "objective assessment of young stutterers' speech production will necessitate a compromise between the realities of what youngsters can and will do and the ideal procedures for collecting speech production data" (p. 132).

In conclusion, more research needs to be done with this group of children and it is hoped that the future will bring about a greater number of studies which integrate the behavioral, acoustical, and physiological areas. Specifically, we might be able to investigate the relationship between linguistic variables and speech motor behavior in young stutterers. As Starkweather (1987) suggested, "a major challenge for those who would explain stuttering as a motoric disorder is to explain the linguistic variations of stuttering in motoric terms" (p. 13). Perhaps we will be able to meet that challenge in the years ahead.

REFERENCES

Adams, M.R. (1977). A clinical strategy for differentiating the normally nonfluent child and the incipient stutterer. *Journal of Fluency Disorders, 2,* 141–148.

Adams, M.R. (1985). The speech physiology of stutterers: Present status. *Seminars in Speech and Language, 6,* 177–196.

Adams, M.R. (1987). Voice onsets and segment durations of normal speakers and beginning stutterers. *Journal of Fluency Disorders, 12,* 133–139.

Adams, M.R., Freeman, F., & Conture, E. (1984). Laryngeal dynamics of stutterers. In R. Curlee & W. Perkins (Eds.), *Nature and treatment of stuttering: New directions.* San Diego: College-Hill Press.

Andrews, G., Craig, A., Feyer, A., Hoddinott, S., Howie, P., & Neilson, M. 1983. Stuttering: A review of research findings and theories circa 1982. *Journal of Speech and Hearing Disorders, 48,* 226–245.

Bloodstein, O. (1987). *A handbook on stuttering.* Chicago: Easter Seal Society.

Caruso, A., Conture, E., & Colton, R. (1988). Selected temporal parameters of coordination associated with stuttering in children. *Journal of Fluency Disorders, 13,* 57–82.

Conture, E. (1987). Studying young stutterers' speech productions: A procedural challenge. In H. Peters & W. Hulstijn (Eds.), *Speech motor dynamics in stuttering.* New York: Springer-Verlag.

Conture, E., Colton, R., & Gleason, J. (1988). Selected temporal aspects of coordination during fluent speech of young stutterers. *Journal of Speech and Hearing Research, 31,* 640–653.

Conture, E., Rothenberg, M., & Molitor, R. (1986). Electroglottographic observations of young stutterers' fluency. *Journal of Speech and Hearing Research, 29,* 384–393.

Hubbard, C., & Yairi, E. (1988). Clustering of disfluencies in the speech of stuttering and nonstuttering preschool children. *Journal of Speech and Hearing Research, 31,* 228–233.

Langlois, A., Hanrahan, L., & Inouye, L. (1986). A comparison of interactions between stuttering children, nonstuttering children, and their mothers. *Journal of Fluency Disorders, 11,* 263–273.

Meyers, S., & Freeman, F. (1985). Mother and child speech rates as a variable in stuttering and disfluency. *Journal of Speech and Hearing Research, 28,* 436–444.

Myers, F., & Wall, M. (1982). Toward an integrated approach to early childhood stuttering. *Journal of Fluency Disorders, 7,* 47–54.

Pindzola, R., and White, D. (1986). A protocol for differentiating the incipient stutterer. *Language, Speech, Hearing Services in the Schools, 17,* 2–15.

Schwartz, H., & Conture, E. (1988). Subgrouping young stutterers: Preliminary behavioral observations. *Journal of Speech and Hearing Research, 31,* 62–71.

Starkweather, W. (1987). Laryngeal and articulatory behavior in stuttering: Past and future. In H. Peters & W. Hulstijn (Eds.), *Speech motor dynamics in stuttering.* New York: Springer-Verlag.

Winkler, L.E., & Ramig, P.R. (1986). Temporal characteristics in the fluent speech of child stutterers and nonstutterers. *Journal of Fluency Disorders, 11,* 217–230.

Yairi, E., & Lewis, B. (1984). Disfluencies at the onset of stuttering. *Journal of Speech and Hearing Research, 27,* 154–159.

Zebrowski, P.M., Conture, E.G., & Cudahy, E.A. (1985). Acoustic analysis of young stutterers' fluency: Preliminary observations. *Journal of Fluency Disorders, 10,* 173–192.

Disfluencies at the Onset
of Stuttering

Ehud Yairi
Barbara Lewis

Objective data concerning the speech characteristics of young children at the time when they were first diagnosed as having begun stuttering are virtually unavailable. Investigators cannot plan to be in the natural home environment to obtain speech samples at the critical moment. Additionally, parents, who are usually the first to notice the "beginning of stuttering," often wait several, if not many, months before bringing the child to a clinician/researcher so that speech can be recorded.

Because it is all but impossible to conduct direct observations during the alleged onset of stuttering, reports made by parents were used as the prime indirect means to extrapolate the desired information (Glasner & Rosenthal, 1957; Johnson et al., 1959; Johnson & Leutenegger, 1955). Such second-hand information concerning events which took place long in the past led the latter investigators to conclude that, at the time of "stuttering onset," disfluencies of children just regarded as "stutterers" were essentially indistinguishable from those of normally speaking children. The diagnosis of stuttering, therefore, was assumed to be erroneous. This assumption has been questioned by several scientists, including Bloodstein (1958), McDearmon (1968), Van Riper (1971), and Wingate (1962).

Johnson's long-term reliance on parent accounts reflected a genuine belief that the behaviors regarded by listeners as the first stuttering are not likely to be recorded and may be altered in character rather quickly. It was only at a later time that his attention turned toward the speaking behavior of the children he studied. To date, the only substantial speech-based data on disfluency characteristics of young beginning stutterers were reported by Johnson et al. (1959) for eighty-nine 2–8-year-old children who were subjects in the last phase of the landmark Iowa studies. Findings showing stutterers to be considerably more disfluent than control nonstutterers did not dissuade the investigators from emphasizing overlaps between the two groups and from pressing the hypothesis that the two groups were less, or not at all, distinguishable at the time of their stuttering onsets.

Although the speech data of Johnson et al. (1959), unlike their interview-based data, are objective, they suffer from at least two serious limitations. First is the age range of the subjects. The meaning of any speech/language data pooled together and averaged for the ages specified above is questionable because of vast differences between 2- and 8-year-olds in almost all respects. The second limitation is the interval, 18 months on the average, from the first indication of a stuttering problem perceived by the parents to the time when speech samples were recorded for the study. Although these data were never viewed as representing speech at onset, such a prolonged interval makes it difficult to view them as a true representation even of the "early" or "incipient" stage of stuttering. Other sources reporting quantified data on disfluencies in early young stutterers (e.g., Bloodstein & Grossman, 1981) bear similar limits to the studies just mentioned. Furthermore, they provide no controls. Individual case studies (Conture, 1982; Wyatt, 1969) have contributed important insight into early stuttering but not disfluency data.

Between the improbable ideal data from the actual moment of onset (if such can indeed be established) on the one hand, and poorly defined data gathered a year and a half past that event on the other hand, there lies a large gap that can be filled with obtainable and carefully assembled information. The general goal of this investigation, therefore, was to study disfluency characteristics of young children very shortly after they were diagnosed by parents as having begun stuttering in comparison to disfluencies of children who were not viewed by parents as exhibiting stuttering. Analysis of speech recorded from a cohesive age group close to the time when its members were identified as "stutterers" can provide a useful basis to evaluate theoretical positions like the ones made by Johnson and his colleagues. That is, would objective analyses of such early speech samples substantiate parents' judgments of children in the two groups? Observations made by other investigators concerning the loci of early stuttering and their implications concerning the nature of stuttering (Bloodstein & Grossman, 1981) can also be reevaluated. From a clinical point of view, data on speech characteristics of young children just beginning to stutter are needed

Reprinted from *Journal of Speech and Hearing Research, 27, no. 1, 154–159.* Copyright © 1984 American Speech-Language-Hearing Association.

to develop meaningful norms that can be used in refining and validating differential diagnostic schemes of early childhood stuttering (Adams, 1977). The present study is based on these assumptions and was made possible after several years during which uncommon speech samples of young children in the incipient stage of stuttering were collected at the Stuttering Research Program at the University of Illinois.

METHOD

Subjects

Two groups of ten 2- and 3-year-old children, each consisting of five boys and five girls, took part in the study. The children lived in a medium-sized community (pop. 100,000) in the midwest or in smaller nearby communities and represented primarily the middle and low-middle socioeconomic class. Children in the Experimental group were seen at the University of Illinois Speech and Hearing Clinic upon parental complaints concerning stuttering. To be included in the group each subject had to

1. be judged as a stutterer but otherwise as developmentally normal by at least one parent;[1]
2. exhibit stuttering for no more than two months prior to participation in this study; and
3. be 2 or 3 years of age.

To ascertain the time of stuttering onset, mothers of the Experimental group subjects were encouraged to consult records, recall concurrent events or proximity to other dates, and so forth. Only children whose mothers' reports (that onset occurred within the preceding two months) were deemed valid with a high degree of certainty were accepted. Judgments of validity were based on the availability of records and/or confidence expressed by parents in giving specific dates or in specifying onset time in relation to concurring events.

Subjects in the Control group were located in several nursery schools and daycare centers. They were regarded by parents as being developmentally normal and had no history of stuttering. Children were 2 or 3 years old and were matched individually to the Experimental subjects according to sex and age within 2 months in either direction. For six experimental subjects there were two matching controls to choose from. To reduce the possible bias of selecting unusually fluent children, the more disfluent of the two was included.

Although parental diagnosis of their child as a "stutterer" or a "nonstutterer" was sufficient for placement in one of the two groups (Johnson et al., 1959), in all cases one investigator and a second speech-language pathologist independently agreed with these parental judgments. It should also be noted that the subjects actually had a narrower age range, only 15 months, than the predetermined 24-month span. The Experimental group's age range was 25–39 months. The mean was 29.0 months (median = 29.0), with a standard deviation of 4.0. They were tape-recorded 2–8 weeks after their reported stuttering onset. The mean interval was 6 weeks. The Control group's age range was 24–39 months. The mean was 29.0 months (median = 29.0 months), with a standard deviation of 4.1.

Procedure

Spontaneous speech samples were audiotape-recorded during play activities in the presence of an adult who also interacted verbally with the subjects. A standard set of pictures, toys, and questions was used to increase the uniformity of testing conditions. Experimental subjects were recorded during their diagnostic evaluations in the Speech and Hearing Clinic. Control subjects were recorded in quiet rooms made available in daycare centers or homes. According to Silverman (1971), the different recording settings for the controls were expected to effect only slight changes in their numbers of disfluencies. In fact, she reported somewhat higher numbers at home than at a clinical setting. Recording sessions lasted 25–45 min with the goal of obtaining approximately 500-syllable samples per subject.

One investigator orthographically transcribed the speech samples verbatim. Unintelligible utterances were deleted. Because the child-adult interaction involved frequent questions, all isolated "yes" and "no" responses were deleted to prevent inflating samples with single-syllable word utterances. "Yes" or "no" followed immediately by another word or phrase, however, was retained.

Disfluencies in the speech samples were analyzed according to a modified scheme outlined in Williams, Silverman, and Kools (1968) and in Williams, Darley, and Spriestersbach (1978).[2] The following categories of disfluency were employed in this study: (a) part-word repetition; (b) single-syllable word repetition; (c) multisyllable word repetition; (d) phrase repetition; (e) interjection; (f) revision-incomplete phrase; (g) dysrhythmic phonation (primarily sound prolongations within words, unusual stress or broken words); and (h) tense pause (barely audible heavy breathing and other tense sounds between words).

Each investigator listened to the recordings of the speech samples to identify locations and classify types of all instances of disfluency. For the first five categories listed above, counts were made of the number of times a disfluency was repeated. The number of repetitions was designated as Repetition Units (RU). A self-agreement index (Sander, 1961), calculated for the combined factors of location, type, and extent of disfluency, was 0.95 for the first author and 0.97 for the second author. The initial interjudge agreement index was 0.93. Later, instances of discrepancies between the authors were resolved through repeated simultaneous listening until a perfect agreement (1.0) was achieved.

RESULTS

Frequency of Disfluency

Table 1 presents means, standard deviations, and ranges of disfluencies for the stutterers and nonstutterers as well as the breakdowns for males and females. The mean total number of disfluencies per 100 orthographic syllables for the stuttering group was 21.54 ($SD = 15.20$), with a median of 21.03. In the nonstuttering group the mean was 6.16 ($SD = 3.04$), with a median of 5.61. Thus, overall, stutterers were three and a half times more disfluent than control subjects.

The most frequent disfluencies in the speech of stutterers, in ranked order, were part-word repetitions, dysrhythmic phonation, and single-syllable word repetition. For the nonstutterers the most frequent disfluencies were, in ranked order, interjection, part-word repetition, and revision-incomplete phrase.

An analysis of variance test (group × disfluency type × sex) was performed. A significant[3] interaction of group and disfluency type ($F = 4.24$; $df = 7, 112$) indicated that the two groups were different in their distribution of disfluencies among the eight types. A significant main effect

TABLE 2. Ranges of frequency of occurrence per 100 syllables of disfluency types for the experimental and control groups.

Disfluency type	Group	
	Experimental	Control
PWR	1.86–10.83	0.57–2.22
SSWR	0.42–9.32	1.19–2.59
MSWR	0.00–1.15	0.00–0.14
PhR	0.00–1.95	0.27–0.92
I	0.63–5.86	0.00–5.23
R-IC	0.51–2.89	0.15–2.06
DP	0.63–29.92	0.15–2.19
TP	0.00–1.73	0.00–0.14
Total	6.51–46.79	2.36–11.06

of group ($F = 11.89$; $df = 1, 16$) showed that the difference between stutterers and nonstutterers in the total number of disfluencies as indicated above was statistically meaningful. Although Table 1 shows that stutterers were more disfluent than controls on all types of disfluency, a post hoc Tukey test (Winer, 1971) indicated that significant differences between the two groups occurred only for part-word repetition and dysrhythmic phonation. The difference between the two means for part-word repetition was 5.74, whereas the critical value for significance was 3.73. The difference between the two means for dysrhythmic phonation was 4.46, whereas the critical value for significance was 3.39.

The analysis of variance also yielded a significant main effect of disfluency type ($F = 7.14$; $df = 7, 112$). It indicated that the eight types occurred at different frequencies (when data are not separated by groups), a finding not particularly meaningful in relation to the goals of this study. There was no significant main effect of sex ($F = 0.28$; $df = 1, 16$). In other words, the tendency for males to be more disfluent than females was not strong enough to consider the two sexes distinguishable on this aspect of speech.

Inspection of Table 1 shows that standard deviations were relatively large. It appears that both groups were quite heterogeneous in respect to disfluent speech behavior. Indeed, in spite of differences in means for stutterers and nonstutterers, the individual data revealed a certain overlap between subjects of the two groups in the distribution of disfluency. This is also seen in the data on ranges presented in Table 2. The total number of disfluencies per 100 syllables for the individual stutterers ranged from 6.51 to 46.79. The range was 2.36–11.06 disfluencies for the normally speaking children. The overlap can be seen in that the three most disfluent nonstutterers exhibited more disfluencies than the three least disfluent stutterers. The degree of overlap, however, varied according to the type of disfluency. Large

TABLE 1. The mean frequency (M) and standard deviation (SD) of each disfluency type and total disfluency per 100 syllables spoken for the experimental and control groups.[b]

Disfluency type[a]		Experimental			Control		
		EF	EM	EG	CF	CM	CG
PWR	M	6.53	7.44	6.99	1.39	1.24	1.32
	SD	2.99	4.38	3.57	0.59	0.69	0.61
SSWR	M	3.86	3.26	3.57	1.05	0.79	0.92
	SD	3.29	2.05	2.61	0.84	0.57	0.69
MSWR	M	0.03	0.03	0.03	0.00	0.03	0.01
	SD	0.06	0.06	0.06	0.00	0.06	0.04
PhR	M	0.93	0.96	0.95	0.58	0.55	0.57
	SD	0.60	0.42	0.48	0.28	0.23	0.24
I	M	3.45	1.46	2.45	0.94	1.91	1.42
	SD	2.50	0.54	2.00	0.79	1.83	1.43
R-Ic	M	1.69	1.50	1.60	1.07	1.26	1.16
	SD	1.10	0.56	0.83	0.47	0.79	0.61
DP	M	2.30	8.06	5.21	0.65	0.85	0.75
	SD	1.88	11.79	8.51	0.42	0.78	0.60
TP	M	0.76	0.55	0.66	0.03	0.03	0.03
	SD	0.60	0.36	0.47	0.06	0.06	0.06
Total	M	19.55	23.26	21.46	5.71	6.66	6.18
	SD	11.35	15.10	12.74	2.04	3.92	2.98

[a](PWR) part-word repetition; (SSWR) single-syllable word repetition; (MSWR) multisyllable word repetition; (PhR) phrase repetition; (I) interjection; (R-Ic) revision/incomplete phrase; (DP) dysrhythmic phonation; (TP) tense pause.
[b](EF) experimental females; (CF) control females; (EM) experimental males; (CM) control males; (EG) combined experimental group; (CG) combined control group.

overlaps occurred between the two groups in interjection and revision-incomplete phrase. Only one stutterer was outside the range for the nonstutterers on interjection, and only two stutterers were outside the range for the nonstutterers on revision-incomplete phrase. Considerably smaller overlaps were noticed in three other disfluency types. Six stutterers were outside the range for nonstutterers in single-syllable word repetition and on phrase repetition. Seven stutterers had more dysrhythmic phonations than the maximum observed among the nonstutterers. The overlap was very minimal in part-word repetition and tense pause. For both types, nine stutterers exhibited more disfluencies than the maximum observed in nonstutterers. Generally, overlap decreased for disfluencies most common in speech of the stutterers. It was difficult to evaluate overlap on multisyllable word repetition because it was exhibited by only three stutterers and one nonstutterer.

Extent of Disfluency

Disfluencies were also analyzed in relation to the number of repetition units (number of times a segment was repeated) per instance of disfluency. This analysis could only be applied to the five types of disfluency involving repetitions of some speech segment, namely, part-word repetition, single-syllable word repetition, multisyllable word repetition, phrase repetition, and interjection. Group means and standard deviations are shown in Table 3. In four of the five disfluency types, stutterers exceeded nonstutterers in the number of times a segment of speech was repeated. The two groups were equal for phrase repetition. Data on part-word repetition, the most common type in the speech of stutterers, are particularly interesting. The range for the stutterers was 1–11 units and for the nonstutterers, 1–2 units. Stutterers repeated a part-word repetition segment on the average 1.72 times, whereas the nonstutterers repeated the segment only 1.12 times. Three stutterers had an average of over two repetition units per instance of part-word repetition, whereas for the nonstutterers instances of more than two repetitions were extremely rare.

TABLE 3. Group means and standard deviations of repetition units (RU) per instance of repetition for five types of disfluency.

Disfluency type		Experimental group RU per instance	Control group RU per instance
PWR	M	1.72	1.12
	SD	0.48	0.58
SSWR	M	1.34	1.09
	SD	0.45	0.17
MSWR	M	2.00	1.00
	SD	0.82	0.32
PhR	M	1.10	1.10
	SD	0.17	0.04
I	M	1.19	1.04
	SD	0.18	0.35

The three-factor analysis of variance yielded a pattern of significant F ratios identical to the one described above in relation to frequencies of disfluencies. Most pertinent to our interest was the significant main effect of classification ($F = 8.27$; $df = 1$, 16), which meant that stutterers and controls differed in terms of the number of times a segment of disfluency was repeated. A post hoc Tukey test revealed that only differences in part-word repetition and single-syllable word repetition significantly differentiated the two groups. The difference between the two means for part-word repetition was .60 while the critical value for significance was .19. The difference between the two means for single-syllable word repetition was .26 while the critical value for significance was .18. Multisyllable word repetition was not included in this analysis because there were only four instances of this type in the speech samples of all 20 subjects.

DISCUSSION

Although we did not obtain the present data precisely on the first day the parents observed the stuttering, our data are closer to the perceived onset of stuttering than any reported thus far. From this point of view, the fact that the experimental subjects were more than three times as disfluent as the control children (21.5 disfluencies and 6.2 disfluencies per 100 syllables, respectively) is perhaps the most important finding of this investigation. In spite of large variability within each group and a certain overlap in their disfluency distributions, it can be clearly recognized that, *as groups*, stutterers and nonstutterers emerged as representing two fairly distinctive population samples. In other words, the data provide strong indications that marked differences exist between the general level of disfluent speech output of most children regarded by their parents as having just developed a stuttering problem and most children regarded as normal speakers by their parents. These results substantiate Yairi's (1983) conclusion that the parents of many young stutterers described their children's speech at the time of onset as different from that of other children.

Other investigators (i.e., Johnson et al., 1959) also have found rather large differences in the number of disfluencies between stuttering and nonstuttering children. Their data showed a mean number of 17.9 disfluencies per 100 words for stutterers as compared to 7.3 for nonstutterers, but they emphasized the overlap and similarities of the two groups. What is important to the present study is that those investigators suggested that when the children were first (erroneously) regarded as stutterers, such differences were actually small or nonexistent. This led them to conclude that stuttering began in the parent's perception, not in the child's speech.

To test this hypothesis, the speech samples in this study were collected at a much earlier time than the 18-month postonset interval used in the past. Yet, substantial differences, perhaps even larger than those reported by Johnson et al. (1959),[4] were still found at or very close to the reported onset of stuttering. The present findings, then, do not support the assertion that the disfluent speech behavior of children just regarded as stutterers is basically similar to the disfluent speech of those children not regarded as stutterers. Although other researchers, particularly Wingate (1962), objected to Johnson's diagnosogenic theory of the onset of stuttering, this study provides more direct evidence which calls the theory into question.

The present data show that normally speaking 2- and 3-year-olds exhibit all recognized types of disfluency although certain types are very rare. Mostly, they exhibit interjections, revisions, and single-unit part-word repetitions and show a relatively even distribution of disfluencies (the top three types varying by only 0.21 in mean number). Overall, the data are comparable to those obtained in previous investigations (Davis, 1939; Johnson et al., 1959; Yairi, 1981; Yairi & Clifton, 1972), a fact that adds validity to the present findings.

Important changes, generally in line with Wingate's (1962) conclusions, appear to have occurred in the disfluency patterns of children at or very soon after the time when they were diagnosed as having developed a stuttering problem. Apparently, this event was associated with a substantial overall increase in the number of disfluencies in the speech of many of the experimental subjects which, justifiably, caught listeners' attention. However, the increase was not uniform across the range of the various disfluencies. Rather, the increase above normal was most significant for part-word repetition and dysrhythmic phonation. The largest difference in absolute terms occurred on part-words. Furthermore, the dispersion data showed that this type was a more consistent characteristic than dysrhythmic phonation (standard deviations were approximately 50 percent and 158 percent of the means, respectively).

Part-word repetition was also outstanding in terms of its extent. When stutterers repeated part words, they frequently did so twice or more per instance. Nonstutterers rarely repeated a speech segment more than once. The fact that almost no overlap occurred in this aspect (extent) of disfluency indicates that it is a more powerful discriminant between the disfluencies of stutterers and nonstutterers than the mere number of instances. The present findings question the validity and utility of Adams's statement (1977, p. 143) that one sign of incipient stuttering involves the occurrence of "at least three iterations of the unit being repeated." Three repetition units is too stringent a criterion and appears to surpass most disfluent productions of young incipient stutterers. Interestingly, whole-word repetitions, which were identified by Bloodstein and Grossman (1981) as the central feature of early stuttering, had only secondary importance in the speech of the present experimental group.

Because of the narrow age range of the subjects and the short interval between the original diagnosis of stuttering and tape recording of the child's speech, the present data may be considered as a nucleus of disfluency norms for beginning stutterers 2 and 3 years old. As always, interpretations of findings should be made with caution considering possible sampling or procedural errors. One reservation that may be raised regarding the present study is that early referrals of young stutterers could be a function of the children's stuttering being more severe than that of the typical beginning stutterer. Early referrals, however, may simply reflect strong parental concerns regardless of severity, alertness of referral sources, and visibility of speech services. In any event, although there was a tendency for our stuttering subjects to be more disfluent than those of Johnson et al. (1959), the difference between the means was only one-half standard deviation.

The present data showed important differences between the disfluent speech of stutterers and the disfluency of children regarded as normal. It still remains unclear if these are mainly quantitative differences or if there are more discrete attributes that distinguish between disfluencies of normals and stutterers. To answer this question, more precise methods such as acoustical and physiological analyses of individual instances of disfluency should be used. It is important, however, that such research continue to be age specific and to be based on data that reasonably can be viewed as early stuttering.

ACKNOWLEDGMENTS

Portions of this report are based on B. Lewis's master's thesis directed by E. Yairi at the University of Illinois. The advice and assistance of Drs. Robert Bilger, John Nuetzel, and Elaine Paden in the execution of this study are greatly appreciated.

NOTES

1. Interviews were conducted with mothers who, in all cases, made the diagnosis of stuttering. However, all fathers concurred with their judgments.
2. The original category of word repetition was subdivided in the present study into single-syllable word repetition and multi-syllable word repetition.
3. Significance of all statistical tests results was determined at the .05 level of confidence.
4. For direct comparison of the two studies, recalculation of the present data from frequency of disfluency per 100 syllables to frequency per 100 words was necessary. This conversion showed the stutterers in the present study as having a mean number of 24.6 disfluencies per 100 words compared with 17.9 disfluencies in the Johnson et al. (1959) study. However, given the small size of the present sample and large standard deviation figures, such differences may not be sustained.

REFERENCES

Adams, M.R. (1977). A clinical strategy for differentiating the normally nonfluent child from the incipient stutterer. *Journal of Fluency Disorders, 2,* 141–148.

Bloodstein, O. (1958). Stuttering as anticipatory struggle reaction. In J. Eisenson (Ed.), *Stuttering: A symposium*. New York: Harper & Row.

Bloodstein, O., & Grossman, M. (1981). Early stutterings: Some aspects of their form and distribution. *Journal of Speech and Hearing Research, 2,* 298–302.

Conture, E. (1982). *Stuttering*. Englewood Cliffs, NJ: Prentice-Hall.

Davis, D.M. (1939). The relation of repetitions in the speech of young children to certain measures of language maturity and situational factors. Part I. *Journal of Speech Disorders, 4,* 303–318.

Glasner, P.J., & Rosenthal, D. (1957). Parental diagnosis of stuttering in young children. *Journal of Speech and Hearing Disorders, 22,* 288–295.

Johnson, W., Boehmler, R., Dahlstrom, G., Darley, F., Goodstein, L., Kools, J., Neelley, J., Prather, W., Sherman, D., Thurman, C., Trotter, W., Williams, D., & Young, M. (1959). *The onset of stuttering*. Minneapolis: University of Minnesota Press.

Johnson, W., & Leutenegger, R.R. (Eds.). (1955). *Stuttering in children and adults*. Minneapolis: University of Minnesota Press.

McDearmon, J.R. (1968). Primary stuttering at the onset of stuttering: A reexamination of data. *Journal of Speech and Hearing Research, 11,* 631–637.

Sander, E.K. (1961). Reliability of Iowa Speech Disfluency Test. *Journal of Speech and Hearing Disorders Monograph Supplement, 7,* 21–30.

Silverman, E. (1971). Situational variability of preschoolers' disfluency: Preliminary study. *Perceptual and Motor Skills, 33,* 1021–1022.

Van Riper, C. (1971). *The nature of stuttering*. Englewood Cliffs, NJ: Prentice-Hall.

Williams, D., Darley, F., & Spriestersbach, D. (1978). Appraisal of rate and fluency. In F. Darley & D. Spriestersbach (Eds.), *Diagnostic methods in speech pathology*. New York: Harper & Row.

Williams, D., Silverman, F., & Kools, J. (1968). Disfluency behavior of elementary-school stutterers and nonstutterers: The Adaptation effect. *Journal of Speech and Hearing Research, 11,* 622–630.

Winer, B.J. (1971). *Statistical principles in experimental design*. New York: McGraw-Hill.

Wingate, M. (1962). Evaluation and stuttering: III. Identification of stuttering and the use of a label. *Journal of Speech and Hearing Disorders, 27,* 368–377.

Wyatt, G. (1969). *Language learning and communication disorders in children*. New York: Free Press.

Yairi, E. (1981). Disfluencies of normally speaking two-year-old children. *Journal of Speech and Hearing Research, 24,* 490–495.

Yairi, E. (1983). The onset of stuttering in two- and three-year-old children: A preliminary report. *Journal of Speech and Hearing Disorders, 48,* 171–178.

Yairi, E., & Clifton, N.F., Jr. (1972). Disfluent speech behavior of preschool children, high school seniors, and geriatric persons. *Journal of Speech and Hearing Research, 15,* 714–719.

Clustering of Disfluencies in the Speech of Stuttering and Nonstuttering Preschool Children

Carol P. Hubbard
Ehud Yairi

The distribution of disfluencies in speech has been of major scientific interest since Johnson & Knott (1936) began an intensive research program concerning the "moment of stuttering." Numerous studies have been published on the overall frequency of such disfluencies, the frequency of specific disfluency types, the consistency and variation of their occurrence, and the linguistic factors that influence their appearance (Bloodstein, 1981). Most of these reports were based on studies of adults. In the past decade, however, there has been a surge of scientific activities concerned with disfluency of stuttering and normally speaking children during the early years of life. For example, new data have been reported that pertain to disfluency norms (Yairi & Lewis, 1984), relationships between disfluencies and language skills (Colburn & Mysak, 1982), loci of disfluencies (Bloodstein & Grossman, 1981; Wall, Starkweather, & Cairns, 1981), acoustical features (Wasowicz, Yairi, & Gregory, 1985) and secondary characteristics associated with disfluencies (Schwartz, Zebrowski, & Conture, 1986).

In spite of this concentrated research effort, one aspect, the clustering of disfluencies within or on adjacent words, has received very limited attention. In fact, there are only two studies of disfluency clustering in the speech of young children, and both included only nonstuttering children (Colburn, 1985; Silverman, 1973). Each investigator reported that disfluencies occurred in clusters more often than would be expected by chance. Similar studies of adult stutterers (Fein, 1970; Still & Griggs, 1979; Still & Sherrard, 1976; Taylor & Taylor, 1967) have yielded conflicting or ambiguous results. Nevertheless, clustering of disfluencies has not been investigated in the speech of young stutterers.

Several investigators have suggested that information on clustering may be useful in assessing or developing

theoretical models of stuttering. Still and Sherrard (1976) showed how anxiety, conflict, and feedback theories can be stated as mathematical models based on the sequential characteristics of moments of stuttering. For example, they reasoned that Sheehan's (1958) conflict theory would predict moments of stuttering to be followed immediately by segments of fluency because of the sharp drop in fear during stuttering. Mysak's (1960) feedback theory, by contrast, implies that stuttering will tend to appear in clusters during periods when the stutterer is monitoring speech feedback.

Although the theoretical potential of clustering remains of interest, priority should be given to developing appropriate methods for studying this phenomenon and to gathering sufficient basic data about its characteristics in children and adults. Information relevant to the classical problem of identifying stuttering and stutterers is one possible outcome of such research. Present data show that the frequency, type, and severity of disfluencies exert considerable influence on listener judgments (Young, 1984). It may be, however, that the "density" of the distributions of disfluencies in speech is another factor. Also, the possible discovery of different clustering patterns could expand the base of current strategies for differentiating incipient stutters from normally nonfluent speakers that also rely heavily on analyses of frequency and type of disfluencies (Adams, 1977; Pindzola & White, 1986). Thus, there are a number of issues that could be influenced by the addition of systematic data on clustering.

The present research compared the clustering of disfluencies in speech of preschool children regarded as stutterers with the clustering of children regarded to be nonstutterers. The underlying goal was to identify those aspects of clustering that are associated with, and might influence, parental distinction between the two groups. In addition to answering the basic question of whether or not clustering occurs significantly above chance, we also focused on group differences in terms of the extent of clustering and its possible relationship to specific disfluency types.

Reprinted from *Journal of Speech and Hearing Research*, 31, no. 2, 228–233. Copyright © 1988, American Speech-Language-Hearing Association.

METHOD

Subjects

Two groups of 15 children participated. Each group consisted of 10 boys and 5 girls ranging in age from 2 to 4 years. Subjects in one group were judged as stutterers by at least one parent and two certified speech clinicians and were, on the average, 5½ months past the reported stuttering onset. They were required to exhibit disfluency on *no less than 5 percent* of the syllables in their speech to ensure sufficient samples for analysis. Mean age was 34.07 months with a standard deviation of 5.98. Subjects in the other group were nonstuttering children and exhibited a disfluency rate of at least 3 percent. They were matched in pairs to the stuttering subjects according to sex, age (within 3 months), and language development. Mean age was 33.87 months with a standard deviation of 4.78.

Because a 2-year age range in early childhood involves a substantial range in verbal skills, and because those skills could possibly affect subjects' disfluency (Colburn & Mysak, 1982; Murray & Reed, 1977; Wall, 1980), including clustering, subjects were also matched using the Developmental Sentences Scoring (DSS) procedure (Lee, 1974). For a pair of subjects to be matched, the differences between their DSS scores had to be within the standard deviation reported by Lee for their respective age level and sex. The mean DSS score for the stuttering subjects was 5.96 with a standard deviation of 1.19. The mean for the nonstuttering subjects was 5.99 with a standard deviation of 1.36.

Speech Samples and Procedures

A spontaneous speech sample of approximately 500 syllables was audiotaped for each subject during free play interaction with an adult. Standard sets of toys and pictures were used to elicit a sufficient amount of verbal output.

The first author listened to the tapes and orthographically transcribed the childrens' speech samples verbatim. Unintelligible utterances were deleted from the samples. Because frequent questions were asked in these adult-child interactions, all isolated "yes" or "no" responses were also deleted to limit the number of single-syllable word utterances in the samples. When "yes" or "no" was followed immediately by another word or phrase, the response was retained. On this basis the mean length of the speech samples for the stuttering group was 680.9 syllables in 604.1 words while the mean length for the comparison group was 615.8 syllables in 555.9 words.

Following transcription, the first author listened again to the tape-recorded speech samples to identify and mark disfluencies. An 8-category disfluency scheme (Yairi, 1981) was employed. It included: (a) Part-Word Repetition; (b) Single-Syllable Word Repetition; (c) Multiple-Syllable Word Repetition; (d) Phrase Repetition; (e) Interjection; (f) Revision-Incomplete Phrase; (g) Dysrhythmic Phonation (primarily sound prolongations or broken words); (h) Tense Pause (audible tense vocalization between words). The first author's overall point-by-point self-agreements for the combined factors of disfluency type and location in 20 percent of the speech samples was 0.80. Overall interjudge agreement between the first and second authors was 0.82. Interjudge agreement for specific types of disfluency was as follows: Interjection: 0.80; Part-Word Repetition: 0.59; Single-Syllable Word Repetition: 0.92; Multiple-Syllable Word Repetition: 0.93; Phrase Repetition: 0.88; Revision Incomplete Phrase: 0.87; Dysrhythmic Phonation: 0.65; Tense Pause: 0.67. The greatest number of disagreements occurred on conflicting identification of Part-Word Repetition and Dysrhythmic Phonation. Although the percent of disagreement on Tense Pause was similar, that type of disfluency occurred rarely.

In the last step of the analysis, the marked transcripts were examined for instances of clustering defined as the occurrence of two or more disfluencies on the same word and/or adjacent words. For example, in the utterance: "Wwwha-What big box?" a within-word cluster occurred consisting of Dysrhythmic Phonation and Part Word Repetition. The sentence "You can . . . you can . . . p-p-put that here" contains a cluster of Phrase Repetition and Part-Word Repetition. The overall numbers of disfluencies occurring as singles and in clusters, and the occurrences of single and clustered disfluencies according to each of the eight types of disfluency were determined for each subject. The percentages of each child's total disfluencies that occurred as singles and in clusters were also calculated.

To determine whether disfluencies occurred greater than chance in clusters, the observed percentages of clustered and single disfluencies were compared using expected percentages derived by the Monte Carlo method (National Bureau of Standards, 1951). This method entailed selecting as many numbers as the total number of disfluencies produced from a set of one trillion random numbers. The selected numbers were placed within the limits of the total number of words in the speech sample. A computer program generated a random distribution of the numbers for each subject's speech sample with the simulation being seeded by the number of words, the number of disfluencies, and a different random number selected by the experimenter each time. When provided with an individual subject's data, the program repeated the simulation process 30 times and averaged the results to obtain expected values. Values were thus generated for the expected number of clusters, the expected number of disfluencies in clusters, the expected number of disfluencies as single instances, the expected sizes of clusters from 2 to 13 disfluencies, and the expected number of clusters on a word surrounded by fluent words.

RESULTS

Frequency of Disfluency

Group data based on the frequency of disfluency per 100 words and 100 syllables are reported in Table 1. Yairi (1981) has argued that the latter data are a more accurate measure of

TABLE 1. The mean frequency (M) and standard deviation (SD) of each disfluency type and total disfluency per 100 words and per 100 syllables spoken for the stuttering and control groups.

Disfluency type		Stutterers Disfluencies per		Control Disfluencies per	
		words	syllables	words	syllables
I	M	3.23	2.83	1.08	0.97
	SD	2.54	2.15	1.02	0.91
PWR	M	6.32	5.64	1.11	0.99
	SD	3.56	3.22	0.70	0.61
SSWR	M	5.04	4.48	1.26	1.14
	SD	4.22	3.80	0.50	0.46
MSWR	M	0.28	0.24	0.11	0.09
	SD	0.33	0.30	0.20	0.17
PhR	M	1.38	1.24	0.73	0.65
	SD	0.87	0.80	0.52	0.48
R-Ic	M	1.41	1.26	1.52	1.36
	SD	0.68	0.61	1.11	0.96
DP	M	6.57	5.99	0.60	0.53
	SD	6.10	6.05	0.36	0.31
TP	M	0.89	0.77	0.17	0.16
	SD	1.26	1.06	0.35	0.32
Total	M	25.10	22.45	6.57	5.90
	SD	12.53	11.56	2.06	1.74

Note: (I) Interjection; (PWR) Part-Word Repetition; (SSWR) Single Syllable Word Repetition; (R-Ic) Revision-Incomplete Phrase; (DP) Dysrhythmic Phonation; (TP) Tense Pause; (MSWR) Multiple-Syllable Word-Repetition; (PhR) Phrase Repetition.

TABLE 2. Observed and expected mean proportions of clustered and single disfluencies for 15 stutterers and 15 nonstuttering preschool children.

Groups and disfluency conditions	Observed	Expected
Stutterers		
Clustered disfluencies	0.57	0.50
Single disfluencies	0.43	0.50
Control		
Clustered disfluencies	0.34	0.17
Single disfluencies	0.66	0.83

disfluencies in speech of young children. The table presents means and standard deviations for stutterers and nonstutterers on each of the eight disfluency types, as well as on the total number of disfluencies. A paired t test indicated that the difference between the mean number of disfluencies was statistically significant [$t(14) = 5.50$, $p < .05$]. The two groups of subjects, then, were clearly different in respect to the number of disfluencies.

Proportions of Disfluencies Occurring in Clusters

To determine whether disfluencies occurred in clusters more than would be expected by chance, the proportions of clustered disfluencies in the speech samples were compared with expected values obtained from computer simulations. The means from these analyses are presented in Table 2.

These data suggest that disfluencies occurred in clusters more frequently than could have been expected by chance for stutterers and controls. The differences were significant for both groups [stutterers: $t(14) = 2.99$; $p < .05$; controls: $t(14) = 5.87$, $p < .05$]. In addition, the proportion of disfluencies occurring in clusters in the speech of the stutterers was substantially higher than that of the nonstuttering subjects. The 23-point difference was statistically significant [$t(14) = 6.44$, $p < .05$].

Number of Clusters

The next step in the analysis concerned the number of clusters. In terms of observed values, it can be seen in Table 3 that stutterers had more than six times as many clusters as nonstutterers. The difference between the two groups was statistically significant [$t(14) = 5.11$, $p < .05$]. However, when the observed values were compared to the numbers of clusters expected by chance, statistical analysis indicated that the difference was significant only from the nonstuttering group [$\chi^2(14, N = 15) = 36.77$, $p < .05$]. The χ^2 value for the stutterers was 12.41.

Sizes of Clusters

The clusters exhibited by stutterers ranged from two to ten disfluencies per cluster while the range for the comparison subjects was only two to five disfluencies. (The expected cluster size was up to 12 disfluencies per cluster for stutterers and 5 for controls.) The mean numbers of clusters of different sizes and the proportion of clusters of each size are reported in Table 4. Because large-size clusters were infrequent, clusters larger than four were combined. It is obvious that stutterers not only generated more clusters that were considerably longer than those exhibited by control subjects, but that clusters longer than two disfluencies occurred in greater proportions in their total clusters than among controls (40% and 19%, respectively.) A paired t test indicated that this difference between groups was significant [$t(14) = 4.41$, $p < .05$].

Types of Disfluency

The next analysis dealt with the question of whether some of the eight disfluency types occurred in clusters more often

TABLE 3. Means (M) and standard deviations (SD) for observed and expected numbers of clusters in the speech of stutterers and control speakers.

Group	Observed number of clusters		Expected number of clusters	
Stutterers	M	35.53	M	34.32
	SD	23.06	SD	22.91
Control	M	5.53	M	3.67
	SD	2.85	SD	2.15

TABLE 4. Mean numbers, standard deviations (in parentheses) and proportions of clusters occurring in different cluster sizes.

Group	2-Disfl. Clusters		3-Disfl. Clusters		4–12 Disfl. Clusters	
	Number	Proportion	Number	Proportion	Number	Proportion
Stutterers	21.40 (13.20)	0.60	7.73 (6.33)	0.22	6.40 (5.40)	0.18
Controls	4.46 (2.23)	0.81	0.60 (0.91)	0.11	0.47 (0.64)	0.08

than as isolated instances. Table 5 displays the numbers of each type of disfluency produced in clusters and as singles, and the adjusted mean proportions of each type of disfluency.

The two groups exhibited different trends. For the stutterers, all eight types of disfluencies occurred in clusters more often than as singles, whereas for the control subjects, all types of disfluencies, except Tense Pause, occurred less often in clusters. For the stutterers, the three disfluency types with the highest clustering proportions were Phrase Repetition, Multiple-Syllable Word Repetition and Interjection. For the controls, the three types with the highest proportions were Tense Pause (6 of only 12 instances), Phrase Repetition, and Dysrhythmic Phonation.

For each group, a separate one-way within-subjects ANOVA (Linton & Gallo, 1975) was used to compare the clustered proportions of the eight disfluency types. If zero disfluencies had been recorded for a given subject's disfluency type, a hypothetical figure was assigned using computer estimates that were derived from residual data (Snedecor & Cochran, 1980). These estimates were the basis for adjustments in the mean proportions reported for each type of disfluency (see Table 5). The proportions of disfluency type did not differ significantly for the stutterers [$F(7,90) = 0.56$, $p > .05$], but did for the controls [$F(7,90) = 2.28, p < .05$]. Follow-up comparisons between all possible pairs of the nonstutterers' disfluency types using the Newman-Keuls test indicated no significant differences between proportion means. These data, however, should be viewed with some caution because the reliability for several disfluency types was not high.

Clustering and Word Boundary

A final analysis examined the question of whether clustering occurs within the boundaries of a single word surrounded by fluent words more or less often than on two or more consecutive words. Group means and standard deviations for the number of clusters that occurred on single words and the number of clusters occurring across two or more adjacent words are presented in Table 6. The paired t test comparisons of the number of disfluencies in these two types of clusters failed to reach statistical significance at the .05 level for the stutterers [$t(14) = .76, p > .05$] or for the control subjects [$t(14) = 1.32, p > .05$].

TABLE 5. The absolute numbers and adjusted proportions of each of the eight disfluency types occurring in clusters and as singles for each subject group.

Disfluency type		Number in clusters	Proportion in clusters	Number as singles	Proportion as singles
I	—Stutterers	200	.68	93	.32
	—Control	33	.29	56	.71
PWR	—Stutterers	339	.54	235	.46
	—Control	32	.34	61	.66
SSWR	—Stutterers	279	.61	187	.39
	—Control	31	.33	76	.67
MSWR	—Stutterers	17	.66	10	.34
	—Control	3	.33	5	.66
PhR	—Stutterers	93	.67	34	.33
	—Control	27	.47	31	.53
R-Ic	—Stutterers	86	.60	47	.40
	—Control	36	.23	93	.77
DPh	—Stutterers	396	.63	184	.37
	—Control	21	.43	28	.57
TP	—Stutterers	54	.60	27	.40
	—Control	6	.53	6	.47

Note: (I) Interjection; (PWR) Part-Word Repetition; (SSWR) Single Syllable Word Repetition; (R-Ic) Revision-Incomplete Phrase; (DP) Dysrhythmic Phonation; (TP) Tense Pause; (MSWR) Multiple-Syllable Word Repetition; (PhR) Phrase Repetition.

TABLE 6. Means (M) and standard deviations (SD) for the numbers of clustered disfluencies on single words and across adjacent words.

	Stutterers		Control	
	Clustered disfl/ single words	Clustered disfl/ adjacent words	Clustered disfl/ single words	Clustered disfl/ adjacent words
M	39.00	59.53	5.07	7.67
SD	29.06	43.87	4.51	4.37

DISCUSSION

To our knowledge, this is the first study to compare clustering of disfluencies in the speech of stutterers and normal speakers directly. It is also the first attempt to examine clustering of disfluencies in the speech of preschool stutterers and is larger in scope than previous investigations of the phenomenon.

The data demonstrate that both stuttering and nonstuttering children produce higher percentages of disfluencies in clusters than expected by chance. This outcome substantiates previous reports regarding the presence of such clustering in the speech of normal preschool children (Colburn, 1985; Silverman, 1973) and that of adult stutterers (Fein, 1970; Still & Griggs, 1979; Still & Sherrard, 1976). The close similarity between the 33 percent figure for clustered disfluency produced by normal children in the current study to figures reported by Colburn (1985), for 2-year-olds (36%), and Silverman (1973), for 4-year-olds (38%), strengthen the validity of the data. Thus, the main conclusion of the present study is that clustering is a significant factor in disfluent speech, normal as well as abnormal, for which there must be made an account.

One of the more important outcomes of the present study is the substantial distinction between the clustering shown by stutterers and control subjects. This distinction is apparent in two important ways. First, there is a large and statistically significant difference between the two groups in the proportions of total disfluencies occurring in clusters. For stutterers, most disfluencies (57%) are clustered. Moreover, clustering spread across all eight categories of stutterers' disfluencies, each of which appeared in clusters over 50 percent of the time. Conversely, single disfluency instances usually prevailed in the speech of control subjects. Although clusters occur in nonstutterers' speech more frequently than expected by chance, only a third of the disfluencies, 33 percent, were clustered. For this group all of the disfluency types, except for Tense Pause, appear less than 50 percent of the time in cluster formations.

A second feature of the differentiation of the two groups

of subjects is cluster size. Generally, stutterers produce longer clusters than do nonstuttering subjects. On the average, strings of more than two disfluencies comprised 40 percent of the clusters of stutterers, but only 20 percent of the clusters of controls. Also, although many stutterers produce clusters of four or more disfluencies, comparison speakers exceeded two-disfluency clusters infrequently. Thus, cluster concentrations encompassing 50 percent or more of all disfluencies in a speech sample, and/or the frequent occurrence of clusters of three or more disfluencies, may be useful indicators of early childhood stuttering.

At present, the slowly accumulating evidence of the sequential relationship among disfluencies is still in initial phases and is open to diverse interpretations. A psychological orientation could lead one to hypothesize that disfluencies beget disfluencies by serving as stimulus cues that elicit the responses of anxiety, physical tension, and further stuttering (Fein, 1970). This explanation, however, is more applicable to stutterers and presumes some features of advanced stuttering symptomatology (anxiety).

A different view of clustering, with implications for normal speakers as well, can be developed relative to Zimmermann's (1980) organically oriented disfluency model. He postulated that when speech musculature exceed certain movement thresholds, afferent feedback to the brainstem throws the speech system into oscillation or tonic behavior (disfluency). If the system is not stabilized immediately to restore afferent-efferent balance, then the stimulation derived from oscillatory and tonic activity causes more maladaptive, hypertonic escape behaviors. Clusters of disfluencies then, especially those composed of Part-Word Repetition and Dysrhythmic Phonation, can be conceived of as resulting from such overflowing, unchecked reflex-induced tonic activities. This model, though, does not readily explain clusters consisting of Revisions and Interjections that appear to reflect uncertainties in formulating and planning utterances rather than disintegration of movement. Better understanding of the differences among various disfluency types and additional information on the internal composition of clusters could be extremely important in resolving these as well as other theoretical alternatives.

The present findings encourage further research on clustering of disfluencies in children and adults. Additional attention to cluster composition, including comparisons of stuttering versus normal disfluencies, and investigation of the relationship of clustering characteristics to the severity of stuttering, might be particularly useful. Future work should also attempt to improve the simulation model that did not take into consideration that clusters across adjacent words could not have occurred at any place in the speech sample where one utterance ended and another began. Simulation programs should be designed with breaking points corresponding to utterance length. It can be predicted that such modifications would decrease the number of expected clusters, thereby increasing the magnitude of the clustering phenomenon.

ACKNOWLEDGMENTS

The advice and assistance of Dennis Jennings and Mike Mathieson of the University of Illinois Department of Statistics, in developing the computer simulation program, is greatly appreciated.

REFERENCES

Adams, M. (1977). A clinical strategy for differentiating the normally nonfluent child and the incipient stutterer. *Journal of Fluency Disorders, 2*, 141–148.

Bloodstein, O. (1981) *A handbook on stuttering*. Chicago: National Easter Seal Society.

Bloodstein, O., & Grossman, M. (1981). Early stutterings: Some aspects of their form and distribution. *Journal of Speech and Hearing Research, 24*, 298–302.

Colburn, N. (1985). Clustering of disfluency in nonstuttering children's early utterances. *Journal of Fluency Disorders, 10*, 51–58.

Colburn, N., & Mysak, E. (1982). Developmental disfluency and emerging grammar. I: Disfluency characteristics in early syntactic utterances. *Journal of Speech and Hearing Research, 25*, 414–420.

Fein, L. (1970). Stuttering as a cue related to the precipitation of moments of stuttering. *Asha, 12*, 456. Abstract.

Johnson, W., & Knott, J. (1936). The moment of stuttering. *Journal of Genetic Psychology, 48*, 475–479.

Lee, L. (1974). *Developmental sentence analysis*. Evanston, IL: Northwestern University Press.

Linton, M., & Gallo, P. S. (1975). *The practical statistician: Simplified handbook of statistics*. Belmont, CA: Wadsworth.

Murray, H., & Reed, C. (1977). Language abilities of preschool stuttering children. *Journal of Fluency Disorders, 2*, 171–176.

Mysak, E. (1960). Servo theory and stuttering. *Journal of Speech and Hearing Disorders, 25*, 188–195.

National Bureau of Standards (1951). *Monte Carlo Method*. Washington, DC: U.S. Government Patents Office.

Pindzola, R., & White, D. (1986). A protocol for differentiating the incipient stutterer. *Language Speech and Hearing Services in the Schools, 17*, 2–15.

Schwartz, H., Zebrowski, P., & Conture, E. (1986). Behavior at the onset of stuttering. *Asha, 28*, 110. Abstract.

Sheehan, J. (1958). Conflict theory of stuttering. In J. Eisenson (Ed.), *Stuttering: A symposium* (pp. 121–166). New York: Harper.

Silverman, E. (1973). Clustering: A characteristic of preschooler's speech disfluency. *Journal of Speech and Hearing Research, 16*, 578–583.

Snedecor, G. W., & Cochran, W.G. (1980). *Statistical Methods* (7th ed.). Iowa City: Iowa University Press.

Still, A., & Griggs, S. (1979). Changes in the probability of stuttering following a stutter: A test of some recent models. *Journal of Speech and Hearing Research, 22*, 565–571.

Still, A., & Sherrard C. (1976). Formalizing theories of stuttering. *The British Journal of Mathematical and Statistical Psychology, 29*, 129–138.

Taylor, I., & Taylor, M. (1967). Test of predictions from the conflict hypothesis of stuttering. *Journal of Abnormal Psychology, 72*, 431–433.

Wall, M. (1980). Comparison of syntax in young stutterers and nonstutterers. *Journal of Fluency Disorders, 5*, 345–352.

Wall, M., Starkweather, W., & Cairns, J. (1981). Syntactic influence on stuttering in young children. *Journal of Fluency Disorders, 6*, 283–298.

Wasowicz, J., Yairi, E., & Gregory, H. (1985). Acoustical and perceptual analysis of stuttering and nonstuttering children's disfluency. *Asha, 27*, 186. Abstract.

Yairi, E. (1981). Disfluencies of normally speaking two-year-old children. *Journal of Speech and Hearing Research, 24*, 490–495.

Yairi, E., & Lewis, B. (1984). Disfluencies at the onset of stuttering. *Journal of Speech and Hearing Research, 27*, 154–159.

Young, M. (1984). Identification of stuttering and stutterers. In R. Curlee & W. Perkins (Eds.), *Nature and treatment of stuttering: New directions* (pp. 13–30). San Diego: College-Hill Press.

Zimmermann, G. (1980). Stuttering: A disorder of movement. *Journal of Speech and Hearing Research, 23*, 122–136.

Nonfluencies of Preschool Stutterers and Conversational Partners: Observing Reciprocal Relationships

Susan C. Meyers

It has been posited that a stutterer's amount and type of nonfluency may fluctuate depending upon the listener and the situation (Ainsworth, 1987; Bloodstein, 1949, 1950a, 1950b). Adult stutterers recount that certain authority figures or impatient listeners are more difficult to talk to than other listeners such as pets or young children (Ainsworth, 1987; Johnson, 1959; Van Riper, 1982). However, investigations to support assumptions that preschool stutterers react differently to specific speaking situations or listeners have not been found (Meyers, 1986).

Studies have also reported that nonfluent speech increases in normal school-age and adult speakers when the speaker feels communicative pressure to talk (Bloodstein, 1949, 1950a, 1950b). Several studies have observed preschool nonstutterers interacting with various partners and in different speaking situations. Conflicting results, however, have been reported (Martin, Haroldson, & Kuhl, 1972a, 1972b; Meyers, 1986; Silverman, 1972).

Silverman (1972) found that nonstuttering children were 8 percent to 10 percent nonfluent during a structured interview situation and 6 percent nonfluent talking in a classroom setting. The structured interview situation in the Silverman study may have been more conversationally demanding for the children for two reasons. First, the examiner was unfamiliar to the children. Second, the structured interview situation was undertaken in a less familiar room, and the topics to be discussed were selected by the unfamiliar examiner. Silverman posited that situational differences were the primary contributors to nonfluent behavior. Notice, however, that embedded in the two situations were different conversational partners. Thus, this latter variable might also have had a significant impact on the child subjects' level of fluency.

Other studies have identified listener variables that consistently fail to elicit different levels of fluency breakdown in normally nonfluent young children. For example,

Martin et al. (1972a, 1972b) observed that nonstuttering children exhibited similar levels of nonfluency when talking with various listeners (their mothers, unfamiliar adults, unfamiliar children, and puppets). The researchers concluded that the children produced 2 percent to 3 percent nonfluency per conversation and did not vary the amount of nonfluency they emitted per play session with the different partners.

Whether or not young stutterers' nonfluency levels vary when talking to certain listeners is a question that remains unanswered. There has apparently been just one study investigating the fluency levels of young stutterers as they spoke to different listeners. Specifically, Meyers (1986) found preschool stutterers and nonstutterers talked to their own mother, a mother of a stuttering child, and a mother of a nonstuttering child with minimal variability. The stutterers produced more nonfluency (about 15% nonfluent speech) when talking to different listening partners than did the nonstutterers (about 3% nonfluent speech). These are similar findings to those of Martin et al. (1972a). Interestingly, the nonfluencies of the stutterers and the nonstutterers did not increase or decrease as a result of verbally interacting with a particular partner. The partners' nonfluency levels were also not statistically different.

The existing research into the fluency levels of normally developing nonstuttering children has operated from a unidirectional perspective instead of a theoretical framework that would include the nonfluency of a child as part of a bidirectional or reciprocal process in the partner-child interaction. The one study by Meyers observing reciprocal relationships of stutterers and nonstutterers interacting with different mothers suggested that the children's nonfluency levels were not influenced by the mothers' nonfluency levels. There have been no investigations observing the fluency levels of young stutterers interacting with different partners such as fathers of stutterers and peers.

It is possible that certain speakers influence fluency failure in stutterers (Knepflar, 1965). We do know from research in normal social interaction that fathers are qualitatively different from mothers in their interactions (Clarke-

Reprinted from *Journal of Speech and Hearing Disorders*, 54, no. 1, 106–112. Copyright © 1989, American Speech-Language-Hearing Association.

Stewart, 1977; Lamb, 1977), and peers may offer additional forms of interactions compared to parents (Vandell & Wilson, 1982). The question remains as to whether talking to a specified listener (such as mother, father, or a peer) influences nonfluency levels in stutterers. The purpose of this study was to determine if the nonfluencies of preschool stutterers vary significantly when talking to different listeners. A second focus of the study was to determine whether stutterers' listening partners differed in their own levels of nonfluency when talking to a stutterer.

METHOD

Subjects

Twelve 2–6-year-old stutterers were videotaped while playing with their mothers, fathers, and familiar peers. The mean age for the stutterers was 4 years 5 months. Seven of the parents reported that their children had been nonfluent less than 1 year (1–9 months reported onset of stuttering). Five of the parents reported that their children had been nonfluent more than 2 years (2–3½ years reported onset of stuttering).

Stutterers were selected to participate in the study from Temple University's Stuttering Prevention Clinic program. Parents were contacted and asked if they would participate in a research project prior to their child receiving therapy. None of the children had ever had a stuttering evaluation or therapy prior to the study.

A peer was defined as a familiar child who played with the stutterer at least 10 hours per week. Parents of stutterers were interviewed and allowed to select a playmate who was familiar to their child. The parents were then asked to estimate how many hours the children played together per week. Parents of the peer were then contacted, informed of the nature of the study, and asked if their child could participate. The peer was not matched according to the chronological age or sex of the stutterer. The mean age for the nonstuttering peer-partner was 6 years 1 month.

All children in the study (stutterers and peers) scored within normal limits on a battery of tests that measured language, articulation, and hearing status. The tests included in the screening were the Peabody Picture Vocabulary Test (Revised edition, Form M, Dunn & Dunn, 1981), informal language sample analysis (Miller, 1981), the Templin-Darley Screening Test of Articulation (Templin & Darley, 1969), and a pure-tone audiometric screening at 20 db HL for frequencies 250, 500, 1000, 2000, and 4000 Hz in both ears (ANSI, 1972). Two stuttering subjects out of 14 were excluded from the study because they failed to meet the screening criteria.

In order to be classified as a stutterer, a child had to receive a severity rating of mild, moderate, or severe on both the Stocker-Probe Technique (Stocker, 1977) and the Stuttering Prediction Instrument for Young Children (Riley, 1981). The child also had to be considered a stutterer by two certified speech-language pathologists. Test results revealed that four stutterers were considered "mild," four were considered "moderate," and four were considered "severe" stutterers.

None of the peer playmates had ever been suspected of having a communication disorder, and none had previously had a speech-language evaluation. Nonstutterers scored less than two stuttering types of disfluency on the Stocker-Probe Technique and the Stuttering Prediction Instrument (considered normal as defined by the test authors).

Instrumentation and Data Collection

Data collection took place at a university clinic in a laboratory setting. Two rooms separated by a one-way mirror were used. The first room (the activity room where the participants interacted) contained two mounted Sony video cameras (GBC Model TC-5000). One camera was equipped with a zoom lens and had the capability of following participants as they interacted. A second stationary camera viewed the participants in specified corners that were out of range of the first camera.

The activity room contained either two play telephones, puppets, or hats; a bucket with small toys (i.e., Fisher-Price people, bus, tractor, airplane, and animals); shoe box-sized blocks from Constructive Playthings; a tool set (consisting of a hammer, saw, wrench, and pliers); and housekeeping objects (broom, mop, dustpan, and ironing board).

The second room (an instrumentation room) held a Panasonic VCR video recorder (Model NV 8420) for recording the sessions, a Marantz Superscope audio recorder (Model CD-320) for ensuring audio quality for the videotaping, and a time-generator (Vicon 11, Model VAS 50/60 Hz) for timing the sessions. The person video recording the sessions operated the cameras via a Special Effects Generator (SEG Model RS 10A).

Ten minutes of free-play interaction between alternated partner-stutterer dyads were video recorded from behind the one-way mirror. The session was then immediately repeated with a different partner interacting with the stutterer. Partners were inserted into the play situation in a random order. All three partners were familiar to the stutterer. Twelve dyads (the stutterer and partner) were observed in the three different conditions, for a total of 36 observations. Each dyad was instructed to go into the room and play as they would at home.

Coding Procedures and Measures

The videotape and the written transcriptions were used for coding nonfluencies. A trained coder transcribed exact conversations into longhand records from the videotaped play periods. Nonfluencies were included in the longhand records. After the transcriptions were completed, the total number of words were tabulated. Words were counted according to Brown's (1973) rules. These measurements have been previously defined and described by Meyers (1986).

The video recordings were again played and replayed so the coder could classify the nonfluent behaviors as stuttering types or normal types. Nonfluencies were categorized according to the systems developed by DeJoy and Gregory (1985) and Williams, Silverman, and Kools (1968). Part-word repetitions, prolongations, tense pauses, broken words, and the total of these categories were coded as stuttering types of nonfluencies. Whole-word and phrase repetitions, revisions and incomplete phrases, interjections, unfilled pauses, and the total of these categories were coded as normal nonfluency types. There were a total of 12 dependent nonfluency variables.

Percentages of nonfluent words were calculated by dividing the number of nonfluencies (of a given type) by the total number of words spoken. For example, all part-word repetitions were added together for a 10-min interaction and divided by the total number of words in that sample produced by the speaker whose fluency was being assessed. This was done for each of the nonfluency types.

Reliability Measures

All nonfluencies were coded verbatim in the longhand records by the transcriber. In order to ensure that nonfluencies were not counted as words, brackets (e.g., [ ]) and two periods (e.g., ..) were used to code the exact location of the nonfluency within an utterance. Following the two periods, the type of nonfluency was identified in parentheses. For example, in the utterance, "[Luh..Luh..Look..Luh..(PW)] Look Mommy," the information enclosed in brackets would be counted as one nonfluency for the attempted word *Look*. Although the child produced multiple iterations of the first sound and added a whole-word repetition, only one nonfluency type is coded. As previously defined by Williams et al. (1968), [Luh..Luh..Look..Luh..] would be considered one nonfluency for the word *Look,* and the most severe type of nonfluency (e.g., the part-word repetition) is scored.

The coder then listed each nonfluency type on a separate summary form so interobserver reliability could be obtained in two ways. First, interobserver reliability was calculated by counting as agreements those occasions where both observers described the nonfluency as occurring at the same location. The total nonfluencies for each observer were then compared. If one coder classified the utterance "[Luh-..Luh..PW)] Look [Luh..(PW)] Look Mommy" as two part-word repetitions in the three-word utterance "Look Look Mommy" and the other coder classified the utterance "[Luh..Luh..Look..Luh..(PW)] Look Mommy" as one part-word repetition in a two-word utterance, the coders would be in disagreement concerning the frequency of nonfluency. Second, interobserver reliability was calculated for each specific nonfluency type by counting as agreements those occasions where both observers described the nonfluency as having the same topography. In order to be in agreement on

the example "[Luh..Luh..Look..Luh] Look Mommy," the coders had to categorize the nonfluency as a part-word repetition. If one coder classified the example as a whole-word repetition instead of a part-word repetition, the coders would be in disagreement in correctly classifying the nonfluency.

One-third of the 36 conversations were randomly selected for use in examining interjudge reliability. Percentages of agreement were used to compare interjudge agreement. That is, agreements/agreements + disagreements × 100 determined reliability (Sackett, 1978). A total of 12 videotaped observations, 10 min in duration, were included in the reliability checks.

Two judges were responsible for independently transcribing the longhand records and analyzing the nonfluencies. The first judge was the investigator of this experiment, a certified speech-language pathologist. She took responsibility for training the second judge. The second judge was a first-year graduate student in speech pathology who spent a semester (3 hours per week for 15 weeks) training to code the different types of nonfluencies. Four tapes of stutterers (including three 10-min interactions per tape, for a total of 12 dyads) were independently transcribed and coded by the two judges to obtain reliability. The two judges were in 96.63 percent agreement for the transcription coding, 96.04 percent agreement for the frequency calculation of nonfluency, and 95.33 percent agreement for the types of nonfluency. The lowest interobserver reliabilities were for revisions-incomplete phrases (90.58%) and unfilled pauses (91.66%). The average ratings assigned by the judges were not statistically different.

Data Analysis

A biomedical program (BMD:P2V) (Dixon, 1981) was selected to perform a series of analyses of variance measures (ANOVAS). First, a series of one-factor repeated measure ANOVAS (three levels of type of partner) were done to determine if stutterers produced more nonfluency and/or different types of nonfluency with different partners. Second, independent one-way ANOVAS were done to determine if the different partners produced the same amount and/or similar types of nonfluency when talking to a stutterer.

RESULTS

Words Spoken and Nonfluency for Stutterers

Table 1 presents the mean values and standard deviations for the stutterers interacting with different partners. There was a significant difference in the number of words spoken by the stutterers [$F(1, 22) = 4.11, p < .05$] under various conditions. The Duncan Range Test (Winer, 1971) revealed that stutterers used more words when talking to their mothers than they did talking to their fathers or peers. Stutterers were not

TABLE 1. Means, standard deviations, and F values for total words and percentage of nonfluency for stutterers interacting with various partners.

Variable	Stutterers with			$F(1, 22)$ value
	Mother	Father	Peer	
Number of words	319.42	248.25	255.00	4.11*
	(90.98)	(75.59)	(85.83)	
Total nonfluency	14.43	15.51	14.36	0.58
	(4.34)	(6.38)	(7.03)	
Stuttering	12.37	13.47	13.23	0.37
	(4.54)	(5.39)	(7.12)	
Normal nonfluency	2.06	2.04	1.13	2.57
	(1.08)	(1.41)	(0.90)	
Stuttering types				
Part-word repetition	5.55	6.48	5.97	0.53
	(2.16)	(3.33)	(4.17)	
Prolongation	5.15	5.53	5.72	0.25
	(4.49)	(5.47)	(5.85)	
Tense pause	1.58	1.32	1.54	0.34
	(0.90)	(0.90)	(1.13)	
Broken words	0.10	0.15	0.00	1.55
	(0.15)	(0.31)	(0.00)	
Normal types				
Whole-word repetition	0.40	0.47	0.26	0.68
	(0.29)	(0.63)	(0.30)	
Phrase repetition	0.12	0.14	0.08	0.36
	(0.15)	(0.22)	(0.16)	
Revision–incomplete phrase	0.75	0.69	0.48	1.11
	(0.62)	(0.58)	(0.53)	
Interjections	0.56	0.61	0.21	1.35
	(0.79)	(1.12)	(0.33)	
Unfilled pause	0.23	0.13	0.10	0.75
	(0.27)	(0.21)	(0.29)	

Note: Standard deviations are shown in parentheses below mean values.
*$p < .05$.

significantly different in their use of words with the father partners or the peer partners.

There were no significant differences in the total amount or types of nonfluencies emitted by stutterers when talking to the various partners. The means for each nonfluency type produced by the stutterers were quite similar indicating that there was little variability within the 12 stutterers' conversations as they talked to the three listening partners. This consistency for nonfluency types was clearly observed in the total percentage of stuttering and the total percentage of normal nonfluency categories. Consistent totals for percentage of stuttering were observed in 8 of the 12 stutterers. In the four stutterers who showed some variability, three subjects produced a low percentage of stuttering when talking to the peer playmate, and one child stuttered less when talking to his father. Stutterers produced a mean of 12.37 percent stuttering talking to mothers, 13.47 percent talking to their fathers, and 13.23 percent talking to a peer. These results were very similar to findings reported by Meyers in 1986. Stutterers in this latter study emitted 12.8 percent stuttering with their own mother, 13.3 percent

stuttering with an unfamiliar mother of another stutterer, and 14.4 percent stuttering with an unfamiliar mother of another nonstutterer.

For normal nonfluency types, stutterers produced a mean of 2.06 percent when talking to their mothers, 2.04 percent when talking to their fathers, and 1.13 percent when talking to a peer. There were 9 of the 12 stutterers who were consistent in the amount of normal nonfluency they produced. There were two stutterers who produced no normal nonfluency when talking to the peer playmate and one stutterer who emitted more normal nonfluency talking with his mother. The overall results reported in this study indicate that the amount and type of nonfluencies produced by these young stutterers when talking to various listening partners were quite similar.

Words Spoken and Nonfluency of Stutterers' Partners

There was a significant difference in the amount of words spoken by the different partners, $F(1, 22) = 10.12$,

$p < .001$. The Duncan Range Test revealed that fathers used significantly more words than mothers or peers, $p < .01$. The difference between the mothers and peers was not significant.

As shown in Table 2, parents were also consistent in the amount and type of nonfluency they exhibited. The lack of variability was observed in 11 of the 12 mother and father partners in total percentage of stuttering and total percentage of nonfluency. There was, however, a significant difference in terms of the total amount of nonfluency that characterized peer speech, $F(1, 22) = 3.93$, $p < .05$. Peers had significantly more stuttering and normal nonfluency types than mothers or fathers (Duncan Range Test, $p < .05$). The difference between the mothers and the fathers was not significant.

In terms of the stuttering types of nonfluency, the peers produced a greater proportion of part-word repetitions than mothers or fathers, $F(1, 22) = 4.71$, $p < .05$. Peers also produced tense pauses, which was a category not exhibited by either the mothers or the fathers, $F(1, 22) = 3.48$, $p < .05$.

In terms of normal nonfluency, peers produced a larger proportion of whole-word repetitions than did mothers and fathers, $F(1, 22) = 4.07$, $p < .05$. There were no significant differences between the mothers and fathers.

There was also a significant difference in the use of interjections, $F(1, 22) = 6.13$, $p < .01$. The Duncan Range Test revealed that peers used a greater proportion of interjections than mothers and fathers ($p < .01$). There were no significant differences between the mothers and fathers.

DISCUSSION

Several authorities have reported that in order to effectively remediate stuttering in young children, clinicians must observe directly those environmental factors that contribute to a child's increased disfluency (Costello, 1983; Gregory & Hill, 1984; Williams, 1987). The present study found similarities in the total numbers and types of nonfluency produced by preschool stutterers when talking with three different, highly familiar partners. As could have been expected,

TABLE 2. Means, standard deviations, and F values for total words and percentage of nonfluency for adults and peers interacting with stutterers.

Variable	Mother	Father	Peer	F(1, 22) value
Number of words	514.25	710.25	474.50	10.12***
	(109.34)	(146.71)	(145.62)	
Total nonfluency	1.26	1.43	2.63	3.93*
	(0.79)	(0.88)	(1.14)	
Stuttering	0.11	0.05	0.41	6.39**
	(0.19)	(0.10)	(0.46)	
Normal nonfluency	1.15	1.38	2.22	4.96*
	(0.72)	(0.88)	(0.83)	
Stuttering types				
Part-word repetition	0.11	0.05	0.35	4.71*
	(0.19)	(0.10)	(0.44)	
Prolongation	0.00	0.00	0.00	0.00
	(0.00)	(0.00)	(0.00)	
Tense pause	0.00	0.00	0.06	3.48*
	(0.00)	(0.00)	(0.11)	
Broken words	0.00	0.00	0.00	0.00
	(0.00)	(0.00)	(0.00)	
Normal types				
Whole-word repetition	0.14	0.25	0.59	4.07*
	(0.17)	(0.30)	(0.53)	
Phrase repetition	0.13	0.29	0.20	1.11
	(0.29)	(0.29)	(0.20)	
Revision–incomplete phrase	0.68	0.63	0.71	0.12
	(0.46)	(0.43)	(0.46)	
Interjections	0.10	0.08	0.44	6.13**
	(0.17)	(0.09)	(0.45)	
Unfilled pause	0.11	0.14	0.28	1.34
	(0.16)	(0.21)	(0.36)	

Note: Standard deviations are shown in parentheses below mean values.
*$p < .05$.
**$p < .01$.
***$p < .001$.

the stutterers exhibited more part-word repetitions and pro-longations than any other type of nonfluency. They also did not differ in the amount of nonfluency produced across listeners. Because children are more nonfluent than adults, it was not surprising that the peer partners were significantly more nonfluent when talking to the stutterer than were the parents. Peers used a larger proportion of part- and whole-word repetitions, tense pauses, and interjections than the parents. The nonfluency levels of the parent partners were quite similar when talking to the stutterers.

The results of this investigation suggest that different, familiar listeners do not affect the nonfluency levels of preschool stutterers. However, Bloodstein (1987) reported that stutterers' fear of listeners occurs during later phases of stuttering development. It is possible that the mild, moderate, and severe preschool stutterers observed in the present experiment were not advanced enough in terms of the history of their disorder to be influenced by a listening partner's reaction, given that listeners do indeed display reactions. What is more, present findings do not rule out the possibility that strangers or specific situations may affect the nonfluency levels of preschool stutterers (Davis, 1940; Silverman, 1972). This study did not address quantitative and qualitative aspects of nonfluency in various speaking situations where demands on the length and complexity of an utterance may influence the variability of stuttering. Additional investigations into situations that may influence nonfluency levels in young children are still warranted.

It has previously been reported in many investigations that normally developing children produce several nonfluency types that diminish with age (DeJoy & Gregory, 1985; Kowal, O'Connell, & Sabin, 1975). Because children are considered more nonfluent than adults, it was not surprising that the peer partners in this study had more hesitant speech than parent partners. Given that the peers were considered normal speakers, it was interesting to note that their percentage levels were low (2.63% total nonfluency) and very similar to those levels reported in the Martin et al. (1972a, 1972b) studies and in a previous investigation by Meyers (1986). As observed in previous experiments and the current study, peers produced a higher percentage of normal nonfluency than stuttering.

One clinical implication arises from the results of the current investigation. Many clinicians make it a practice to try to stabilize a preschool stutterer's fluency with different listening partners. However, if levels of nonfluency do not differ across partners, as suggested by the results reported here, preschool stutterers are not likely to benefit from such a treatment approach. Indeed, this step would be unnecessary. In a similar vein, many practitioners routinely suggest to parents that certain interactions may precipitate stuttering development in young children (Culp, 1984; Gregory & Hill, 1984; Guitar, 1982; Riley & Riley, 1984; Shine, 1984; Starkweather, 1987). Results of this study indicate that the preschool stutterer subjects did not differ in the amount and type of nonfluency they produced regardless of probable

differences in interactional style between adult (mother and father) and peer listeners.

Further research into the reciprocal relationship of the parent-stutterer or peer-stutterer verbal interactions is still necessary. Locating situations within the parent-child interactions, in the child's utterance length, or in the child's rate of speech that alter the frequency and type of a child's nonfluencies may be better indicators of how stuttering develops than observing if the presence of a talking partner influences stuttering behavior.

ACKNOWLEDGMENTS

A portion of this paper was presented at the American Speech-Language-Hearing Association Annual Convention in 1987. This work was supported by Psi Iota Xi, the ASHA Foundation, and the U.S. Department of Education, Special Education Department (G008400756). Special thanks to C.W. Starkweather and Sheryl Gottwald at Temple University for providing subjects for this project. Many thanks to Brenda Loyd for statistical consulting and to Lisa LaSalle and Emily Hall at the University of Virginia for assisting in the data collection.

REFERENCES

Ainsworth, S. (1987). *If your child stutters* (2nd ed.). Memphis, TN: Speech Foundation of America.

American National Standards Institute. (1972). *American National Standards Specifications for audiometers* (ANSI S3.6-1969). New York: Author.

Bloodstein, O. (1949). Conditions under which stuttering is reduced or absent: A review of literature. *Journal of Speech and Hearing Disorders, 14*, 295–302.

Bloodstein, O. (1950a). Hypothetical conditions under which stuttering is reduced or absent. *Journal of Speech and Hearing Disorders, 15*, 142–153.

Bloodstein, O. (1950b). A rating scale study of conditions under which stuttering is reduced or absent. *Journal of Speech and Hearing Disorders, 15*, 29–36.

Bloodstein, O. (1987). *A handbook on stuttering* (4th ed.). Chicago: National Easter Seal Society for Crippled Children and Adults.

Brown, R. (1973). *A first language: The early stages*. Cambridge, MA: Harvard University Press.

Clarke-Stewart, A. (1977, March). *The father's impact on mother and child*. Paper presented at the biennial meeting of the Society for Research in Child Development, New Orleans.

Costello, J. (1983). Current behavioral treatments for children. In D. Prins & R. Ingham (Eds.), *Treatment of stuttering in early childhood* (pp. 69–112). San Diego: College-Hill Press.

Culp, D. (1984). The preschool fluency development program: Assessment and treatment. In M. Peins (Ed.), *Contemporary approaches in stuttering therapy* (pp. 39–69). Boston: Little, Brown.

Davis, D. (1940). The relation of repetitions in the speech of young children to certain measures of language maturity and situational factors: Parts II and III. *Journal of Speech Disorders, 5,* 235–246.

DeJoy, D., & Gregory, H. (1985). The relationship between age and frequency of disfluency in preschool children. *Journal of Fluency Disorders, 10,* 107–122.

Dixon, W. (1981). *BMPD statistical software* [Computer program]. Los Angeles: University of California Press.

Dunn, L., & Dunn, L. (1981). *Peabody Picture Vocabulary Test* (rev. ed.). Circle Pines, MN: American Guidance Service.

Gregory, H., & Hill, D. (1984). Stuttering therapy for children. In W. Perkins (Ed.), *Stuttering disorders* (pp. 77–93). New York: Thieme-Stratton.

Guitar, B. (1982). Fluency shaping with young stutterers. *Journal of Childhood Communication Disorders, 6,* 50–59.

Johnson, W. (1959). *The onset of stuttering.* Minneapolis: University of Minnesota Press.

Knepflar, K. (1965). Speaking fluency in the parents of stutterers and nonstutterers. *Asha, 7,* 391.

Kowal, S., O'Connell, D., & Sabin, E. (1975). Development of temporal patterning and vocal hesitations in spontaneous narratives. *Journal of Psycholinguistic Research, 4,* 195–207.

Lamb, M. (1977). Father-child and mother-child interaction in the first year of life. *Child Development, 48,* 167–181.

Martin, R., Haroldson, S., & Kuhl, P. (1972a). Disfluencies in child-child and child-mother speaking situations. *Journal of Speech and Hearing Research, 15,* 753–756.

Martin, R., Haroldson, S., & Kuhl, P. (1972b). Disfluencies of young children in two speaking situations. *Journal of Speech and Hearing Research, 15,* 831–836.

Meyers, S. (1986). Qualitative and quantitative differences and patterns of variability in disfluencies emitted by preschool stutterers and nonstutterers during dyadic conversations. *Journal of Fluency Disorders, 11,* 293–306.

Miller, J. (1981). *Assessing language production in children: Experimental procedures.* Austin, TX: Pro-Ed.

Riley, G. (1981). *Stuttering Prediction Instrument for Young Children.* Tigard, OR: C.C. Publications.

Riley, G., & Riley, J. (1984). A component model for treating stuttering in children. In M. Peins (Ed.), *Contemporary approaches in stuttering therapy* (pp. 123–171). Boston: Little, Brown.

Sackett, G. (1978). *Observing behavior: Vol. 1. Theory and applications in mental retardation.* Baltimore: University Park Press.

Shine, R. (1984). Assessment and fluency training with the young stutterer. In M. Peins (Ed.), *Contemporary approaches in stuttering therapy* (pp. 173–216). Boston: Little, Brown.

Silverman, E. (1972). Generality of disfluency data collected from preschoolers. *Journal of Speech and Hearing Research, 15,* 84–92.

Starkweather, C. (1987). *Fluency and stuttering.* Englewood Cliffs, NJ: Prentice-Hall.

Stocker, B. (1977). *The Stocker-Probe Technique.* Tulsa, OK: Modern Education Program.

Templin, M., & Darley, F. (1969). *The Templin-Darley Test of Articulation.* Iowa City: University of Iowa.

Vandell, D., & Wilson, K. (1982). Social interactions in the first year: Infants: Social skills with peers versus mother. In K. Rubin & H. Ross (Eds.), *Peer relationships and social skills in childhood* (pp. 156–174). New York: Springer-Verlag.

Van Riper, C. (1982). *The nature of stuttering* (2nd ed.). Englewood Cliffs, NJ: Prentice-Hall.

Williams, D. (1987). *Counseling stutterers.* Memphis, TN: Speech Foundation of America.

Williams, D., Silverman, F., & Kools, J. (1968). Disfluency behavior of elementary school stutterers and nonstutterers. The adaptation effect. *Journal of Speech and Hearing Research, 11,* 622–630.

Winer, B. (1971). *Statistical principles in experimental design* (2nd ed.). New York: McGraw-Hill.

Subgrouping Young Stutterers: Preliminary Behavioral Observations

Howard D. Schwartz
Edward G. Conture

Numerous investigators have speculated that speech and nonspeech differences among stutterers, particularly young stutterers, may be as important as speech and nonspeech differences between stutterers and their normally fluent peers (e.g., Adams, 1982; Andrews & Harris, 1964; Clutter & Freeman, 1984; Daly, 1981; Preus, 1981; Van Riper, 1982; Yairi, 1972; Yairi, 1983; Yairi & Lewis, 1984). Such speculation appears related to the fact that various differences in speech and nonspeech associated[1] behaviors exist among stutterers themselves (e.g., Douglass & Quarrington, 1952; Froeschels, 1943; Prins & Lohr, 1972) as well as to the theories that stuttering may have multiple etiologies (Berlin, 1955; St. Onge, 1963; Van Riper, 1982). Examination of differences among stutterers has led investigators to suggest that these differences may be accounted for by identifying and describing subgroups of stutterers (Andrews & Harris, 1964; Blood & Seider, 1981; Cross & Luper, 1979; Preus, 1981; Prins & Lohr, 1972; Riley & Riley, 1979; St. Onge & Calvert, 1964).

As Preus (1981) points out in his recent subgrouping study of 100 stutterers, "the subgroup hypothesis has neither been proved nor disproved, but has found partial support in some studies. The need for new and better empirical investigations of this hypothesis is strong" (pp. 39–40). Thus, while many studies suggest the presence of subgroups, conclusions drawn from these studies are limited because of a lack of empirical data and clearly specified methodology. Typically, investigations of subgroups of stutterers have either focused on the characteristics of *stutterers* (e.g., articulation problems, intelligence, birth order, handedness etc.) or the characteristics of their *stutterings* (e.g., the type of speech disfluency, associated speech and nonspeech behaviors). Although stutterers appear to differ among themselves when their characteristics are examined (e.g., Andrews & Harris, 1964; Blood & Seider, 1981; Daly, 1981; Preus, 1981), many of these examinations have involved the use of unclearly and/or qualitatively defined variables. Furthermore, for many of these studies, there is little relation

between these variables and the stutterers' stuttering behavior itself. In contrast, examination of variables that characterize the stutterers' stuttering (e.g., speech disfluency type, associated speech and nonspeech behaviors) would appear to provide a more quantifiable and objective means of studying differences among these individuals.

As early as 1940, Barr suggested that nonspeech behavior should be considered when evaluating a stutterer's speech. Subsequently, Johnson (1955) mentioned that it is the speech behavior itself that appears to differentiate stutterers from their normally fluent peers, rather than intelligence, birth order, etc. Prins and Lohr (1972) reported that by identifying audible and visible behaviors associated with instances of stuttering, they were able to identify behavioral similarities supporting the presence of "behavioral subtypes" in adult stutterers. Thus, there is reason to believe that by objectively assessing stuttering and its associated behavior as suggested by Prins and Lohr, it may be possible to differentiate quantitatively and more precisely among youngsters who stutter.

Identifying and describing subgroups of young stutterers has at least three important clinical and research implications. First, identifying and describing the behaviors that characterize subgroups may help to explain disparate published findings (e.g., Adams, 1982; St. Onge, 1963). That is, if an investigator knew the criteria for subgroup membership, then he or she could, on an a priori basis, group or categorize subjects and experimentally investigate differences among the subgroups as well as their normally fluent peers. This would make it possible to determine potential sources of within- as well as between-group variability. Second, knowing the specific behaviors that characterize subgroups could assist in the diagnosis of young stutterers. With such knowledge, the examining clinician might be able to provide more specific, perhaps more accurate, diagnostic information based upon the behaviors and problems specific to the subgroup, rather than the entire population of young stutterers. Third, knowing the specific subgroup within which a child falls could provide prognostic information relative to therapeutic intervention. With this sort of information, it might be possible for a clinician to implement

Reprinted from *Journal of Speech and Hearing Research, 31,* no. 1, 62–71. Copyright © 1988, American Speech-Language-Hearing Association.

specific therapeutic strategies specially designed for a subgroup's unique problem behaviors (Adams, 1982; Riley & Riley, 1979) that should enhance both the efficacy as well as economy of the child's rehabilitation.

Although the foregoing review highlights past as well as present interest in studying the presence of subgroups of stutterers, it also suggests that few if any investigations have attempted or been able to quantify the variables or behaviors necessary to establish criteria for subgroup membership, particularly in young children. We assumed that one reasonable means of determining the nature and number of subgroups of young stutterers would be to examine their stuttering and associated behavior objectively. Possibly, this sort of examination might provide a more quantifiable and perhaps more sensitive means of differentiating among stutterers than would an examination of more general characteristics such as socioeconomic status or birth order. Therefore, the purpose of the present investigation was to describe the behaviors associated with the production of young stutterers' stuttering and to use these behaviors in an initial attempt to discern and/or describe subgroups of these individuals.

METHOD

Subjects

Forty-three young stutterers from the Central New York region, took part in the present investigation. All children were referred to the Syracuse University Gebbie Speech and Hearing Clinic because of known or suspected stuttering. Referral was made by either of the child's parents, school personnel, or a speech-language pathologist within the child's nursery or elementary school. These 43 young stutterers (10 girls and 33 boys) had a mean age of 5:11 (years:months, range: 3:10 to 9:4). All subjects exhibited stutterings in the forms of sound/syllable repetitions and sound prolongations. Their mean stuttering frequency was 9.4 stutterings per 100 words of conversational speech (range = 3 to 42 stutterings per 100 words of conversation). Fifteen of these 43 young stutterers simultaneously participated in a study designed to describe the temporal aspects of speech production associated with their stuttering (Schwartz, 1987). Analysis of these 15 youngsters' behaviors associated with stuttering indicated no differences from the other 28 subjects, and thus, their data were added to the data corpus and included in the overall analysis.

To be included in this study a subject had to have (a) three or more stutterings per 100 words of conversational speech; (b) people in the child's environment who expressed concern about the child's speech fluency; and (c) no known hearing, neurological, developmental, academic/intellectual, or emotional problems. In addition to the 43 children used in the present study, 7 boys with a mean age of 4:5 were not included because of their failure to meet the above criteria. All 43 subjects were paid volunteers who were unaware of the purpose and the method of the study.

Speech Samples and Conditions

Within-word speech disfluencies and the associated behaviors that characterized the child's stuttering problem were identified during two different speaking tasks: (a) conversational speech and (b) structured speaking activities. Two speaking tasks were used because pilot work had shown that for some children, conversational interaction with the examiner would fail to produce a sufficiently large data corpus from which to identify within-word disfluencies. In view of this fact, repetition of phrases (for example, "Say Pete again"), sequential story strips (Developmental Learning Materials), and items from the *Stocker Probe Technique* (Stocker, 1976) were used to elicit additional speech from the child. A mean sample size of 304 words was obtained from the 43 subjects (range: 81 to 655 spoken words per child).

Behavioral Data: Collection, Measurement, and Analysis

To analyze the data, it was necessary to: (a) video/audio record each subject; (b) locate and determine the specific type of disfluency; (c) categorize and quantify associated behaviors; (d) form speech and behavioral indices; and (e) complete appropriate statistical analyses.

Video/Audio Recording of 43 Subjects. The entire verbal interchange between the examiner and each of the 43 subjects was video/audio recorded. A stationary video camera (Sony, Model AVC 3200) was placed in the recording room and positioned at a constant distance (74 cm) from each child to provide a clear, adequately illuminated view of the youngster's head, arms, and torso. The audio signal was obtained using a lapel microphone (Sony ECM-50) or a headset microphone (Unex HS-1 A101) placed within 18 cm of the subject's lips. The video and audio signals were led to a video monitor (Sony, Trinitron) and videotape recorder (Sony, Model BVU 200A) located in the aforementioned laboratory. Prior to actual recording, the investigators determined the appropriateness of the camera position and adequacy of the audio and video signals. The video signal was recorded at 30 frames per sec (60 video fields per sec) on ¾-inch video cassette for later analysis. The audio signal was recorded simultaneously on the same cassette.

Location of Stuttering and Determination of Disfluency Type. After data collection but prior to the behavioral data analysis, the following preliminary procedures were implemented to insure an accurate description of the speech and nonspeech behaviors associated with specific within-word disfluencies: (a) identification of the beginning and end of a sample of conversational speech from video/audio recording; (b) notation of the approximate beginning and end of each stuttering using a video editor's digital tape footage counter (min:sec:frames); (c) determination of type of stuttering (sound/syllable repetition, sound prolongation); and (d) visibility of behavior associated with each individual stuttering.

Visibility of each stuttering was determined to be satisfactory if the first author was able to obtain a frontal view of the subject on the video monitor throughout the entire duration of the stuttering.

Similar research by Prins and Lohr (1972) and Riley (1980) as well as preliminary work of Conture and Schwartz (1984) has suggested that there are at least 44 audible or visible behaviors that occur in association with stuttering. The Appendix provides a description of the 14 different behaviors that were extracted, for the purposes of this study, from the 44 behaviors. The 14 behaviors selected were obviously not the only behaviors available for analysis. However, these 14 behaviors appeared to have the highest likelihood (Conture & Schwartz, 1984) of being observed both within and between stutterers (these behaviors were not idiosyncratic to a minority of stutterers) as well as being unambiguously measured with an acceptable degree of inter-judge and intrajudge reliability.

Quantification of Associated Behaviors.   The associated behaviors coincident with 10 stutterings for each of the 43 youngsters were identified and quantified (430 stutterings selected from the total sample of 1,094 stutterings). These 10 stutterings were selected so that any stuttering (anywhere within a subject's data corpus) was equally likely to be selected for analysis. The selection of 10 stutterings per subject was judged to be a reasonable compromise between oversampling the relatively infrequent stutterings of less severe stutterers and undersampling the relatively frequent stutterings of more severe stutterers.

To quantify the 14 possible behaviors associated with each of the 10 stutterings, it was necessary to:

1.   Locate and record the beginning and end of each stuttering by visual/auditory means. The video editor (Sony, BVE 200A) allowed the investigator to note the tape footage (minutes:seconds:frames) as well as to view the video-tape from stop motion through real time.
2.   View each stuttering from its apparent beginning to its end. This viewing of the stuttering occurred as many times as necessary to record all associated behaviors.

Statistical Analysis: Cluster Procedures

Because the goal of this investigation was to use behaviors associated with stuttering in attempts to describe and develop subgroups of young stutterers, it was thought that cluster analysis procedures would provide one of the best methods for statistically differentiating among the subjects. Numerous investigations have demonstrated the usefulness of cluster analysis procedures in speech articulation disorders (Arndt, Shelton, Johnson, & Furr, 1977; McNutt & Hamayan, 1984), aphasia (Kertesz & Phipps, 1977), and clinical depression (Andreasen, Grove, & Maurer, 1980). In

brief, when using cluster analysis procedures one accepts the observed variables at face value and attempts to consider the union of every possible pair of clusters in order to divide the sample into subgroups based on the similarity of these observed variables (Romesberg, 1984). Three speech and behavioral indices (to be discussed later) were submitted to a Ward's Hierarchical cluster analysis procedure (SAS Manual, 1982) that was used to form clusters on the basis of the 43 subjects' speech and behavioral data. This clustering procedure is used to group subjects so that within-cluster variability is minimized while between-cluster variability is maximized. It should be recognized that cluster analysis procedures always result in the creation of clusters. As McKinney and Speece (1985) point out:

> Empirical classification techniques, such as cluster analysis provide methods of grouping individuals who show a similar pattern of response on a given set of variables; they do not insure that they (the clusters) are psychologically or educationally meaningful or predictive. (p. 4)

Thus, for the purpose of this study, the cluster analysis procedure was chosen as a starting point toward investigating subgroups of stutterers, a preliminary investigation of possibly significant behavioral differences among youngsters who stutter.

Formation of Speech and Behavioral Indexes and Completion of Cluster Analysis.   A series of reiterative cluster analyses of the speech and behavioral data was completed. During these procedures, measurable characteristics of stuttering and its associated behaviors were grouped into various categories to create these clusters. These categories were selected on the basis of (a) reasonable frequency of occurrence both within and among stutterers, (b) their ability to be quantified as well as unambiguously measured, and (c) clinical observation and literature suggestions that these categories may significantly vary among stutterers. These categories included:

1.   Three most frequently occurring associated behavioral events occurring across all 10 stutterings.
2.   Total associated behavioral events occurring across all 10 stutterings.
3.   Frequency of occurrence of all instances of stuttering.
4.   Frequency of occurrence of instances of stuttering immediately followed by an instance of stuttering.
5.   Average duration of all sound/syllable repetitions.
6.   Average duration of all sound prolongations.
7.   Frequency of occurrence of all sound prolongations.
8.   Average number of nonspeech behaviors per stuttering.
9.   Average number of different behaviors per stuttering.

Results of the cluster analyses were examined to determine which combination of categories could be related meaningfully to behaviors typically produced by young stutterers, as well as to our present knowledge of stuttering in children. This examination led to the formulation of three indices chosen to reflect suggestions that differences in speech disfluency type, as well as number and variety of associated behaviors, reflect changes in the development of stuttering (Bloodstein, 1981; Conture 1982).

Sound Prolongation Index (SPI).

This is the total number of sound prolongations divided by the total number of stutterings in the conversational sample. For example, a youngster who produces 25 sound prolongations in a corpus of 100 stutterings would exhibit an SPI = 25 percent. For all subjects, increases in the number of sound syllable repetitions resulted in a lower SPI while an increase in the number of sound prolongations resulted in a higher SPI.

Nonspeech Behavior Index (NBI).

The average number of nonspeech behaviors per 10 measured stutterings is the NBI. For example, a youngster who exhibits 30 head turns during 10 stutterings would exhibit a NBI = 30/10 or an average of 3.0 nonspeech behaviors per stuttering.

Behavioral Variety Index (BVI).

The BVI is the average number of different behavior types per 10 measured stutterings. The BVI deals with only the type rather than the quantity of behavior produced. For example, a young stutterer who produces two eye blinks, two head turns, and two torso movements for each of the 10 stutterings, would exhibit three different behaviors per stuttering. Thus, three different behaviors per each of the 10 stutterings results in a BVI = 30/10 or an average of 3.0 different behaviors per stuttering.

Determining the Number of Clusters.

There are no universally accepted quantitative or qualitative procedures for determining the number of clusters or subgroups within a given sample (Everitt, 1981; SAS Manual, 1982; Seber, 1981). For this and other reasons (McKinney, Short, & Feagans, 1985), there is no one correct solution for any given clustering problem. Experimenters typically rely on a variety of objective procedures as well as their own knowledge of the data to determine the *minimum* number of meaningful, relatively cohesive clusters within a sample. Likewise, we relied on graphical representation of the hierarchical clustering (dendrograms, Seber, 1981), plots of individual data against their cluster means for each cluster solution, and our own knowledge of the behavior and subjects under investigation to determine the number of clusters that would most appropriately account for subject similarities and differences within the sample.

Intrajudge and Interjudge Reliability

Intra- and interjudge measurement reliability were assessed for (a) judgments of stuttering frequency and type of disfluency; and (b) behavioral indices.

Frequency and Type of Disfluency.

To assess the intrajudge and interjudge reliability for measuring the frequency of occurrence of within-word disfluencies and the identification of speech disfluency type (SPI), 10 randomly selected conversations (2,947 words) were selected from two subjects in each of the five behavioral subgroups (see Results). Three hundred and thirty-nine stutterings were remeasured. The two authors viewed the audio/video recordings of these 10 conversational samples and remeasured the percentage of within-word disfluencies per total number of words (frequency), as well as the percentage of sound prolongations per total number of within-word disfluencies (SPI) within each conversational sample. For the percentage of within-word disfluencies, there was a mean interjudge difference of 2.5 percent ($SE = 0.65\%$) and a mean intrajudge difference of 2.4 percent ($SE = 0.62\%$). For the SPI there was a mean interjudge difference of 5.9 percent ($SE = 3.35\%$) and a mean intrajudge difference of 6.6 percent sound prolongations ($SE = 2.82\%$).

Behavioral Measures.

One within-word disfluency was randomly selected for each subject to determine intra- and interjudge reliability of behavioral measures. The two authors reevaluated each of the 43 within-word disfluencies. These 43 disfluencies consisted of 22 sound prolongations and 21 sound/syllable repetitions, a ratio that closely approximated the ratio of 224 sound prolongations to 206 sound/syllable repetitions that existed for the entire corpus of 430 stutterings. Behaviors associated with each of the 43 stutterings were reduced to form the NBI and the BVI for all 43 stutterings. The mean difference value for interjudge agreement was a 0.49 NBI ($SE = 0.16$ NBI) and a 0.53 BVI ($SE = 0.17$ BVI). Intrajudge difference values were a 0.42 NBI ($SE = 0.14$ NBI) and a 0.37 BVI ($SE = 0.14$ BVI).

RESULTS

Inspection of clustering results suggested that five clusters was the minimum number of meaningful, relatively cohesive clusters within this sample of 43 young stutterers' associated behaviors. The experimenters made this determination by initially studying the graphic representations (dendrograms) of the cluster analysis which suggested that four to six clusters provided cohesive clustering solutions for the 43 subjects' behavior. The relative cohesiveness of each of these clustering solutions was assessed in part by comparing the root-mean-square standard deviation (*RMS SD*) of each cluster solution. The Ward's clustering procedure begins with each subject representing an individual cluster where the *RMS SD* is at a minimum. As every possible cluster combination is considered, the Ward's procedure forms clusters so that the *RMS SD* gradually increases to a maximum—representing the total variance both within and between cluster across all three indices—when all 43 subjects are grouped in a single cluster. Noting those cluster solutions where the *RMS SD* began to appreciably change from its maximum, and then exhibit little change with further clustering, it was found that the *RMS SD* appreciably decreased (from 0.98) to 0.50 with the four cluster solution, to 0.53 for the five cluster solution, to 0.45 for the six cluster solution, and thereafter changing minimally following the six cluster solution. These changes suggest that the four, five, and six cluster solution could potentially account for subject similarities and differences but required further analysis.

To further assess the relative cohesiveness of each of three clustering solutions, we next studied plots of individual values of the three indices around the cluster means for the four, five, and six cluster solutions. Assessment of these plots suggested that the five cluster solution was the most relatively cohesive clustering schema because individual data were closely associated with cluster means but were clearly differentiated from other cluster means. Finally, each of these cluster solutions was examined for interpretability and meaningfulness relative to the examiner's understanding of the speech and nonspeech behaviors associated with the stutterings of young stutterers.

Examination of the behavioral differences between the four and five cluster solutions indicated that the number and variety of associated behaviors of three children within the fourth cluster of the four cluster solution were highly similar to one another and relatively dissimilar to others within this fourth cluster. Thus, as indicated in the five cluster solution, these three subjects were grouped as a separate, fifth cluster. Furthermore, when examining differences between the fifth and sixth cluster solutions, it was noted that in the sixth cluster solution, the number and variety of youngsters' behavior in clusters 1 ($n = 12$) and 2 ($n = 5$) appeared more similar than dissimilar and, as indicated in the five cluster solution, they could be meaningfully grouped together as one cluster. Therefore, on the basis of considering graphic and numeric aspects of the cluster analysis dendrograms, plotting individual data against the cluster means for each cluster solution, and using knowledge of young stutterers and their behavior, it was determined that five was the minimum number of subgroups that could most appropriately account for subject similarities and differences within this sample.

Figure 1 depicts a three-dimensional representation of the results of the five cluster solution from the aforementioned Ward's Hierarchical cluster analysis. This three-dimensional representation (see Figure 1) illustrates the differences among and within the five clusters based upon the SPI, BVI, and NBI. Results of the cluster analysis will be discussed for each of the five clusters in terms of central

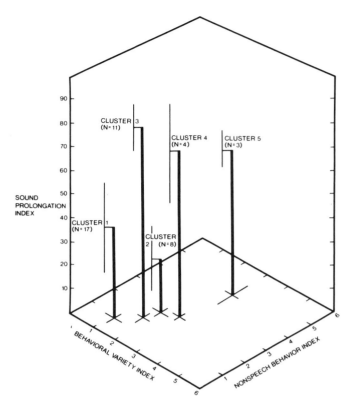

Figure 1. A three-dimensional representation of the cluster analysis results based on a Ward's hierarchical cluster analysis procedure for three indices of behavior (Sound Prolongation Index = percentage of sound prolongations per total number of stutterings determined from conversational sample; Behavioral Variety Index = number of different behaviors per stuttering; and Nonspeech Behavior Index = number of nonspeech behaviors per stuttering) characterizing 43 young stutterers. The average values of the SPI are represented by the top of each thick vertical line, while the bottom of these thick lines represents the average value for the BVI and NBI for each cluster. The thin vertical line represents + or − one standard deviation for the Sound Prolongation Index while the thin crossed lines at the base of each cluster represent + or − one standard deviation for the Behavioral Variety Index and Nonspeech Behavior Index respectively.

tendencies (means, *M*) and dispersion of scores (standard deviations, *SD*).

Cluster 1

Cluster 1 contained 17 subjects. The average SPI was 36.3 percent (*SD* = 19.0) indicating that the within-word disfluencies were primarily sound/syllable repetitions for subjects in this cluster. It should be recalled that the higher the percentage of sound/syllable repetitions within the conversational sample, the lower the SPI and vice versa. This cluster also exhibited an average BVI of 1.17 (*SD* = 0.31) and an average NBI (*SD* = 0.36) of 0.81. These results indicated that this cluster's stutterings were associated with a relatively small number and variety of associated behaviors.

Cluster 2

Cluster 2 consisted of eight subjects who also exhibited a relatively large number of sound/syllable repetitions as indicated by their average SPI of 23 percent ($SD = 14.0$). The BVI for Cluster 2 was 2.01 ($SD = 0.34$), and the NBI for Cluster 2 was 2.07 ($SD = 0.31$). Thus, Cluster 2 was primarily differentiated from Cluster 1 in terms of the higher NBI and BVI scores.

Cluster 3

Cluster 3 consisted of 11 subjects who exhibited an average SPI of 78.2 percent ($SD = 10.0$). In addition, this group exhibited a BVI of 1.75 ($SD = 0.26$) and a NBI of 1.46 ($SD = 0.29$). Thus, Cluster 3 primarily differed from Clusters 1 and 2 in terms of SPI.

Cluster 4

Cluster 4 contained four subjects and produced a relatively high frequency of sound prolongations (SPI = 67.3%, $SD = 21.0$) as well as a large number of associated behaviors per disfluency (BVI average = 2.6, $SD = 0.29$; NBI = 2.3, $SD = 0.27$). Cluster 4, therefore, primarily differed from Cluster 3 in terms of the two behavioral indexes.

Cluster 5

Cluster 5 consisted of three subjects whose average SPI of 69.6 percent ($SD = 8.0$) was similar to that of Cluster 4 (67.3%). Cluster 5 produced the greatest number of behaviors per stuttering among all five clusters. This cluster exhibited, on the average a 3.0 BVI ($SD = 0.26$) and 4.47 NBI ($SD = 0.80$). It seems reasonable to assume, therefore, that the tendencies of three subjects of Cluster 5 differ from the central tendencies exhibited by the other 40 subjects.

Cluster Membership, Age, and Frequency of Disfluency

Because it was considered possible that cluster membership merely reflected differences in the young stutterers' chronological age or stuttering severity (which can be reliably represented by stuttering frequency, Bloodstein, 1981), the mean ages for each of the five clusters as well as stuttering frequency, in each cluster were examined. Visual inspection of Table 1 shows little apparent difference among the five behavioral clusters in terms of chronological age although the frequency of stuttering varies from a mean of 6.8 percent for Cluster 4 to a mean of 13.8 percent for Cluster 2.

Additional examination of the possible relationship among age, frequency of disfluency, and cluster indices was completed by computing a Pearson product-moment correla-

TABLE 1. Means (years:months), standard deviation (in parenthesis), range of the mean age (years:months), and frequency of disfluency (based upon the number of stutterings observed in conversational sample (range = 86 to 655 words) for 43 young stutterers in five behavioral clusters determined by Ward's hierarchical cluster analysis.

Cluster		Age	Frequency of Disfluency
1 ($n = 17$)	Mean:	5:10 (1:7 months)	7.0% (3.6)
	Range:	3:10–8:9 months	
2 ($n = 8$)	Mean:	5:9 (1:7)	13.8% (6.8)
	Range:	3:10–8:0	
3 ($n = 11$)	Mean:	5:11 (1:7)	10.3% (11.3)
	Range:	3:10–9:4	
4 ($n = 4$)	Mean:	5:11 (1:5)	6.8% (1.7)
	Range:	4:5–7:10	
5 ($n = 3$)	Mean:	6:8 (0:2)	11.7% (4.6)
	Range:	6:7–6:10	

tion for these variables. Table 2 lists the result of this statistical procedure which suggests that age and frequency of disfluency do not correlate highly with the various speech or behavioral indices.

DISCUSSION

General Considerations

In the present investigation, three findings regarding subgroups of young stutterers appear particularly salient. (a) Subgroups of young stutterers could be identified based upon

TABLE 2. Pearson Product-Moment Correlations among the three behavioral indexes: (Sound Prolongation Index (SPI) = percentage of sound prolongations determined from obtained conversational sample; Behavioral Variety Index (BVI) = average number of different behaviors per stuttering; and Nonspeech Behavior Index (NBI) = the average number of nonspeech behaviors per stuttering) used to cluster (Ward's hierarchical cluster analysis) youngsters who stutter ($N = 43$) and the chronological age (Age, in months) and frequency of within-word disfluencies (Freq Dis, per 100 words of conversational speech) of these children.

	Freq Dis	NBI	BVI	SPI
Age	−.093	.110	.042	.254
Freq Dis	—	.252	.129	−.081

within-word speech disfluency type and associated speech and nonspeech behavior. (b) Regardless of how developed a young stutterer's problem appeared, every child in this investigation produced, to greater or lesser degrees, associated speech and nonspeech behaviors. (c) Neither a young stutterer's chronological age nor overall frequency of stuttering appear to be correlated with the number and variety of associated behaviors or number of sound prolongations produced. In the following section we will discuss these three results, their relationship to other investigations, and some of their clinical/theoretical implications.

Subgrouping Young Stutterers on the Basis of Behavioral Data.   The first of the three major findings was that subgroups of young stutterers could be determined based upon these youngsters' speech disfluency type and associated behaviors. As already mentioned, many previous investigations of subgroups were focused on the stutterers' characteristics (Andrews & Harris, 1964; Blood & Seider, 1981; Preus, 1981) and the exact relation of these characteristics to the problem of stuttered speech is often difficult to interpret or specify. In the present study, by using quantifiable characteristics of stutterers' stuttering, five subgroups were identified.

The issue of quantifying behavioral characteristics associated with stuttering is certainly not new (cf., Barr, 1940; Brutten, 1975; Riley, 1972, 1980). For example, Riley (1980) attempted to deal with both stuttering frequency and behaviors exhibited by stutterers in his *Stuttering Severity Instrument (SSI)*. Riley's protocol does not, however, appear to require quantification of individual behaviors produced by the young stutterer but rather the development of an overall "impression" of the number of behaviors produced. This derived impression is used to assist in developing the overall SSI score. Present findings suggest that by quantifying young stutterers' speech disfluency types and their associated behaviors, young stutterers within a specific subgroup may be more similar to each other in terms of speech disfluency type and associated behaviors than they are to other young stutterers in other subgroups. Thus, it appears that by quantifying behaviors associated with stuttering, we may begin to consider within-group similarities and between-group differences as important issues when viewing the onset and development of stuttering.

Young Stutterers Exhibit Associated Behaviors.   The second of the three major findings was that regardless of how developed a youngster's stuttering appeared, all of the young stutterers, to greater or lesser degrees, produced speech and nonspeech behaviors in association with their stuttering. Previous investigators have suggested or reported that the behaviors produced in association with stuttering are: (a) most likely exhibited only *after* the stuttering problem itself has become more advanced in its development (e.g., Brutten & Shoemaker, 1967); (b) are most likely to be produced in later stages of the development of the stuttering problem as

reactions to sound prolongations (e.g., Conture, 1982); and (c) are associated with adult stutterers' stutterings (Prins & Lohr, 1972). If, for the sake of argument, we believe reports that the early stages of stuttering are characterized primarily by sound/syllable repetitions (Bloodstein, 1981; Bluemel, 1932, Brutten & Shoemaker, 1967; Conture, 1982; Froeschels, 1921; Johnson & Associates, 1959; Van Riper, 1982; Yairi, 1983; Yairi & Lewis, 1984), then the children in Clusters 1 and 2 would seem to fit that description most closely. Interestingly, however, even children in Clusters 1 and 2, who appear to be in the earliest stages of the development of the stuttering problem, were producing *some,* albeit few, behaviors associated with their within-word disfluencies. Thus, the children in this investigation exhibited associated behaviors as did adult stutterers reported by Prins & Lohr (1972) although it is relatively safe to assume that the number and variety of associated behaviors are typically greater for the adult stutterer. Thus, it appears that from the onset, or at least near the onset of their problem, youngsters who stutter exhibit behaviors that heretofore were regarded as characterizing only more advanced or established stuttering problems.

Chronological Age and Stuttering Frequency as Indicators of the Development of Stuttering.   The third of the three findings was that a young stutterer's chronological age was not strongly correlated to the number and variety of associated behaviors or to stuttering frequency. In view of the lack of a relationship found among age, frequency of stuttering, and behaviors associated with stuttering, it may be time to reconsider the common clinical notion that changes in stuttering and associated behavior merely reflect changes in the child's chronological age. Riley and Riley 91982) have also suggested that "frequency (of stuttering) is not the most useful predictor of chronic stuttering." Perhaps a better method of approaching the development of stuttering in children would be to use the nature, number, and variety of young stutterers' speech disfluency types and their associated behaviors to determine some index of stuttering development.

Five Clusters Reduced to Two

It may be possible to consider the behavioral clusters as something other than five separate entities. As an alternative, we considered the possibility that there are only two groups of young stutterers that are differentiated by speech disfluency type and their subsequent behavioral reactions to their stuttering. Similarly, Froeschels (1943) suggested that stutterers could be divided into two groups based upon the type of speech disfluency they exhibited; that is, clonic-repetitive muscle movement versus tonic-sustained muscle contraction. Although this concept has received its share of criticism over the years (Van Riper, 1982), the notion that stutterers may be differentiated based upon the type of disfluency they most frequently exhibit, finds some support in the present investigation. At the same time, our data cannot be readily taken as lending support to Froeschels' concept of tonic versus clonic stutterers, which are in essence two seemingly exclusive and distinctly different clinical entities. Rather, we agree with Van Riper who said:

> Most of those who have conducted research with clonic and tonic stutterers have had to use the adverbial phrases "predominantly clonic" and "predominantly tonic" in defining different groups of subjects since they were unable to isolate any pure types. (p. 253)

In the present investigation, it was evident that few children exclusively produced one type of stuttering. However, if, in fact, we only have two groups of stutterers, then quantifying the most frequently occurring speech disfluency type can still provide an investigator with an objective method of grouping stutterers in a manner that could have important clinical and research implications.

Behavioral Indices and Young Stutterers' Reactions

To further assist in the differentiation of young stutterers, one may examine the Nonspeech Behavior and Behavioral Variety indices across behavioral clusters. Brutten and Shoemaker (1967) have suggested that many behaviors associated with instances of stuttered speech occur as escape and avoidance responses to the noxious stimulation associated with stuttering. Van Riper (1982, p. 122) suggested that associated behaviors "are learned and habituated reactions to the experience or fear of having repetitions and prolongations." Perhaps those children who exhibit the fewest number and variety of associated behaviors (Cluster 1 and Cluster 3) represent those youngsters who react the least behaviorally, are least aware of their stuttering, and therefore, have the greatest potential for recovering from stuttering without therapeutic intervention. On the other hand, those children who exhibit the largest number and variety of behaviors (Clusters 2, 4, & 5), may be signaling to the trained observer, a keener awareness of their stuttering as well as more frequent and varied attempts to adjust or to respond to the problem, and therefore, are more in need of direct therapeutic intervention.

Future Research and Some Cautions

Although cluster analysis procedures seem to be one ideal means of resolving heterogeneity among stutterers, various caveats should be kept in mind (for further discussion of such concerns see McKinney, Short, & Feagans, 1985; Speece, McKinney, & Applebaum, 1985). First, as mentioned previously, cluster analysis procedures are designed to produce clusters and there is no certainty that obtained clusters have any theoretical or therapeutic meaningfulness or predictability to the data under investigation. It is the investigator's task to determine whether the number and nature of obtained

clusters make sense, on any level, given the knowledge of the population and variables under consideration. Second, there is the issue of internal validation or "stability" of the clusters. This stability may be determined by using different cluster analysis procedures on the same data or randomly selecting a subsample of the original and reclustering "these subjects to determine the concordance in membership between the original and replication clusters when the sample had been altered" (McKinney, Short, & Feagans, 1985, p. 10). In the present study, the clustering procedure was employed reiteratively on the whole as well as on portions of the data corpus until the number and nature of derived clusters were consistent and interpretable given the authors' knowledge of stuttering and related behaviors in young stutterers. However, one of the better tests of internal stability, which was not possible with the present study, would require longitudinal study whereby cluster analysis was performed on different samples of the same subjects collected at different times. It is our speculation, based upon present findings, that if we had completed such a longitudinal study with our subjects, then certain subjects might have shifted cluster membership but the nature and number of clusters themselves would have remained relatively intact. Third, there is the matter of external validation that involves trying to determine whether the clusters or subtypes also differ on variables not related to those used to define the original clusters (Schwartz, 1987). Indeed, it is hoped that this third issue, external validation, will receive extensive future investigation once there is reasonable agreement among independent researchers about the number and nature of clusters or subtypes among young stutterers.

In conclusion, these findings support the notion that there are significant behavioral differences among youngsters who stutter. However, it should be noted that these findings are preliminary in nature. These findings are probably most appropriately viewed as pointing the way toward, not arriving at, a final destination in terms of our understanding of how young stutterers vary among themselves. We hope that these results will provide a touchstone to which future investigations of stuttering subgroups can be compared, expanded upon, and eventually refined.

ACKNOWLEDGMENTS

This research is based on the first author's doctoral dissertation and supported in part by NINCDS contract (NO1-N-0-2331) to Syracuse University. Special thanks is extended to Dr. John R. Gleason for his valuable statistical consultation and assistance and to Dr. John H. Saxman for his support and insights during the dissertation process. Special thanks is offered to Richard Reppert and Patricia Zebrowski who assisted in all stages of this project, Richard Molitor for his insightful editorial comments, and Drs. Sally Peterson-Falzone, Martin Adams, and Martin Young for their editorial assistance during the review process. We are especially thankful to all of the young subjects and their parents who participated in this investigation.

NOTES

1. For the purposes of this discussion, associated behaviors are those speech (e.g., phrase repetitions) and nonspeech (e.g., head movement) events associated with the production of an instance of stuttering.

REFERENCES

Adams, M. R. (1982). Fluency, nonfluency, and stuttering in children. *Journal of Fluency Disorders, 7,* 171–185.

Andreasen, N. C., Grove, W. M., & Maurer, R. (1980). Cluster analysis and the classification of depression. *British Journal of Psychiatry, 137,* 256–265.

Andrews, G., & Harris, M. (1964). *The syndrome of stuttering.* London: Spastics Society Medical Education and Information Unit in Association with Wm. Heinemann Medical Books Ltd.

Arndt, W., Shelton, R. L., Johnson, A. F., & Furr, M. L. (1977). Identification and description of homogeneous subgroups within a sample of misarticulating children, *Journal of Speech and Hearing Research, 20,* 263–292.

Barr, H. (1940). A quantitative study of the specific phenomena observed in stuttering. *Journal of Speech Disorders, 5,* 277–280.

Berlin, A. J. (1955). An exploratory attempt to isolate types of stuttering. *Speech Monographs, 22,* 196–197.

Blood, G. W., & Seider R. S. (1981). The concomitant problems of young stutterers. *Journal of Speech and Hearing Disorders, 46,* 31–33.

Bloodstein, O. (1981). *A handbook on stuttering.* Chicago: National Easter Seal Society.

Bluemel, C. S. (1932). Primary and secondary stuttering. *Quarterly Journal of Speech, 18,* 187–200.

Brutten, G. J. (1975). Stuttering: Topography, assessment, and behavior-change strategies. In J. Eisenson, (Ed.), *Stuttering: A second symposium* (pp. 199–262). New York: Harper & Row.

Brutten, E. J., & Shoemaker, D. J. (1967). *The modification of stuttering.* Englewood Cliffs, NJ: Prentice-Hall.

Clutter, M. H., & Freeman, F. J. (1984). Stuttering: The six blind men revisited. *Journal of Fluency Disorders, 9,* 89–92.

Conture, E. G. (1982). *Stuttering.* Englewood Cliffs, NJ: Prentice-Hall.

Conture, E. G., & Schwartz, H. D. (1984). Children who stutter: Diagnosis and remediation. *Communicative Disorders, 9(1),* 1–18.

Cross, D., & Luper, H. (1979). Voice reaction time of stuttering and nonstuttering children and adults. *Journal of Fluency Disorders, 4,* 59–77.

Daly, D. A. (1981). Differentiation of stuttering subgroups with Van Riper's developmental tracks: A preliminary study. *Journal of National Student Speech and Hearing Association, 9,* 89–101.

Douglass, E., & Quarrington, B. (1952). The differentiation of interiorized and exteriorized secondary stuttering. *Journal of Speech and Hearing Disorders, 17,* 377–385.

Everitt, B. S. (1981). *Cluster analysis* (2nd ed.). Exeter, NH: Heinemann Educational Books.

Froeschels, E. (1921). Beitrage zur symptomatologie des stotterns. *Monatsschr Ohrenheilk, 55,* 1109–1112.

Froeschels, E. (1943). Pathology and therapy of stuttering. *Nervous Child, 2,* 148–161.

Johnson, W. (1955). A study of onset and development of stuttering. In W. Johnson & R. R. Leutenegger (Eds.), *Stuttering in children and adults* (pp. 37–73). Minneapolis: University of Minnesota Press.

Johnson, W., & Associates (1959). *The onset of stuttering.* Minneapolis: University of Minnesota Press.

Kertesz, A., & Phipps J. B. (1977). Numerical taxonomy of aphasia. *Brain and Language, 4,* 1–10.

McKinney, J., Short, E., & Feagans, L. (1985). Academic consequences of perceptual-linguistic subtypes of learning disabled children. *Learning Disabilities Research, 1,* 6–17.

McKinney, J., & Speece D. (1985, April). *Academic consequences and longterm stability of subtypes of learning disabled children.* Paper presented at annual meeting of American Educational Research Association, Chicago.

McNutt, J. C., & Hamayan, E. (1984). Subgroups of older children with articulation disorders. In R. Daniloff (Ed.), *Articulation assessment and treatment issues* (pp. 51–70). San Diego: College-Hill Press.

Preus, A. (1981). *Identifying subgroups of stutterers.* Oslo, Norway: Universitetsforlaget.

Prins, D., & Lohr, F. (1972). Behavioral dimensions of stuttered speech. *Journal of Speech and Hearing Research, 15,* 61–71.

Riley, G. D. (1972). A stuttering severity instrument for children and adults. *Journal of Speech and Hearing Disorders, 37,* 314–321.

Riley, G. D. (1980). *Stuttering severity instrument: For children and adults.* Tigand, OR: C.C. Publishing.

Riley, G. D., & Riley, J. R. (1979). A component model for diagnosing and treating children who stutter. *Journal of Fluency Disorders, 4,* 279–293.

Riley, G. D., & Riley, J. R. (1982). Evaluating stuttering problems in children. In H. L. Luper (Ed.), (Special issue) *Intervention with the young stutterer* (pp. 15–25). *Journal of Childhood Communicative Disorders, 6.*

Romesburg, H. C. (1984). *Cluster analysis for researchers.* Belmont, CA: Lifetime Learning Publications.

St. Onge, K. R. (1963). The stuttering syndrome. *Journal of Speech and Hearing Research, 6,* 195–197.

St. Onge, K. R., & Calvert, J. J. (1964). Stuttering research. *Quarterly Journal of Speech, 50,* 159–165.

SAS Institute (1982). *SAS users guide: Statistics.* Cary, NC.

Schwartz, H. D. (1987). Subgrouping young stutterers: A physiological perspective. In H. F. M. Peters & W. Hulstijn (Eds.), *Speech motor dynamics in stuttering.* (pp. 212–228). Wien: Springer-Verlag.

Seber, G. (1981). *Multivariate observations.* New York: John Wiley.

Speece, D., McKinney, J., & Applebaum, M. (1985). Classification of behavioral subtypes of learning-disabled children. *Journal of Educational Psychology, 77,* 67–77.

Stocker, B. (1976). *The Stocker probe technique manual.* Tulsa, OK: Modern Education.

Van Riper, C. (1982). *The nature of stuttering* (2nd ed). Englewood Cliffs, NJ: Prentice-Hall.

Yairi, E. (1972). Disfluency rates and patterns of stutterers and nonstutterers. *Journal of Communication Disorders, 5,* 225–231.

Yairi, E. (1983). The onset of stuttering in two- and three-year-old children: A preliminary report. *Journal of Speech and Hearing Disorders, 48,* 171–178.

Yairi, E., & Lewis, B. (1984). Disfluencies at the onset of stuttering. *Journal of Speech and Hearing Research, 27,* 154–159.

APPENDIX

A description of the 14 behavioral events obtained through frame-by-frame audio/video observation of stutterings exhibited by 43 young stutterers. For the purposes of this study, these behaviors have been defined as either nonspeech or speech associated behaviors.

Associated Nonspeech Behavior

1. Eyelid Open & Close
   Visually perceived downward and upward movement of both eyelids from the open to closed to open position was recorded as one event. Incomplete eyelid closure (eyeball still visible) with subsequent opening of eye was recorded as one event.

2. Eyeball Lateral & Vertical Movement
   Visually perceived movement of both eyeballs from their initial gaze position to a new horizontal or vertical position was recorded as one event.

3. Head Movement
   Visually perceived movement of the head from its initially viewed position to a second position, for example, tilted backward, forward, to the side or turned from its initial position was recorded as one event.

4. Limb Movement
   Visually perceived movement of one or both of the subject's arms, legs, or combination of arm and leg together, during production of a stuttering was recorded as one event.

5. Torso Movement
   Visually perceived movement of the subject's torso from its initially viewed position to a second position where it was leaned or twisted laterally, or moved up and down vertically, was recorded as one event.

Associated Speech Behaviors

6. Whole-Word Repetition (WWR)
   Audible perception of a whole-word repetition immediately prior to, during, or immediately following the production of a stuttering (for example, "—T Tom Tom Tom went. . ."). In this case the subject began by producing an inaudible sound prolongation and then produced two whole-word repetitions before fluently producing "Tom went." For this subject two WWR were recorded.

7. Phrase Repetition
   Audible perception of a phrase repetition immediately prior to, during, or immediately following the production of a stuttering (for example, "IIII, I have to, I have to, I have to go now.") For this subject an audible sound prolongation was followed by two phrase repetitions that are followed by the fluent production of the sentence. Two phrase repetitions would be recorded for this subject.

8. Interjection
   Audible perception of an interjection immediately prior to, during, or immediately following the production of a stuttering (for example, "y-y-y ah yesterday"). In this example the subject produced a sound/syllable repetition of the "y" in yesterday and then included an interjection before fluently producing "yesterday." For this subject one interjection was recorded.

9. Revision
   Audible perception of a revision immediately prior to, during, or immediately following the production of a stuttering (for example, "I have ttt(o) . . . I went home.") In this example the subject prolonged the "t" sound in attempts to produce the word "to." The subject then revised the word and produces a new phrase "I went home." One revision was recorded in this example.

10. Audible Inhalation
    Auditory perception of an inhalation immediately prior to, during, or immediately following the production of a stuttering.

11. Audible Exhalation
    Auditory perception of an exhalation immediately prior to, during, or immediately following the production of a stuttering.

12. Vocal Intensity Changes
    Auditory perceptible changes in the subject's loudness/intensity during, or immediately following the production of a stuttering.

13. Lip Movement
    Visible perception of movement of one or both lips (for example, protruding or retracting) in ways not integral to the production of the specific sound, syllable, or monosyllabic whole-word being examined.

14. Other Speech/Nonspeech Behavior
For some subjects, specific, unique, behaviors were produced (for example, tongue clicks). These behaviors were categorized as speech or nonspeech and recorded.

No Observable Behaviors

If no speech or nonspeech behaviors are perceptible during the production of a stuttering, the stuttering was categorized as containing no behavior.

CHAPTER 2 ADDITIONAL READINGS

Adams, M. R. (1987). Voice onsets and segment durations of normal speakers and beginning stutterers. *Journal of Fluency Disorders, 12,* 133–139.

Anderson, J.M., Hood, S. B., & Sellers, D. E. (1988). Central auditory processing abilities of adolescent and preadolescent stuttering and nonstuttering children. *Journal of Fluency Disorders, 13,* 199–214.

Blood, G. W. (1985). Laterality differences in child stutterers: Heterogeneity, severity levels, and statistical treatments. *Journal of Speech and Hearing Disorders, 50,* 66–72.

Blood, G. W., & Blood, I. M. (1984). Central auditory function in young stutterers. *Perceptual and Motor Skills, 59,* 699–705.

Blood, G. W., Blood, I. M., & Hood, S. B. (1987). The development of ear preferences in stuttering and nonstuttering children: A longitudinal study. *Journal of Fluency Disorders, 12,* 119–131.

Bloodstein, O., & Grossman, M. (1981). Early stutterings: Some aspects of their form and distribution. *Journal of Speech and Hearing Research, 24,* 298–302.

Brutten, G. J., & Trotter, A. C. (1986). A dual-task investigation of young stutterers and nonstutterers. *Journal of Fluency Disorders, 11,* 275–284.

Caruso, A. J., Conture, E. G., & Colton, R. H. (1988). Selected temporal parameters of coordination associated with stuttering in children. *Journal of Fluency Disorders, 13,* 57–82.

Colcord, R. D., & Gregory, H. H. (1987). Perceptual analyses of stuttering and nonstuttering children's fluent speech productions. *Journal of Fluency Disorders, 12,* 185–195.

Cullinan, W. L., & Springer, M. T. (1980). Voice initiation and termination times in stuttering and nonstuttering children. *Journal of Speech and Hearing Research, 23,* 344–360.

Dejoy, D. A., & Gregory, H.H. (1985). The relationship between age and frequency of disfluency in preschool children. *Journal of Fluency Disorders, 10,* 107–122.

Devore, J. E., Nandur, M. S., & Manning, W. H. (1984). Projective drawings and children who stutter. *Journal of Fluency Disorders, 9,* 217–226.

Gordon, P. A., Luper, H. L., & Peterson, H. A. (1986). The effects of syntactic complexity on the occurrence of disfluencies in 5-year-old nonstutterers. *Journal of Fluency Disorders, 11,* 151–164.

Homzie, M. J., & Lindsay, J. S. (1984). Language and the young stutterer: A new look at old theories and findings. *Brain and Language, 22,* 232–252.

Horsley, I. A., & Fitzgibbon, C. T. (1987). Stuttering children: Investigation of a stereotype. *British Journal of Disorders of Communication, 22,* 19–35.

Krikorian, C. M., & Runyan, C. M. (1983). A perceptual comparison: Stuttering and nonstuttering children's nonstuttered speech. *Journal of Fluency Disorders, 8,* 283–290.

Langlois A., Hanrahan, L. L., & Inouye, L. L. (1986). A comparison of interactions between stuttering children, nonstuttering children, and their mothers. *Journal of Fluency Disorders, 11,* 263–273.

Long, K. M., & Pindzola, R. H. (1985). Manual reaction time to linguistic stimuli in child stutterers and nonstutterers. *Journal of Fluency Disorders, 10,* 143–149.

McKnight, R. C., & Cullinan, W. L. (1987). Subgroups of stuttering children: Speech and voice reaction times, segmental durations, and naming latencies. *Journal of Fluency Disorders, 12,* 217–222.

Merits-Patterson, R., & Reed, C. G. (1981). Disfluencies in the speech of language-delayed children. *Journal of Speech and Hearing Research, 24,* 55–58.

Meyers, S. C. (1986). Qualitative and quantitative differences and patterns of variability in disfluencies emitted by preschool stutterers and nonstutterers during dyadic conversations. *Journal of Fluency Disorders, 11,* 293–306.

Meyers, S. C., & Freeman, F. J. (1985). Are mothers of stutterers different? An investigation of social-communicative interaction. *Journal of Fluency Disorders, 10,* 193–209.

Meyers, S. C., & Freeman, F. J. (1985). Mother and child speech rates as a variable in stuttering and disfluency. *Journal of Speech and Hearing Research, 28,* 436–444.

Meyers, S. C., & Freeman F. J. (1985). Interruptions as a variable in stuttering and disfluency. *Journal of Speech and Hearing Research, 28,* 428–435.

Palen C., & Peterson, J. M. (1982). Word frequency and children's stuttering: The relationship to sentence structure. *Journal of Fluency Disorders, 7,* 55–62.

Pitluk, N. (1982). Aspects of the expressive language of cluttering and stuttering school children. *South African Journal of Communication Disorders, 29,* 77–84.

Riley, G., & Riley, J. (1980). Motoric and linguistic variables among children who stutter: A factor analysis. *Journal of Speech and Hearing Disorders, 45,* 504–513.

Riley, G., & Riley, J. (1986). Oral motor discoordination among children who stutter. *Journal of Fluency Disorders, 11,* 335–344.

Riley, G., & Riley, J. (1988). Looking at a vulnerable system. *Asha, 30,* 32–33.

Stocker, B., & Gerstman, L. J. (1983). A comparison of the probe technique and conventional therapy for young stutterers. *Journal of Fluency Disorders, 8,* 331–340.

St. Louis, K. O., Hinzman, A. R., & Hull, F. M. (1985). Studies of cluttering: Disfluency and language measures in young possible clutterers and stutterers. *Journal of Fluency Disorders, 10,* 151–172.

Till, J. A., Reich, A., Dickey, S., & Seiber, J. (1983). Phonatory and manual reaction times of stuttering and nonstuttering children. *Journal of Speech and Hearing Research, 26,* 171–180.

Wall, M. J. (1980). A comparison of syntax in young stutterers and nonstutterers. *Journal of Fluency Disorders, 5,* 345–352.

Wall, M. J., & Myers, F. L. (1982). A review of linguistic factors associated with early childhood stuttering. *Journal of Communication Disorders, 15,* 441–449.

Westby, C. E. (1979). Language performance of stuttering and nonstuttering children. *Journal of Communication Disorders, 12,* 133–145.

Winkler, L. E., & Ramig, P. (1986). Temporal characteristics in the fluent speech of child stutterers and nonstutterers. *Journal of Fluency Disorders, 11,* 217–230.

Yovetich, W. S. (1984). Message therapy: Language approach to stuttering with children. *Journal of Fluency Disorders, 9,* 11–20.

Zebrowski, P. M., Conture, E. G., & Cudahy, E. A. (1985). Acoustic analysis of young stutterers' fluency: Preliminary observations. *Journal of Fluency Disorders, 10,* 173–192.

CHAPTER THREE

The Physiology of Stuttering

In the past two decades there has been a renewed interest and a number of empirical investigations in the physiology of stuttering. A major portion of this line of research has focused on comparisons of stutterers' and nonstutterers' fluency and stuttering as measured by speech acoustic, physiological, aerodynamic, and neurophysiologic techniques. The articles in this chapter provide the reader with a sample of research that has been conducted in this area. A list of readings has been provided at the end of this chapter for those who would like to pursue a more in-depth study of the physiology of stuttering.

Historically, researchers have been interested and intrigued by the notion that stuttering results from some form of physiological anomaly. In the early years of the twentieth century, Lee Travis was instrumental in initiating some of the first research on the physiology of stuttering. He is most remembered for his contributions to the field in the development of the cerebral dominance theory of stuttering with Orton (Wingate, 1986). Briefly, the cerebral dominance theory proposed that stutterers lacked the necessary dominant hemisphere for the execution and processing of neural information to the peripheral speech musculature. If one of the cerebral hemispheres failed to become sufficiently dominant over the other, then each hemisphere would tend to act independently. As a consequence, the bilateral musculature of the speech mechanism would be poorly coordinated and a predisposition to stutter would result (Bloodstein, 1987). Although this concept of stuttering had enormous appeal at that time in history, subsequent research showed that the concepts underlying the theory could not be supported.

In the mid-1930s, the physiological orientation to stuttering was beginning to wane in favor of a psychological frame of reference. The shift away from a physiological research emphasis toward a psychological one was due primarily to the development of dynamic psychology by Sigmund Freud and an increased focus on behaviorism (Wingate, 1986). In fact, for about the next 40 years, research interest in stutterers' physiological behaviors lay dormant. However, around 1970, researchers became disenchanted with the psychological and behavioral research in stuttering and a major shift back to the study of stutterers' speech physiology began to emerge. With the advent of modern scientific equipment and refined investigative techniques, some of the first studies conducted in stutterers' speech physiology addressed the issue of laterality differences between stutterers and nonstutterers. A related body of research was devoted to issues of stutterers' speech-timing abilities and neurolinguistic processing abilities (Wingate, 1986).

One impelling force that increased researchers' interest in stutterers' speech physiology was the publication of two articles by Wingate (1969, 1970). In these articles, Wingate critically reviewed the research on various fluency-inducing conditions such as singing, choral recitation, speaking rhythmically, and speaking in the presence of a delayed auditory feedback unit (DAF). He proposed that there was a common theme that would account for the increased fluency that a stutterer experienced under these conditions. Wingate hypothesized that stutterers used their voices in more efficient ways while speaking under these fluency-inducing conditions than when speaking normally. These changes in vocalization were thought to be associated with improvements in the functioning of a stutterers' laryngeal behavior during these novel speech patterns. Thus, it was speculated that a relationship existed between stutterers' fluency and changes in their laryngeal physiology. If this were the case, others hypothesized that disruptions in a stutterers' phonatory behavior might be associated with other perceptually fluent moments that stutterers produced during an utterance.

Direct evidence for aberrant laryngeal activity in stuttering has been provided by Freeman and Ushijima (1978), Freeman (1984), and Shapiro (1980). Through the use of electromyographic techniques, these investigators showed that stutterers' laryngeal muscle activity during episodes of stuttering was characterized by increased levels of the abductory and adductory muscles of the larynx. A co-contraction of these abductory and adductory muscles was directly associated with a stuttering moment. Additionally, it was reported that instances of stutterers' perceptibly fluent responses were found to have heightened levels of laryngeal muscle activity. These findings suggested that stutterers might experience a discoordination of laryngeal behavior during both stuttered and some "fluent" moments.

Research from indirect studies of stutterers' phonatory behavior during fluency has also been reported. Numerous studies have shown that stutterers exhibit slower voice reaction times (Cross, Shadden, and Luper, 1979; Reich, Till, & Goldsmith, 1981), slower voice onset, initiation, and termination times (Adams & Hayden, 1976; Hillman & Gilbert, 1977; Starkweather, Hirschman, & Tannenbaum, 1976) than do nonstutterers. However, there are studies in this area that have revealed few, if any, differences between stutterers' and nonstutterers' vocal behavior during fluency (for example, Healey & Gutkin, 1984; Metz, Conture, & Caruso, 1979; Watson & Alfonso, 1982). Also, recall from the Introduction of Chapter 2 that the results of studies involving acoustic measures of young stutterers' fluent phonatory behaviors have produced equivocal results. The reasons for these equivocal findings are not clear. Perhaps it relates to how "fluency" is defined and identified in a segment of speech. The review article by Finn and Ingham in this chapter provides a comprehensive look at the research that has been conducted on stutterer's "fluent" speech. This article also offers some direction for those interested in pursuing this line of research.

Another contemporary research trend has been the study of performance differences between stutterers and nonstutterers with regard to parts of the speech mechanism other than the larynx. For example, direct measurements of coordination of the articulators were assessed by Zimmermann and Hanley (1983) using cinefluorography. In this article, it was found that stutterers made improvements in the dynamics of articulatory control during repeated fluent productions of the same linguistic material. In an article by Baken, McManus, and Cavallo (1983), the possibility is presented that the delays in voicing onset frequently found in stutterers may be reflected in abnormal patterns in the prephonatory posturing of the respiratory system. Although they found no significant differences in general disorganization of speech-breathing movements between stutterers and nonstutterers, there was a difference between the groups with regard to the manner in which lung volume changed during laryngeal closure prior to phonation. The results of this study supported the notion that stutterers have disrupted phonatory rather than respiratory movement patterns.

One other study that investigated the interaction of respiratory and phonatory activity during stutterers' fluent speech responses is the article by Peters and Boves, which is included in this chapter. These researchers discovered that stutterers produced both deviant patterns of subglottal pressure buildup and glottal waveform tracings during some fluent utterances. These findings suggest that stutterers' perceptually fluent utterances are different from those of nonstutterers.

Another aspect of examining stutterers' perceptually fluent speech involves an analysis of fluent responses that are surrounded by instances of stuttering and those that are surrounded by other fluent utterances. In 1981, Adams and Runyan pointed out that the phonetic environment from which the measurements of stutterers' fluency are taken could help differentiate between the speech-production abilities of stutterers and nonstutterers. A recent test of this notion in terms of relative speech-timing differences between stutterers and nonstutterers was conducted by Prosek, Montgomery, and Walden. As can be seen in this article, Prosek and colleagues found that the articulatory control exhibited by stutterers and nonstutterers during fluency was not different in spite of changes in speech rate and episodes of stuttering surrounding an utterance. Thus, these authors concluded that measures of stutterers' relative speech timing may be one factor that remains intact in order for a stutterer to produce a fluent response. However, as is known, acoustic measures of stutterers' speech behavior are indirect indicators of their underlying physiological patterns. Therefore, as Prosek and colleagues indicate, a measure such as relative timing should be measured in conjunction with other direct, physiological data in order for us to obtain a better understanding of the motor control of stutterers.

One other area of research involving the physiology of stuttering is associated with the neurolinguistic organizational differences between stutterers and nonstutterers. As stated at the beginning of this Introduction, there was a rebirth of interest in stutterers' hemispheric processing of linguistic information in the early 1970s. In this chapter, the article by Rastatter and Dell provides a brief review of the research in this area. This article is also informative in that it shows that both of a stutterer's cerebral hemispheres compete with each other when decoding linguistic information. In some stutterers, it could be hypothesized that the left hemisphere fails to assume control of the processing of linguistic functions as it does for nonstutterers.

The findings from the Rastatter and Dell study also show that this hemispheric processing difference is associated with all levels of stuttering severity. Therefore, these data, along with numerous other studies in this area, suggest that stutterers' inappropriate hemispheric processing of linguistic messages is a common finding and one worthy of continued research.

REFERENCES

Adams, M.R., & Hayden, P. (1976). The ability of stutterers and nonstutterers to initiate and terminate phonation during production of an isolated vowel. *Journal of Speech and Hearing Research, 23*, 457–469.

Adams, M.R., & Runyan, C.M. (1981). Stuttering and fluency: Exclusive events or points on a continuum? *Journal of Fluency Disorders, 6*, 197–218.

Baken, R., McManus, D., & Cavallo, S. (1983). Prephonatory chest wall posturing in stutterers. *Journal of Speech and Hearing Research, 26*, 444–450.

Bloodstein, O. (1987). *A handbook on stuttering.* 4th ed. Chicago: National Easter Seal Society.

Cross, D.E., Shadden, B.B., & Luper, H.L. (1979). Effects of stimulus ear presentation on the voice reaction time of adult stutterers and nonstutterers. *Journal of Fluency Disorders, 4*, 45–58.

Freeman, F. (1984). Laryngeal muscle activity of stutterers. In R. Curlee & W. Perkins (Eds.), *Nature and treatment of stuttering.* San Diego: College-Hill Press.

Freeman, F., & Ushijima, T. (1978). Laryngeal activity during stuttering. *Journal of Speech and Hearing Research, 21*, 538–562.

Healey, E.C., & Gutkin, B. (1984). Analysis of stutterers' voice onset times and fundamental frequency contours during fluency. *Journal of Speech and Hearing Research, 27*, 219–225.

Hillman, R., & Gilbert, H. (1977). Voice onset time for voiceless stop consonants in the fluent reading of stutterers and nonstutterers. *Journal of the Acoustical Society of America, 61*, 610–611.

Metz, D., Conture, E., & Caruso, A. (1979). Voice onset time, frication, and aspiration durations: A comparison of stutterers and nonstutterers. *Journal of Speech and Hearing Research, 22*, 649–656.

Reich, A., Till, J., & Goldsmith, H. (1981). Laryngeal and manual reaction times of stuttering and nonstuttering adults. *Journal of Speech and Hearing Research, 24*, 192–196.

Shapiro, A. (1980). An electromyographic analysis of the fluent and disfluent utterances of several types of stutterers. *Journal of Fluency Disorders, 5,* 203–232.

Starkweather, W., Hirschman, P., & Tannenbaum, R. (1976). Latency of vocalization onset: Stutterers versus nonstutterers. *Journal of Speech and Hearing Research, 19,* 481–492.

Watson, B., & Alfonso, P. (1982). A comparison of LRT and VOT values between stutterers and nonstutterers. *Journal of Fluency Disorders, 7,* 219–242.

Wingate, M. (1969). Sound and pattern in "artificial" fluency. *Journal of Speech and Hearing Research, 12,* 677–686.

Wingate, M. (1970). Effects on stuttering of changes in audition. *Journal of Speech and Hearing Research, 13,* 861–873.

Wingate, M. (1986). Physiological and genetic factors. In G. Shames & H. Rubin (Eds.), *Stuttering then and now.* Columbus, OH: Charles E. Merrill.

Zimmermann, G., & Hanley, J. (1983). A cinefluorographic investigation of repeated fluent productions of stutterers in an adaptation procedure. *Journal of Speech and Hearing Research, 26,* 35–42.

The Selection of "Fluent" Samples in Research on Stuttering: Conceptual and Methodological Considerations

Patrick Finn
Roger J. Ingham

During the past decade a substantial and growing body of research has been directed toward evaluating the characteristics of stutterers' speech that is free of stuttering and/or specified disfluencies. Investigations into this aspect of stutterers' speech have been conducted from various perspectives. Some descriptors for these perspectives, along with some studies that fit those descriptors are as follows: acoustic properties (cf. Borden, Baer, & Kenney, 1985; Healey & Gutkin, 1984; Starkweather & Myers, 1979); temporal characteristics (cf. Adams & Hayden, 1976; Murphy & Baumgartner, 1981; Reich, Till, & Goldsmith, 1981); perceived quality (cf. Colcord & Gregory, 1987; Ingham & Packman, 1978; Krikorian & Runyan, 1983); characteristics during novel stimulation or "fluency-inducing" conditions (cf. Andrews, Howie, Dozsa, & Guitar, 1982; Ingham & Packman, 1979; Ramig, Krieger, & Adams, 1982); and characteristics after treatment (cf. Metz, Samar, & Sacco, 1983; Runyan & Adams, 1978, 1979; Shenker & Finn, 1985). The findings of these studies, which have tended to suggest that the stutter-free and/or disfluency-free speech of stutterers contains unusual characteristics, have also made substantial contributions to many recent propositions concerning the nature of stuttering and the effects of its treatment (see Adams, 1985; Bloodstein, 1987; Curlee & Perkins, 1984; Ingham, 1984, in press). Of equal concern has been the meaning of these findings with respect to stutterers' "fluency." Martin Adams, for example, who has been a prominent researcher in this area, recently concluded that "the greatest weight of evidence provides that stutterers' fluency is significantly different from the matched fluent utterances of normal persons" (Adams, 1985, p. 185). In fact, much of this evidence led him to state that it is tempting to conclude that "the speech production abilities of stutterers are inher-

ently inferior to those of normal persons" (Adams, 1985, p. 186). In regard to treatment, Adams and Runyan (1981) in an earlier review of this research recommended that the

. . . scrutiny of stutterers' fluency is neither academic nor a trivial enterprise. Rather, it is encouraged because that fluency is likely to be flawed, . . . This means, of course, that clinically we must direct our therapeutic intervention not just toward a patient's stuttering, but toward . . . fluency as well (Adams & Runyan, 1981, p. 210).

In the midst of this interest in the so-called fluency of stutterers it is noteworthy that research in this area has proceeded with surprisingly little concern about the definitive or distinguishing features of fluency. Indeed, much of this research has been conducted with the assumption that the absence of stuttering is equivalent to fluency. From one perspective, that assumption should not be surprising, because so few studies have investigated the concept of fluency or attempted to determine whether stutter-free or even disfluency-free speech can also be described as fluent speech. But stutter-free or disfluency-free speech and fluent speech are not necessarily identical and the blurring of this distinction may distort any conclusions drawn from recent studies in this area. That distortion may be even more serious when these studies ignore the obvious differences between speech that is stutter-free and speech that is normally fluent, or the possible difference between "fluent" and "normally fluent" speech. It is somewhat ironic to find that these issues have received little consideration in research concerning a disorder that changes so readily when the speaker uses nonnormal sounding speech.

It is the purpose of this paper to review the concept of fluency and consider the ways in which it has been employed in investigations on the speech of stutterers. In addition, factors will be highlighted that need to be recognized when considering the inferences about stutterers' stutter-free speech that have been made on the basis of many of these

Reprinted from *Journal of Speech and Hearing Research*, 32, no. 2, 401–418. Copyright © 1989, American Speech-Language-Hearing Association.

investigations. The concern about this issue is increasingly important in view of the growing theoretical and clinical significance of this research.

THE CONCEPT OF FLUENCY

Like the concept of stuttering, fluency appears to be an easily understood concept, but one that also resists a straightforward and unambiguous definition. Seemingly, "fluency" refers to certain meaningful and recognizable features of behavior, though it is far from clear that those features can be specified. Adams (1982), for instance, made the following observations regarding "fluency":

> Undoubtedly, all of us have "in our heads," a good idea of what fluency looks and sounds like. That is to say, we can recognize fluency when we see and hear it. But what audible and visible features of the speech act tell us that an individual's utterances are being produced fluently? (1982, pp. 171–172).

However, the concept of fluency alluded to in Adams's quotation actually incorporates some reasons why "fluency" has been hard to define. This is because the meanings that are attached to the term extend far beyond the production of utterances. For instance, Perkins (1971) has suggested that fluency should be viewed as a "barometer for the entire speech system, the limits of which are set by the adequacy of performance of the semantic, syntactic, morphemic, and prosodic dimensions of speech" (Perkins, 1971, p. 92). Others addressing this topic have found it necessary to add even more parameters to this list in order to adequately describe their concept of fluency (Dalton & Hardcastle, 1977; Leeson, 1975; Starkweather, 1987). It is difficult to categorize these parameters, but in general they appear to refer to either speech and/or language behavior. This may also partly explain why it has been difficult to specify the meaning and essential features of fluency.

A completely different orientation to the concept of fluency has been proposed by Hegde (1978) following his review of approaches to the definition, measurement, and modification of fluency. He concluded that fluency is best identified as a response unit "that is devoid of disfluencies, silent prolongations, and silent pauses" (1978, p. 59). This negative definition of fluency—relying as it does on the absence of unspecified disfluencies—appears to have been adopted in one form or another by many researchers. This definition probably refers only to speech behavior, but it is not clear that it necessarily identifies speech that listeners would agree is fluent. It is even less clear that it refers to normally fluent speech.

Webster's Dictionary (1975) defines "fluent" as "flowing; having words at one's command and uttering them with facility and smoothness; voluble" (1975, p. 376). If this respected guide to the meaning and use of English has any validity then this definition should capture the features that most listeners would use when they identify fluent speech or a fluent speaker. In other words, whatever parameters are involved in speaking fluently, they probably cause listeners to judge fluent speech as "flowing" and having "smoothness." But Webster's reference to "having words at one's command" probably refers to language as much as speech. This was also recognized by Starkweather (1984) in reviewing the concept of fluency with respect to stuttering. He suggested that speakers are also labeled fluent if they are able to find words and formulate sentences, presumably readily and easily.

It is reasonably obvious that most recent investigations into stutterers' stutter-free speech have directed their attention to speech fluency rather than language fluency. However, it is entirely possible that language factors may contribute variables that could influence listeners' judgments about stutter-free speech quality. This may be particularly important, for instance, if the samples of spontaneous speech are from a stutterer who is practicing word avoidance, one of the distinguishing features of stuttering (Bloodstein, 1987). Word avoidance by stutterers has not been systematically investigated (Ingham, 1984). Nevertheless, it is generally accepted that skillful word avoidance may produce speech that is free of stuttering, even fluent (Bloodstein, 1987). It seems unlikely, though, that listeners would judge a speaker who uses an awkward, even nonmeaningful, language structure (presumably to avoid stuttering) as a fluent speaker. In all likelihood, therefore, the distinguishing features of such speech would reside at the level of language rather than speech.

Fillmore (1979) is one of very few who have explored the concept of language fluency. He suggests that there are actually four types of language fluency. The first type is the ability to speak at length without having to stop many times to think of what to say or how to say it. Fillmore considers that radio disc jockeys or sports announcers exemplify this type of fluent speaker. A second type of fluency is characterized by the speaker who displays a wide variety of syntactic structures and a wide breadth and depth of meaning. The commentator William Buckley is considered to typify this type of speaker (Fillmore). The third type of fluency is represented by the speaker who is readily able to say whatever is appropriate to a situation or setting. Starkweather (1984) suggests this type of fluency could be called pragmatic fluency. The final kind of fluency is represented by the ability to demonstrate novel and creative language skills through the use of devices such as puns, jokes, and metaphors.

Fillmore (1979) has presented a very broad notion of language fluency; so broad, in fact, that Hieke (1985) has argued that it is not sufficiently restrictive to be useful. Starkweather (1984) notes, however, that Fillmore's linguistic representation of fluency does have the advantage of separating language from motor-based notions of fluency. In regard to stuttering, Starkweather (1984) has also argued that "stuttering is probably not a disorder of language fluency" (Starkweather, 1984, p. 35). That may be true; it is rarely considered to be a distinguishing feature of the disorder (Bloodstein, 1987). Nevertheless, it is entirely possible that this type of fluency is relevant when assessing or depicting certain features of stutterers' stutter-free speech. Indeed, as was mentioned earlier, it is the poor quality of this type of fluency that could be most obvious when stutterers convolute their language in order to avoid expected moments of stuttering.

Several writers suggest that prosody is another parameter of fluency (Crystal, 1971; Dalton & Hardcastle, 1977; Perkins, 1971). Crystal describes the features of this dimension as normal variation in pausing and tempo, pitch range, loudness, rhythm, and intonational patterns. Interestingly, Crystal goes on to suggest that experimental validation of these variables should be tried by presenting "a piece of language to judges, systematically varying certain features of it, and noting variations in terms of fluency (or some synonym)" (p. 51). From informal attempts to do this, Crystal reports that the "avoidance" or restriction of pitch-range, loudness, and rhythmical variation did influence listeners' fluency judgments. It may also be relevant that Perkins (1973) found that listeners' ratings of the fluency of treated stutterers were also positively correlated with their ratings of prosody.

Another dimension of language fluency described in the literature is phonologic fluency (Starkweather, 1984). Leeson (1975) suggests that this type of fluency is characterized by speakers with adequate articulatory precision at normal rates of speech production. Starkweather (1984) suggests that speakers who demonstrate creative use of sounds of the language are displaying this type of fluency as well. This dimension of fluency has not been investigated for its contribution to judgments of fluency, but it is difficult to imagine that a speaker with phonologic deficiencies or difficulties would also be judged normally fluent.

The concept of fluency in the context of stuttering research is generally associated with speech fluency rather than with language fluency. Starkweather (1987) defines speech fluency as "the ability to talk with normal levels of continuity, rate, and effort" (Starkweather, 1987, p. 12). To elaborate on this, he states that a fluent speaker is someone who produces "normally long strings of sounds at a normally rapid rate without pausing or hesitation, and with a normal absence of effort" (Starkweather, 1987, p. 12). There are many problems in stipulating the dimensions of normal rate or effort and then inferring that when they occur speech will be fluent, but these problems multiply when the dimensions are not well defined.

This seems to be the case when Starkweather (1987, chap. 2) argues that a number of findings reported in the psycholinguistic and acoustic analysis literature show that continuity, rate, effort, and perhaps, rhythm are the critical variables that constitute speech fluency. The evidence cited in support of his argument, though, is not entirely satisfactory because the subjects in the cited studies were never judged to be normally fluent speakers. Whenever subject descriptions were provided in these studies the subjects were variously reported to have "normal speech" (Brown & Brandt, 1971; McClean, 1973; Prosek & House, 1975;

Subtelny, Worth, & Sakuda, 1966), to be "native speakers of English" (Gay, Ushijima, Hirose, & Cooper, 1974; Oller, 1973), "speakers of General American Dialect" (Malecot, 1968), to be "free of speech or hearing defects" (Amerman, Daniloff, & Moll, 1970; Grosjean & Collins, 1979; Weismer & Ingrisano, 1979), or have no "peculiarity in pronunciation" (Umeda, 1977). Of course it is likely that most of these subjects did display normally fluent speech. The fact remains, however, that it is yet to be established that these descriptors apply equally to "normally fluent" speech; even "normal speech" could embrace different levels (and types) of fluency (or disfluency). Furthermore, there is no evidence in any of the studies that the speech quality descriptors were independently assessed for their reliability.

Speech fluency has also been described in terms of speech physiology. Thus, Adams (1982) has argued that a fluent utterance starts "promptly and easily" and is "characterized throughout, by the coordination of respiratory, phonatory, and articulatory activity as the speaker moves sequentially from sound to sound and syllable to syllable in a continuous, forward-flowing manner" (p. 174). This account of a fluently produced utterance may describe some of the principal activities associated with such an utterance. But it has yet to be established that the sequential coordination of these activities necessarily results in speech that listeners will always judge to be fluent. It is quite conceivable, for example, that a speaker may produce (promptly and easily) interjections (for example, "like, uh, this, uh, and um, well, um"), yet still have continuous and coordinated speech movements. It is improbable, however, that such a speaker would be described as producing fluent speech—a point also acknowledged by Adams (1982)—though in some instances it might be described as "normally fluent speech."

It is well known that "normally fluent speech" is not free of disfluencies. Such disfluencies, as Wingate (1984; 1987) has pointed out, are usually considered benign, though some may not be easily distinguished from stutterings (Curlee, 1981; MacDonald & Martin, 1973). In any event, there may be substantial differences between speech that is literally fluent—free of disfluency—and speech that is normally fluent. Clearly, many semantic problems, even assessment problems, in this area would diminish if the term "fluent speech" was reserved for speech that is (at the very least) disfluency-free, and the oxymoron "normally fluent speech" was replaced by "normal sounding speech." In the meantime it is clear that there may be fundamental differences between judgments of fluency and normal fluency.

DIMENSIONS OF SPEECH FLUENCY

Two general points appear to have emerged from this overview of concepts of fluency. The first is that fluency appears to be a multidimensional concept; a speaker may be judged as fluent on the basis of performance in quite different and even independent domains. This also suggests that if researchers intend to investigate fluency they should clarify the type of fluency they are investigating. The second point is that there is little evidence that any suggested dimension of fluency has been carefully investigated to establish what contribution it makes to listener-judged normal fluency. Interestingly, the limited amount of research that might address this issue has been conducted on treated stutterers.

As mentioned earlier, Perkins (1973) reported a significant correlation between listeners' judgments of fluency using a 4-point rating scale and their judgments of prosody in the speech of treated stutterers. Perkins (1973) also found a positive relationship between listeners' judgments of fluency and independent measures of speech rate. Positive correlations between listener judgments of fluency and speech rate measures were also reported by Ingham and Packman (1978) in their study on the spontaneous speech of treated stutterers. Harrold and Murdoch (1986), however, failed to obtain significant correlations between their listeners' judgments of fluency and either speech rate or prosody using similar speech samples from treated stutterers.

On the whole, these studies do not provide much help in the search for the constituents of fluency. On the one hand, their findings cannot be easily compared because the subjects used different modes of speech: that is, either monologue or conversational speech. And on the other hand, the 4-point scale used to judge fluency in these studies not only had a restricted range, but it may not have allowed judges freedom to assess fluency independently of stuttering.

To the best of our knowledge, there are virtually no published reports of investigations into the constituents of listener-judged, normally fluent speech. The one possible exception is a study by O'Connell and Kowal (1984), which found positive correlations between (a) listener ratings of fluency in samples taken from native (English) and second language (German) poetry readings and (b) independent measures of phrase length and articulation rate, plus ratings of expressiveness. They also found a significant negative correlation between fluency judgments and a measure of pause duration. In this study, incidentally, the raters evaluated the speakers on a scale from 1 through 5 (*very poor, poor, average, good, very good*), both for expressiveness and for fluency; the reliability of these ratings was not reported. O'Connell and Kowal's findings are of interest, but it would be important to know that the relationships they found apply to more customary speech as well as to poetry recitations.

Without question, further research is needed to identify the contributions that the various hypothesized components make to the concept of fluency. There is a need to investigate the effects of manipulating some of these dimensions (for example, prosody, speech rate, and pause frequency) by observing their separate or interactive effects on listeners' ratings of speech fluency. Until the possibility of an objective definition of fluency is realized, the identification of reliable and valid samples of "fluent speech" will continue to rest on listeners' judgments. In fact, the identification of normal fluency may always rely on listener judgments because

objective measures will probably refer only to speech fluency rather than to speech *and* language fluency.

The search for a valid and objective measure of speech or language fluency may prove to be more problematic than the search for a valid and objective measure of stuttering. Indeed, some obvious parallels exist between the difficulties that face both endeavors. Most problems related to identifying stuttering seem to stem from the difficulties in specifying speech characteristics that unambiguously describe the disorder. Research has shown that defining stuttering in terms of specified behaviors has not been altogether successful, largely because stuttering cannot be identified reliably by referring to disfluency descriptors (Bloodstein, 1987; Young, 1984). Furthermore, the types of speech disfluencies that have been related to stuttering (Johnson & Associates, 1959; Wingate, 1964)—and some that are not—have both qualitative (Huffman & Perkins, 1974) and quantitative (DeJoy & Jordan, 1988; Hegde & Hartman, 1979a; 1979b) characteristics that appear to cause listeners to decide that a speaker is stuttering.

It should not be surprising, therefore, that stuttering is sometimes identified more reliably on the basis of perceptual judgments by listeners (Martin & Haroldson, 1981) rather than on the basis of specified behaviors that some claim define stuttering (Wingate, 1964). That perceptual judgments of stuttering may also be valid judgments is captured by Bloodstein's (1987) conclusion that stuttering is "whatever is perceived as stuttering by a reliable observer who has relatively good agreement with others" (Bloodstein, 1987, pp. 9–10). That statement might apply equally to the search for the definitive features of fluency. Any attempt to identify or define speech fluency, for instance, by reference to variables that correlate with speech fluency ratings may only yield information about speech rate, pausing, or prosody—variables that may be necessary, but not sufficient descriptors of speech fluency.

Meanwhile, it appears that listener judgments will continue to be essential when determining whether speech samples are fluent or normally fluent with respect to speech or language. In turn this means that investigators must control for the many variables that may threaten the reliability and validity of measures that derive from observer judgments or ratings. It is of interest, therefore, to consider how this has been managed or controlled during studies that have investigated stutterers' fluent speech. The methods used to identify fluent speech in these studies are reviewed below.

PROCEDURES USED TO IDENTIFY A FLUENT UTTERANCE OR SPEECH SAMPLE IN STUTTERING RESEARCH

The studies selected for this review are those published in journals that have investigated either stutter-free speech samples or nonstuttered utterances from stutterers. In many cases, these samples and utterances are also purported to be disfluency-free. Most of these studies also claim to have investigated fluent speech samples or utterances. As indicated earlier, these studies extend over a broad area of published research, largely concerning voice onset time, vocal reaction time, judgments of listeners, effects of "fluency-inducing" conditions, and effects of treatment. The studies that were reviewed (N=110) are listed in the Summary Table. Each study was examined and coded according to the criteria that were used to identify a stutter-free and/or disfluency-free event (see below) and whether these criteria were accompanied by reliability procedures.

The studies under review here fall into two broad categories with respect to their methodologies. One category includes studies where a stutterer's "fluent" utterance (for example, an isolated phoneme such as an extended /a/, or a nonsense syllable, or a word) is used either alone or is compared with a nonstutterer's fluent utterance, mainly to measure voice reaction time. The other category includes studies where presumably stutter-free and/or disfluency-free samples from stutterers are compared with "matched" samples from nonstutterers in order to test whether differences occur within stutterer-nonstutterer sample pairs or between groups of samples from both types of speakers. In either group of studies the claim is made that the stutterer's and/or nonstutterer's utterance or speech sample is fluent (see for examples, Adams, 1987; Borden, 1983; Colcord & Gregory, 1987; Conture, Rothenberg, & Molitor, 1986; Hillman & Gilbert, 1977; Metz, Conture, & Caruso, 1979; Prosek, Montgomery, Walden, & Hawkins, 1987; Runyan & Adams, 1978; Shapiro, 1980; Zimmermann, 1980).

In some instances it becomes perfectly obvious that the so-called fluent sample or utterance is, at best, stutter-free and not necessarily normal sounding or normally fluent. For example, when stutterers' speech samples have been obtained under some fluency-inducing conditions, such as 250-msec delayed auditory feedback, listeners rate these samples as significantly more unnatural sounding than nonstutterers' speech samples (Martin, Haroldson, & Triden, 1984). The point that such fluent samples may not sound normal is rarely made explicit in these studies. Often the only test for fluency is a check that the utterance or the sample does not contain stutterings or disfluencies—although even this check occurs with surprising infrequency. Some studies, however, carry a compelling inference in their purpose and methodology that their samples are both stutter-free *and* normally fluent. This is most evident in studies that use normal speakers' samples as a control or point of comparison. In these studies it is assumed that the nonstutterers' speech is the referential standard for either fluency or normally fluent speech. If that were not the case then it would be difficult to understand why samples from nonstutterers were employed.

The most frequently reported method for identifying a "fluent" utterance or speech sample from a stutterer has involved two components. In the first, the researcher speci-

fies the guideline that was followed when identifying the "fluent" speech segment or sample. The segment or sample is identified by reference to a behavioral or a perceptual definition of fluency, or to a behavioral or perceptual definition of disfluency (nonfluency), dysfluency, or stuttering. The second component is the medium used to assess the speech segment or sample. That medium has been either audio-only or audiovisual monitoring and/or recording of the subject's speech. There is, however, considerable variety among methods that are then used to establish that the segment or sample is "fluent," particularly the extent to which these methods make it possible to judge that the segment or sample is *normally fluent*. These matters will become clearer in our later review of these procedures.

The reference to the identification of nonfluencies and dysfluencies among the guidelines mentioned above highlights yet another semantic problem in this area that some authorities, most notably Wingate (1984), have attempted to correct. It is reasonably clear that whenever "nonfluency" is used in any of the studies reviewed here it is a synonym for "disfluency." Fortunately, time and usage seem to be giving preference to disfluency over nonfluency. However, the current prominence of neurophysiological concepts of stuttering appears to have revived the use of the term "dysfluent," presumably to describe stuttering (e.g., Watson & Alfonso, 1982; 1983), though occasionally it is used as a descriptor for nonstuttered disfluencies (e.g., Huffman & Perkins, 1974). As Wingate (1984) has argued, the prefix "dys-" means "abnormal" and for that reason dysfluency should be reserved for abnormal disfluencies. Among the studies reviewed here it is obvious that dysfluency is a synonym for stuttering, although there is no evidence that judgments of stuttering and dysfluency are indistinguishable. On balance, it seems that only confusion is fostered by the continuing use of the term dysfluency, rather than stuttering, unless it is meant to describe abnormal disfluencies that are not necessarily stutterings.

Establishing Guidelines for Identifying a Fluent Segment of Speech

The absence of a generally agreed-upon method of identifying fluency is perhaps the most striking feature of the studies reviewed here. Most researchers simply assume the presence of either fluency or normal fluency by claiming that there was either no stuttering or no disfluency in their target behavior. Some researchers have developed a definition of fluency (e.g., Meyers & Freeman, 1985a), but most have followed the more heavily traveled route of indirectly identifying fluency as the absence of stuttering or disfluency. Of the 93 studies that reported using a guideline for identifying fluency, 71 virtually defined fluency as the absence of stuttering or disfluency (see Summary Table).

It is patently misleading to assume that the absence of stuttering or disfluency means that the resulting behavior must be fluent speech, however it might be defined. In the most extreme circumstance the resulting behavior could be silence, whispering, or singing—behaviors that are rarely, if ever, related to the term fluent speech, or even fluency. For this reason it is important for those who identify fluency essentially by default to establish that (a) stuttering and/or disfluencies were reliably identified, and (b) the resulting behavior is at least related to fluent or normally fluent speech. These issues are most pertinent to studies that use a "fluent (or normally fluent)-by-default" method as their guideline, but they apply equally to all other studies in this area.

The method used to identify the stutterings or disfluencies that have been excluded from samples may give some indication whether those samples contain speech that could be judged as fluent or perhaps normally fluent. One determining factor is whether behavioral or perceptual criteria were used to identify stutterings or disfluencies. When behavioral criteria have been used in the studies reviewed here (regardless of whether it was to identify stutterings or disfluencies) then they were usually confined to specified disfluencies (usually syllable repetitions, prolongations, broken words, or hesitations).

For the purpose of this review, a definition was coded as "behavioral" when the researcher(s) stated explicitly the speech characteristics (e.g., sound repetitions, prolongations, and blocks) that were employed to identify the sample of interest (see Summary Table). A definition was coded as "perceptual" when specific speech characteristics were not prescribed in judging whether a sample was stuttered, disfluent, or fluent. In this case it was assumed that stuttering, disfluency, or fluency was identified on the basis of a listener's judgment. The procedures used to categorize these studies in the Summary Table involved independent assessments by the first and second authors. When disagreements occurred they were either resolved by a subsequent rereading of the study or the category label was marked "not clear."

The use of a behavioral definition means that, at best, the sample did not include specified disfluencies, though it might include nonspecified disfluencies (Wingate, 1987). Consequently, it is unlikely that a methodology that relies on a behavioral definition would procure samples that were literally fluent. Even if a speech sample was free of all disfluencies, however, that does not mean it was normal sounding. The sample might also include nonnormal-sounding prosody or rate characteristics that might cause listeners to judge the speech as not *normally* fluent. Indeed, that is entirely possible because when some investigators have selected samples from stutterers that are presumed to be free of all disfluencies, listeners have been able to distinguish those samples from samples produced by speakers presumed to have normal fluency (Runyan & Adams, 1978; 1979; Runyan, Hames, & Prosek, 1982).

When experimenters use samples that omit perceptually judged stutterings (e.g., Ingham, Gow, & Costello, 1985; Ingham & Packman, 1978) there is an even stronger possibility that the stutter-free sample is not fluent. Listeners to such samples might be expected to hear a sprinkling of nonstuttered disfluencies which, of course, could vary in their frequency. Hence, any differences between these samples and similar samples from nonstutterers might be due to differences in the frequency of nonstuttered disfluencies in the samples from both groups. Because many reviewed studies failed to control for frequency of nonstuttered disfluencies when comparing stutterers' and nonstutterers' samples, any differences between these samples may be confounded by this variable.

One solution to a part of the problem mentioned above is to use criteria for choosing speech samples that are stutter-free, and/or disfluency-free, and other criteria for ensuring that the sample is also fluent. Examples of this approach occur in studies reported by Meyers and Freeman (1985a) and Healey and Ramig (1986). Meyers and Freeman (1985a) accompanied their behavioral definition of stuttering with a definition of a fluent word. Such words, they claimed, should involve a "continuous flow of phonation without disruption or hesitant speech" (Meyers & Freeman, 1985a, p. 429). This definition of a fluent word may be confusing because it appears to suggest that voiceless speech sounds cannot occur in fluent utterances.[1] Healey and Ramig, on the other hand, appear to have favored a perceptually based definition of fluency and a behavioral-based definition of disfluency. They defined fluency as speech that was "perceived as 'normal sounding' as well as motorically and linguistically fluent" (p. 326). This definition seems to carry more face validity than that used by Meyers and Freeman (1985a). A closer examination of both of these studies, however, reveals that the fluent intervals were probably identified through the absence of certain features, rather than the presence of normal-sounding fluency. It is yet to be established that either of these approaches will identify speech samples that listeners judge to be normally fluent.

Some researchers have sought fluent samples or utterances by ensuring that they do not contain variables that are supposed to be either incompatible with fluency or part of stuttering. Thus, Ramig, Krieger, and Adams (1982) consider fluent speech to be free of "unusual accent or timing, incorrect stress or breaks and other irregularities judged to be incompatible with fluency" (p. 372). It is not clear what the "other irregularities" are or whether the variables they list are actually incompatible with speech that is judged to be fluent. This is an even more pertinent issue in the methods reported by Borden, Baer, and Kenney (1985), where they suggest that fluent speech should be free of "abnormal fluctuations in laryngeal impedance" (p. 365) via electroglottograph signals, and Zimmermann (1980), who stipulated that fluent utterances should not include "descriptively aberrant movement patterns" (p. 197). The difficulty with all these descriptors is that there is no evidence that these features are always absent in samples or utterances that are judged to be fluent.

It should be clear by now that researchers cannot be certain which guidelines listeners might use when requested to judge whether a speech sample is "fluent." Those guidelines may be quite diverse, categorically and qualitatively. On the other hand, to date, no study has shown that listeners actually use guidelines specified by experimenters to identify fluent samples or segments. It almost goes without saying, therefore, that research is needed to determine (a) the effect of instructions to assess the fluency of language or speech and (b) whether "fluent" and "normally fluent" evoke different or similar listener responses. It is also unclear whether such instructions yield perceptually and/or acoustically different speech samples.

Among the few studies where stutter-free samples or utterances were judged for fluency (rather than absence of stuttering or disfluencies) there are indications that guidelines were needed to control listener judgments. Virtually all of these studies were concerned with samples no larger than a word, and so elaborate guidelines were probably unnecessary. Nevertheless, among the studies that did investigate judged fluent words or syllables (see Summary Table) there are indicators that the judges were required to focus on phonologic variables. Thus some investigations of the fluent words of young stutterers (Adams, 1987; Conture et al., 1986; Winkler & Ramig, 1986) required that their utterances should be "correctly articulated" as well as perceptually fluent. Actually Adams (1987) also required that the fluent utterance should have "grammatically correct form" and "appropriate pattern of stress." Unfortunately, none of the guidelines employed by Adams were assessed for reliability.

Some studies report that perceptual judgments of a fluent word or syllable were used in conjunction with guidelines to ensure the exclusion of stuttering or disfluency. For example, Klich and May (1982) excluded "perceived stuttering behaviors" whereas Conture et al. (1986) eliminated "within or between-word disfluency." More demanding criteria for the selection of fluent samples were used by Shapiro (1980), who required four listeners, the subject, and the experimenter to agree that a token was "fluent" or "dysfluent." At the same time it is not entirely clear that a fluent token was merely a token that listeners judged to be free of "dysfluency."[2] This would not exclude unusual or nonnormal sounding stutter-free tokens. In fact the only study that reports an attempt to control for this possibility was conducted by Di Simoni (1974). He only used stutter-free multisyllables (/isi/,/isa/) that were also judged to be "natural sounding." Unhappily, the reliability of these judgments was not reported.

The complex issues surrounding judgments of fluency are made even more complex by the size of speech segments that listeners are required to judge. For instance, when experimenters seek "fluent" utterances that are as small as a single vowel or syllable (McFarlane & Shipley, 1981; Reich, Till, & Goldsmith, 1981; Starkweather, Franklin, & Smigo, 1984; Starkweather, Hirschman, & Tannenbaum, 1976; Zimmermann, 1980) the speech fluency criteria that listeners use in their judgments must be very limited. With the qualified exception of Di Simoni's (1974) study there is every indication that the only criterion that judges could use

reliably was the presence or absence of evident disfluency. In these studies it appears to make more sense to label these utterances as stutter-free or disfluency-free rather than "fluent." That is especially true if "fluent" also infers normalcy. It would suggest that these utterances would be produced in the same way during normally fluent speech—a proposition that needs additional verification.

Finally, this review (see Summary Table) identified many studies that used single "fluent" utterances from stutterers, but these studies did not report guidelines for identifying these segments. The majority of these investigations were concerned with measuring stutterers' voice initiation or vocal reaction times. Most of these studies measured the time interval between an external stimulus and the initiation of voicing. It emerges that it is actually necessary to assume that these investigations were concerned with non-stuttered or fluent initiation of voicing because so few confirmed that this was always the case (see for example, Adams & Hayden, 1976). If the initiation of voicing did occur in conjunction with stuttering, or even a disfluent response, then this would place a very different construction on the findings of these studies. It is fair to add, however, that some recent studies have carefully documented that their procedure included confirmation that these utterances were stutter-free. A recent study by Cross and Olson (1987a), for example, provides an illustration of procedural controls that should prevent this confounding.

Medium of Assessment

One interesting feature of the research on stutterers' stutter-free speech is that it is not always clear why the medium used to evaluate that speech was from audio-only or audiovisual recordings. The present paper found that, among the 110 studies reviewed, 59 reported making judgments of fluency on the basis of audio-only information and 22 used both audio and visual information (see Summary Table). Nine out of 110 reports indicated that audio information was used, but it was not clear whether visual information was also used. Finally, there were 20 out of these 110 studies that failed to make clear which medium of assessment was used.

The medium of assessment has considerable importance because not all stuttering events can be identified on the basis of auditory information alone. A number of studies have compared audio and audiovisual assessments of stutterers and shown that judges may identify more stutterings when they have access to both visual and auditory information (Luper, 1956; Coyle & Mallard, 1979; Seymour, Ruggerio, & McEneaney, 1983). It is conceivable, for example, that visually evident stuttering could occur at junctures where normal pauses are either expected or presumed to have occurred. This type of error may be especially problematic for fine-grained acoustic analyses conducted on supposedly stutter-free or disfluency-free samples (see Hillman & Gilbert, 1977; Howell & Vause, 1986; Love & Jeffress, 1971; Zebrowski, Conture, & Cudahy, 1985). Consequently, where investigators have relied on audio-only measures, nonaudible but visible stuttering may have had an influence on their findings. The impact of this factor on conclusions drawn from audio-only studies cannot be too substantial if the findings have been replicated in studies using audiovisual measures. However, this is not true for some areas of this research. For instance, the findings of no differences between audio assessed stutter-free and/or disfluency-free speech samples from stuttering and nonstuttering children (Colcord & Gregory, 1987; Krikorian & Runyan, 1983) have yet to be replicated in studies using audiovisual data.

The differential effects of audio and audiovisual assessment may also turn out to have important implications if judges are instructed to evaluate a sample for fluency rather than for absence of stutterings. At present, the visual components of fluency remain unknown. Nevertheless, it is conceivable that the dimension of "ease," and perhaps of "flow," might have visual correlates that could influence observer judgments of fluency. Whatever the case, it is an aspect of fluency that warrants investigation.

Establishing the Reliability of Fluent Speech Identification Procedures

A crucial step in establishing viable guidelines for selecting stutter-free, disfluency-free or fluent samples in a stutterer's speech is to determine the reliability with which these guidelines are used by the same or different judges. Without this fundamental step it is impossible to be sure that independent judges would select similar speech samples or that the procedures for doing so are in any way replicable.

The present review found that only 54 percent of the published studies listed in the Summary Table reported a procedure for establishing the reliability of the guidelines that their observers used to judge if a sample was stutter-free or disfluency-free. Among those studies that did report reliability, interjudge reliability was reported more frequently than intrajudge reliability (see Summary Table). But for both types of reliability, measures were made more often on judgments of disfluencies or stutterings than on judgments of fluency. That is, the independent judge was asked to assess the presence (or absence) of disfluencies or stutterings but not of fluency. As mentioned above, these appear to be quite different tasks, which may be performed with quite different levels of reliability.

Among the studies included in the Summary Table, six assessed the reliability of both stuttering and fluency judgments (Colcord & Adams, 1979; Healey & Ramig, 1986; Manning, Trutna, & Shaw, 1976; Meyers & Freeman, 1985a; Shapiro, 1980; Zimmerman & Hanley, 1983). There were three studies that reported interjudge reliability on fluency judgments only (Conture et al., 1986; Janssen, Wienke, & Vaane, 1983; Zimmermann, 1980). Finally, there was one study (Robb, Lybolt, & Price, 1985) that reported both intrajudge and interjudge reliability, again on

fluency judgments only. One potential advantage of employing fluency judgments only as a sample selection criterion is that it probably excludes disfluencies that some might judge to be stutterings. That advantage may be lost where the identification of a stutter-free speech sample was based on interjudge agreement that no stuttering occurred in the sample.

Many studies have shown that listeners or observers have considerable difficulty achieving total agreement on point-by-point judgments of stuttering (see Young, 1984). It would be surprising, therefore, if the judges, in studies reviewed here did not have the same difficulties. There is, in fact, some evidence that suggests that this was the case. For example, Metz, Samar, and Sacco (1983) could only report a .50 interclass agreement coefficient between judges for certain stutterings ("broken words"), whereas Samar, Metz, and Sacco (1986) achieved a .88 coefficient for the same agreement index on the same category of stutterings. These coefficients show quite clearly that the judges in these studies could not always agree that a sample was stutter-free. This is even more evident in a study by Hillman and Gilbert (1977), who acknowledged that up to "10% of the judges" in their study could have regarded so-called fluent productions, of /p, t, k/ as not fluent. Given the uncertainty with which judges identify instances of stuttering it seems strange that these researchers would not reduce that uncertainty as much as possible by ensuring that their target utterances were judged unanimously to be stutter-free and/or disfluency-free.

A similar problem is evident in some studies that employed fluency-only judgments. For example, Robb et al. (1985) reported percent agreement on fluency word counts of 89 percent and between 75 percent and 92 percent for interjudge and intrajudge reliability respectively. Similarly, Meyers and Freeman (1985a) reported 99 percent agreement (range: 97–99%) on interjudge reliability of fluent and disfluent word counts. Thus, it appears that some words analyzed in these studies were not unambiguously judged by listeners to be fluent.

Other Methodological Considerations

There are other methodological issues related to the identification of stuttering that have received some consideration by researchers, though there is little agreement on their resolution. These include the relationship of the stutter-free sample to occurrences of stuttering, and the subject's role in judging a sample to be stutter-free or even fluent.

Based on an earlier proposal by Williams (1957), Adams and Runyan (1981) suggested that stuttering and fluency might be viewed as "events along a continuum," and that "as speech flows forward there is a drift, sometimes gradual, sometimes rapid, toward stuttering" (p. 205). For this reason they suggested that "the closer a speaker comes to that overt stuttering event, the more abnormal the speech produced" (p. 205). Presumably this means that nonstuttered utterances immediately adjacent to stutterings are likely to be "contaminated" by stuttering. Given the problem of identifying instances of stuttering reliably, that problem would seem to be magnified if this notion requires the experimenter to establish the point separating stuttering and nonstuttering in a speech sample. Even if that were possible, it is not at all clear where a nonstuttered speech segment should be located in order to avoid contamination by stuttering. These reservations notwithstanding, there would seem to be some justification for ensuring that stutter-free samples do not abut judged stutterings, if only because of the uncertain accuracy of stuttering judgments.

Some investigators (10% of the reports included in the Summary Table) have taken this precautionary step. Not surprisingly, Adams and his colleagues have advocated and employed this sample selection control (see, for examples, Prosek & Runyan, 1982; Ramig, Krieger, & Adams, 1982; Runyan & Adams, 1978, 1979), but they have not been alone (see also, Mallard & Westbrook, 1985; Pindzola, 1986; Wendahl & Cole, 1961). The size of the "buffer zone" between a stuttering event and a sample in these studies ranged from single words (e.g., Ramig, Krieger, & Adams) to as many as four words either side of the sample (e.g., Mallard & Westbrook, Runyan & Adams, 1978; 1979). Shapiro (1980) reported a more rigorous criterion for establishing the size of this "buffer zone." Instead of a linguistic or speech production criterion, he used a time interval in which the fluent utterance was not analyzed if it occurred within 10 sec of a stuttering. The advantage of this criterion is that it can be standardized across subjects, whereas speech-related criteria are subject to variations caused by speaking rate.

The importance of the relationship of instances of stuttering to stutter-free sampling is yet to be demonstrated. There is, as yet, no convincing evidence that the perceptual or acoustic quality of stutter-free speech is influenced by the proximity of moments of stuttering.[3] Even more surprising is the total absence of evidence that variations in the frequency of stuttering, within or between subjects, affect the perceptual or acoustic quality of stutter-free speech. If Adams and Runyan's (1981) contention is true (i.e., abnormal speech is more evident closer to stuttering) then stuttering frequency should influence the quality of stutter-free speech.

A recent proposal by Perkins (1983) presents another consideration in the search for procedures that should be used to identify either a stutter-free or a normally fluent speech sample. Perkins (1983) suggests that stuttering is the result of a temporary and involuntary loss of speech control, an experience that is available only to the stutterer. It is largely for this reason that he contends that the stutterer's judgment of loss of control is the only valid indicator of a moment of stuttering—a contention that Siegel (1987) has suggested is probably better described as a hypothesis at present.

Perkins's proposal has two interesting implications for identifying stutter-free speech samples. The first is that the stutterer's judgments might have additional importance in determining whether a speech sample is fluent. That is a debatable point, though, considering Martin and Harold-

son's (1986) finding that listeners' stuttering counts and stutterers' loss of control counts do not show meaningful differences across repeated oral readings by stutterers. More importantly, their findings were supplemented by descriptions of events that appeared to be almost textbook examples of stuttering, yet their stutterers failed to judge these as events associated with loss of control.

The second implication of Perkins's proposal may be an intriguing extension of his "definition": is it possible that when stutterers, or indeed nonstutterers, speak fluently they also experience an exceptional sense of control over their manner of speech production? It is often suggested that when stutterers speak fluently, especially after therapy, they do so with excessive levels of "control" over their speech (Bloodstein, 1987; Ingham, 1984, chap. 10). In this instance it would seem that an exceptional "sense of control" over speech would be inconsistent with normal fluency. And it may be quite incompatible with the notion that fluent speech is characterized by "ease" or "lack of effort" (Starkweather, 1987).

The major problem with Perkins's definition is the seemingly impossible task of establishing the reliability with which stutterers make loss of control judgments. However, this difficulty should not justify researchers ignoring information from subjects about their speech performance. It is most unlikely that any researcher would find it satisfactory to analyze listener-judged, stutter-free speech that a stutterer had judged to contain stuttering. Probably the safest method for selecting stutter-free samples would be one that ensures that the subject's and the experimenter's judgments on the sample are in agreement. It remains to be seen whether stutterers' judgments of loss of speech control are also important to the sample selection procedure.

Very few studies (11%) reviewed here have included the subject's self-judgment of either stuttering or fluency in their sample selection procedure (see Summary Table). It is hoped that this will become more commonplace in the future. At the same time, it is worth noting that this procedure may require additional research in order to assess its reactive effects. It is entirely possible, for example, that when stutterers are alerted to the experimenter's interest in fluency, this may be sufficient to induce atypical speech.[4] That problem could be solved to some extent by collecting information about the subject's judgments of fluency after the subject's speech has been sampled.

TOWARD THE ASSESSMENT OF FLUENCY

It is not clear what implications flow from the imprecise specification of "fluent" among studies on stutterers' stutter-free speech. This may not be considerable in the case of brief utterances, such as a vowel or word; but that might not be true when stutter-free speech samples (perhaps sentence length or longer) are employed. The pattern of results among studies using longer samples suggests that adult and adolescent stutterers' speech is perceptually and acoustically different from nonstutterers' speech. On the other hand, this difference does not seem to be as evident among samples taken from stuttering and nonstuttering children (Adams, 1985). What is suggested by the studies that have used adult and adolescent stutterers is that their "fluency" is characterized by unusual and distinguishing features.

Thus far, we have learned very little about the nature of these distinguishing features. The listeners in Colcord and Gregory's (1987) study did describe some features that they used to identify the stutter-free speech of 4–9-year-old stutterers, but these features also occurred among samples that the listeners identified incorrectly. Prosek and Runyan (1982, 1983) found that when pauses and rate in stutterers' samples were modified to match those found in nonstutterers' speech, listeners could not distinguish between the samples from both groups. This is consistent with the findings reported by Love and Jeffress (1971), and suggests that pauses and rate may be the distinguishing variables. On the other hand, Prosek and Runyan used only phrase length samples so the variables that listeners could use to distinguish between them were severely restricted. What is not clear is the level of fluency that existed in the nonstutterers' samples; that may be a powerful reason why listeners were able to distinguish between the two samples. This could occur because the nonstutterers' speech was judged to be either exceptionally fluent or perhaps not as fluent as the stutterers' speech. This may be important in trying to explain why the stutter-free speech of children is not distinctive. As Krikorian and Runyan (1983) point out, judges in these studies "may use a standard of fluency that tolerates deviations from and differences in speech production to a greater degree than they would when listening to more mature subjects" (p. 288).[5]

It becomes quite clear that many attempts to identify the sources of difference between the speech of nonstutterers and the stutter-free and/or disfluency-free speech of stutterers may depend on whether the quality of fluency in nonstutterers' speech can be adequately described or measured. The extent to which speech or language fluency can be quantified reliably by listeners is the starting point for any worthwhile discussion about differences between the quality of fluency in stutterers' and nonstutterers' speech. Unfortunately, no study has addressed either this issue or whether listeners do distinguish between the different types of fluency mentioned earlier in this paper. In some respects, these issues are accentuated by recent studies showing that listeners are able to rate speech naturalness with satisfactory levels of inter- and intrajudge reliability (Onslow & Ingham, 1987). The concept of speech naturalness appears to be related to speech and/or language fluency, though that is yet to be established. It will certainly be interesting to learn whether the semantic differences between these labels refer to real differences in speech quality.

One of the few scales for quantifying levels of fluency reported in the stuttering literature comes from treatment outcome valuation studies.[6] Perkins (1973; also reported in Perkins, Rudas, Johnson, Michael, & Curlee, 1974) used a 4-point fluency scale that specified 1 = *severe stuttering or stammering*, 2 = *mild stuttering and stammering*, 3 = *fluent with normal hesitations*, and 4 = *exceptionally fluent* speech. The scale was used by college undergraduates to rate 1-min speech samples from treated stutterers (n=24) and "normal" speakers (n=12). The interjudge reliability of ratings in this scale (by groups of 3–5 listeners) was 0.88, which did suggest that the form of fluency referred to in this scale can be rated with reasonable reliability. This scale has also been used with comparable interjudge reliability in other studies.

Ingham and Packman (1978) presented to a group of undergraduate students eighteen 1-min samples of audio-taped conversational speech of nine treated stutterers and nine "normally fluent" speakers. The percentage agreement for the intragroup judgment reliability on the fluency scale described by Perkins (1973) was 85.0 percent. Even higher levels of agreement have been achieved in studies that have used experienced listeners. Harrold and Murdoch (1986), who also used Perkins's 4-point scale, asked four trained speech-language pathologists to rate 1-min audiotaped samples from monologues given by 10 posttreatment (Mean = 21 months) stutterers and 10 nonstutterers. The percentage self-agreement of ratings (or intragroup reliability) of these listeners was 91.7 percent. Finally, Goldsmith and Anderson (1984) used this scale with five "unsophisticated judges" who watched and heard unspecified length videotaped recordings of "spontaneous speech" of three "successfully therapeutized" stutterers and three normal speakers. The percentage of agreement between their judges' ratings was 90 percent.

These studies strongly suggest that fluency can be reliably rated by different types of judges who are presented with audio or audiovisual samples from various speaking contexts. One obvious drawback to Perkins's (1973) fluency scale, however, is that three of the items refer to stuttering or disfluency, which means that speech which is free of hesitations is, perhaps, exceptionally fluent speech according to this scale. To avoid this suggestion, listeners need to be able to rate fluency within that domain alone; a suitable rating scale for this purpose might be one that runs from "non-normal fluency" to either "normal" or perhaps "exceptional fluency." Another drawback to Perkins's scale is that its 4-point range, when compared with a 7- or 9-point scale range, might restrict the judges' opportunity to discriminate among different levels of fluency.

Findings from investigations of stutterers' speech naturalness via a rating scale provide some useful indications that stutter-free speech quality can be assessed reliably using a 9-point naturalness scale, where 1 represents *highly natural sounding speech* and 9 represents *highly unnatural sounding speech*. Martin, Haroldson, and Triden (1984) demonstrated that relatively unsophisticated listeners could use this scale to rate speech naturalness reliably. Listeners rated audio recordings of 1-min spontaneous speech samples from 10 stutterers, 10 normal speakers, and 10 stutterers speaking under the influence of delayed auditory feedback. Thus, the last two groups provided virtually stutter-free samples. The judges in this study proved to be in fairly good agreement (allowing plus or minus one scale unit difference) with each other (75%) on their ratings of naturalness and in very good agreement with themselves (88%) on their reratings of the same samples 1–3 weeks later. Comparable levels of listener reliability using this 9-point scale have been shown in subsequent studies investigating the speech naturalness of treated stutterers and normal speakers (Ingham, Gow, & Costello, 1985; Ingham, Martin, Haroldson, Onslow, & Leney, 1985).

Other findings from these speech naturalness studies have interesting implications for rating levels of fluency. Among the findings presented by Martin et al. (1984) was the intriguing evidence that a small percentage (4%) of the stutterers' samples were judged as highly natural sounding (scores of 1–2), even though the samples contained some stutterings. It seems difficult to believe that speech fluency and speech naturalness are entirely independent dimensions, but these data would suggest that this may be the case. Thus, it appears that judging a segment of speech to be highly natural does not necessarily mean it is fluent. To some extent that distinction is also evident in Ingham, Gow, and Costello's (1985) finding that some listeners gave ratings of 9 (highly unnatural sounding speech) to a nonstutterer who was considered to be a normally fluent speaker. Similarly, Martin et al.'s (1984) findings also revealed that a small percentage of nonstutterers were judged as somewhat unnatural sounding (scale values of 4–5). These findings suggest that some nonstutterers who are ostensibly normally fluent speakers may also sound unnatural to listeners. The implications of these findings for judgments of fluency are not entirely clear, but they do suggest that ratings of fluency are probably not the same as ratings of speech naturalness.

There are some rather obvious reasons why a reliable scale for rating fluency, especially different types of fluency, could be very useful. It would establish that these different types of fluency can be quantified and thereby provide a basis for more meaningful evaluations of stutter-free samples of fluent speech from stutterers. Thus, we would learn the effects of differing levels and types of fluency on the variables that are reported to characterize stutterers' stutter-free speech (for example, pauses and prosody). Such a scale would also permit more meaningful comparisons between speech samples from stutterers and nonstutterers. These are ripe areas for research.

SUMMARY AND CONCLUSIONS

The overall purpose of this paper was to review the concept of fluency and the application of this concept to recent investigations of the fluent speech of stutterers. It is clear that

researchers have given little consideration to the different meanings that apply to the term "fluent" and the extent to which variations in these meanings may influence the conclusions that can be drawn from investigations of stutterers' fluent speech. It is evident that fluency is a multidimensional concept encompassing at least two broad dimensions: speech fluency and language fluency. It is also clear that there are essential differences between "fluent" and "normally fluent" speech, differences that may also apply to language. In any event, these differences have not been systematically investigated and it is not at all clear what the term "fluent" refers to in view of these differences. In the absence of an adequate definition of fluency or specific types of fluency it is evident that listeners' judgments are essential to determine whether a speech sample or utterance is fluent. In turn, this means that there should be adequate controls to ensure that these judgments are reliable and valid.

This review showed that the most common method used to select a fluent sample is based on a negative definition of fluency, that is, the absence of stuttering or certain types of disfluencies. In fact, 76 percent (71/93) of the reviewed studies that reported the use of any kind of guideline employed a negative definition of fluency. However, this approach does not logically lead to a "fluent" sample of speech, nor indeed to a "normally fluent" sample of speech. In addition, this approach requires adequate controls to ensure that stuttering and/or disfluency can be reliably identified. Two important considerations are the definition of stuttering and/or disfluency that was used and the medium for determining the presence or absence of stuttering (i.e., audio vs. audiovisual). It would seem that, at minimum, a researcher needs to demonstrate that the sample of speech remaining after employing an "absence of stuttering" or "absence of disfluency" definition is also in some way "fluent" and, more to the point, "normally fluent." Of the studies reporting guidelines, only 13 percent (12/93) used an additional procedure that attempted to ensure such a sample was also "fluent." Of the remaining studies that reported guidelines, 11 percent (10/93) used "fluency" as the only sample selection procedure. No study included a procedure to determine whether the fluent sample was also normal sounding speech.

Whatever methodology is employed to identify a "fluent" speech sample, reliability judgments are essential when human observers are asked to make judgments. Only 54 percent (50/93) of those studies reporting any type of guiding criterion also reported any form of reliability on these guidelines. An additional judgment criterion that would appear to aid content validity is the stutterer's judgment that the sample was stutter-free or even fluent. Only 11 percent (12/110) of the studies reported using the stutterer's judgment as to whether a sample was free of stuttering or disfluency.

A final point to emerge from this review is that there has been little evident interest in establishing the level of fluency (however it is defined) of nonstutterers' speech. The development of a reliable and valid method for quantifying fluency would be extremely useful in addressing this concern as well as some of the issues mentioned above.

On the basis of this review, there appear to be some suitable guidelines that researchers should employ when identifying segments of stutterers' speech that are either stutter-free and/or disfluency-free or fluent. First, a generally agreed-upon procedure for identifying either a stutter-free or disfluency-free speech sample is sorely needed. That procedure should be suitable for reliable use by independent listeners. Second, the most appropriate medium for assessing stutter-free samples is audiovisual recordings. Third, in some cases the surrounding context of the stutter-free segment should be examined for the possible influence of stuttering. Fourth, the experimenter's judgment that the sample is stutter-free needs to be verified by independent listeners and, where appropriate, by the stutterer.

Bloodstein (1987) has stated that "we can define stuttering in any way that we agree on, but the question of whether anything is 'really' stuttering or 'really' fluency is unanswerable" (p. 31). The heart of Bloodstein's statement may well be true, but we will never know for certain if we do not examine more carefully the methodologies that are used to select fluent speech samples from stutterers. The tools of science in this area are relatively modest ones but if they are used rigorously and carefully they can be quite powerful.

A relatively new perspective on the nature of stuttering and its treatment is beginning to emerge, in part because of investigations on stutterers' stutter-free utterances or speech samples. It is not at all clear whether these investigations are concerned with speech that is similar to or different from normally fluent speech, but it is certainly the case that it is frequently referred to as "fluent speech." It is clear, however, that no attempt has been made to take account of the vast differences that may occur among speech samples that are described as "fluent." It is hoped that this paper has drawn attention to the possibility that the new perspective on stuttering that is emerging from these studies may be clouded if investigators fail to establish what they mean when they study "fluent speech."

ACKNOWLEDGMENTS

Authorship of this paper is equal. Portions of this paper were completed with support from a Medical Research Council of Canada Studentship awarded to Patrick Finn.

NOTES

1. It is not absolutely clear that Meyers and Freeman (1985a) employed this definition to select fluent words because they also state that "fluent words were derived (from a transcript) by subtracting the disfluent words from the total words" (1985a, p.

429). This is also implied within a report on a similar study by the same experimenters (Meyers & Freeman, 1985b) because "flow of phonation" was omitted from the definition of fluent words.

2. Unfortunately, Shapiro's (1980) description of this procedure also fails to make clear whether the mixed list of fluent and "dysfluent" tokens were presented only via a transcript or via audio or audiovisual presentation.

3. However, Wendahl and Cole (1961) did show that their judges rated samples that were supposedly adjacent to stutterings as having significantly poorer speaking rate, greater force or strain, and less rhythm.

4. Healey and Ramig (1986, p. 326), for example, reported in their acoustic study of stutterers' and nonstutterers' fluency that they "did not provide any verbal or nonverbal clue that would have indicated to subjects that their fluency was being evaluated." The precautionary steps they took to do this, however, were not reported.

5. This issue may be complicated further in some studies [i.e., Caruso, Conture, & Colton (1988)] where the researchers state that "normally fluent" children may produce "two or fewer stutterings per 100 words" (p. 60).

6. Curran and Hood (1977a, 1977b) have described a 15-point scale consisting of values 1 (*fluent*) through 15 (*severe stuttering*), that their listeners used to rate disfluency in children. The scale was divided into 5 nominal categories. The fluent category was represented by the values 1 (*very fluent*) through 3 (*very nearly normal disfluency*). The scale was reported as very reliable among the observations made by 40 listeners.

REFERENCES

Adams, M. R. (1982). Fluency, nonfluency, and stuttering in children. *Journal of Fluency Disorders, 7*, 171–185.

Adams, M. R. (1985). The speech physiology of stutterers: Present status. *Seminars in Speech and Language, 6*, 177–197.

Adams, M. R. (1987). Voice onsets and segment durations of normal speakers and beginning stutterers. *Journal of Fluency Disorders, 12*, 133–139.

Adams, M. R., & Hayden, P. (1976). The ability of stutterers and nonstutterers to initiate and terminate phonation during production of an isolated vowel. *Journal of Speech and Hearing Research, 19*, 290–296.

Adams, M. R., & Ramig, P. (1980). Vocal characteristics of normal speakers and stutterers during choral reading. *Journal of Speech and Hearing Research, 23*, 457–469.

Adams, M. R., & Runyan, C. M. (1981). Stuttering and fluency: Exclusive events or points on a continuum? *Journal of Fluency Disorders, 6*, 197–218.

Adams, M. R., Runyan, C., & Mallard, A. R. (1975). Air flow characteristics of the speech of stutterers and non-stutterers. *Journal of Fluency Disorders, 1*, 4–12.

Adams, M. R., Sears, R., & Ramig, P. (1982). Vocal changes in stutterers and nonstutterers during monotoned speech. *Journal of Fluency Disorders, 7*, 21–35.

Amerman, J. D., Daniloff, R., & Moll, K. L. (1970). Lip and jaw coarticulation for the phoneme/æ/. *Journal of Speech and Hearing Research, 13*, 147–161.

Andrews, G., Howie, P., Dozsa, M., & Guitar, B. (1982). Stuttering: Speech pattern characteristics under fluency-inducing conditions. *Journal of Speech and Hearing Research, 25,* 208–216.

Baken, R. J., McManus, D. A., & Cavallo, S. A. (1983). Prephonatory chest wall posturing in stutterers. *Journal of Speech and Hearing Research, 26,* 444–450.

Bar, A. (1971). The shaping of fluency not the modification of stuttering. *Journal of Communication Disorders, 4,* 1–8.

Bloodstein, O. (1987) *A handbook on stuttering* (4th ed.). Chicago: National Easter Seal Society.

Borden, G. J. (1983). Initiation versus execution time during manual and oral counting by stutterers. *Journal of Speech and Hearing Research, 26,* 389–396.

Borden, G. J., Baer, T., & Kenney, M. K. (1985). Onset of voicing in stuttered and fluent utterances. *Journal of Speech and Hearing Research, 28,* 363–372.

Borden, G. J., Kim, D. H., & Spiegler, K. (1987). Acoustics of stop consonant-vowel relationships during fluent and stuttered utterances. *Journal of Fluency Disorders, 12,* 175–184.

Brayton, E. R., & Conture, E. G. (1978). Effects of noise and rhythmic stimulation on the speech of stutterers. *Journal of Speech and Hearing Research, 21,* 285–294.

Brown, S. L., & Colcord, R. D. (1987). Perceptual comparisons of adolescent stutterers' and nonstutterers' fluent speech. *Journal of Fluency Disorders, 12,* 419–427.

Brown, W. S., & Brandt, J. F. (1971). Effects of auditory masking on vocal intensity and intraoral pressure during sentences production. *Journal of the Acoustical Society of America, 49,* 1903–1905.

Caruso, A. J., Conture, E. G., & Colton, R. H. (1988). Selected temporal parameters of coordination associated with stuttering in children. *Journal of Fluency Disorders, 13,* 57–82.

Ciambrone, S. W., Adams, M. R., & Berkowitz, M. (1983). A correlational study of stutterers' adaptation and voice initiation times. *Journal of Fluency Disorders, 8,* 29–37.

Colcord, R. D., & Adams, M. R. (1979). Voicing duration and vocal SPL changes associated with stuttering reduction during singing. *Journal of Speech and Hearing Research, 22,* 468–479.

Colcord, R. D., & Gregory, H. H. (1987). Perceptual analyses of stuttering and nonstuttering children's fluent speech productions. *Journal of Fluency Disorders, 12,* 185–195.

Conture, E., Rothenberg, M., & Molitor, R. (1986). Electroglottographic observations of young stutterers' fluency. *Journal of Speech and Hearing Research, 29,* 384–393.

Coyle, M., & Mallard, A. R. (1979). Word-by-word analysis of observer agreement utilizing audio and audiovisual techniques. *Journal of Fluency Disorders, 4,* 23–28.

Cross, D., & Luper, H. (1979). Voice reaction times of stuttering and nonstuttering children and adults. *Journal of Fluency Disorders, 4,* 45–58.

Cross, D. E., & Olson, P. L. (1987a). Interaction between jaw kinematics and voice onset for stutterers and nonstutterers in a VRT task. *Journal of Fluency Disorders, 12,* 367–380.

Cross, D. E., & Olson, P. L. (1987b). Articulatory-laryngeal interaction in stutterers and normal speakers: Effects of a bite-block on rapid voice initiation. *Journal of Fluency Disorders, 12,* 407–418.

Cross, D. E., Shadden, B. B., & Luper, H. L. (1979). Effects of stimulus ear presentation on the voice reaction time of adult stutterers and nonstutterers. *Journal of Fluency Disorders, 4,* 49–58.

Crystal, D. (1971). Stylistics, fluency, and language teaching. In *Interdisciplinary approaches to language.* London: Centre for Information on Language Teaching. Occasional paper Number 6, 34–53.

Cullinan, W. L., & Springer, M. T. (1980). Voice initiation and termination times in stuttering and nonstuttering children. *Journal of Speech and Hearing Research, 23,* 344–360.

Curlee, R. F. (1981). Observer agreement on disfluency and stuttering. *Journal of Speech and Hearing Research, 24,* 595–600.

Curlee, R. F., & Perkins, W. H. (1984). *Nature and treatment of stuttering: New Directions.* San Diego: College-Hill Press.

Curran, M. F., & Hood, S. B. (1977a). Listener ratings of severity for specific disfluency types in children. *Journal of Fluency Disorders, 2,* 87–97.

Curran, M. F., & Hood, S. B. (1977b). The effect of instructional bias on listener ratings of specific disfluency types in children. *Journal of Fluency Disorders, 2,* 99–107.

Dalton, P., & Hardcastle, W. J. (1977). *Disorders of fluency.* London, England: Edward Arnold.

DeJoy, D. A., & Jordan, W. J. (1988). Listener reactions to interjections in oral reading versus spontaneous speech. *Journal of Fluency Disorders, 13,* 11–25.

Di Simoni, F. G. (1974). Preliminary study of certain timing relationships in the speech of stutterers. *Journal of the Acoustical Society of America, 56,* 695–696.

Few, L. R., & Lingwall, J. B. (1972). A further analysis of fluency with stuttered speech. *Journal of Speech and Hearing Research, 15,* 356–363.

Fillmore, C. J. (1979). On fluency. In C. J. Fillmore, D. Kempler, & W. S-Y Wang (Eds.), *Individual differences in language ability and language behavior* (pp. 85–102). New York: Academic Press.

Frayne, H., Coates, S., & Marriner, N. (1977). Evaluation of post treatment fluency by naive subjects. *Australian Journal of Human Communications Disorders, 5,* 48–54.

Freeman, F. J., & Ushijima, T. (1975). Laryngeal activity accompanying the moment of stuttering: A preliminary report of EMG investigations. *Journal of Fluency Disorders, 1,* 36–45.

Gay, T., Ushijima, T., Hirose, H., & Cooper, F. S. (1974). Effect of speaking rate on labial consonant-vowel articulation. *Journal of Phonetics, 2,* 47–63.

Goldsmith, T., & Anderson, D. (1984). The enigma of fluency: A single case study. *The South African Journal of Communication Disorders, 31,* 47–52.

Gronhovd, K. D. (1977). A comparison of the fluent oral reading rates of stutterers and nonstutterers. *Journal of Fluency Disorders, 2,* 247–252.

Grosjean, F., & Collins, M. (1979). Breathing, pausing, and reading. *Phonetica, 36,* 98–114.

Halvorson, J. A. (1971). The effects on stuttering frequency of pairing punishment (response cost) with reinforcement. *Journal of Speech and Hearing Research, 14,* 356–364.

Harrold, E. G., & Murdoch, B. E. (1986). Stuttering: a perceptual analysis of speech following treatment. *Australian Journal of Human Communication Disorders, 14,* 75–85.

Hayden, P. A., Adams, M. R., & Jordahl, N. (1982). The effects of pacing and masking on stutterers' and nonstutterers' speech initiation times. *Journal of Fluency Disorders, 7,* 9–19.

Hayden, P. A., Jordahl, N., & Adams, M. R. (1982). Stutterers' voice initiation times during conditions of novel stimulation. *Journal of Fluency Disorders, 7*, 1–7.

Healey, E. C. (1982). Speaking fundamental frequency characteristics of stutterers and nonstutterers. *Journal of Communication Disorders, 15*, 21–29.

Healey, E. C., & Adams, M. R. (1981a). Rate reduction stategies used by normally fluent and stuttering children and adults. *Journal of Fluency Disorders, 6*, 1–14.

Healey, E. C., & Adams, M. R. (1981b). Speech timing skills of normally fluent and stuttering children and adults. *Journal of Fluency Disorders, 6*, 233–246.

Healey, E. C., & Gutkin, B. (1984). Analysis of stutterers' voice onset times and fundamental frequency contours during fluency. *Journal of Speech and Hearing Research, 27*, 219–225.

Healey, E. C., & Howe, S. W. (1987). Speech shadowing characteristics of stutterers under diotic and dichotic conditions. *Journal of Communication Disorders, 20*, 493–506.

Healey, E. C., & Ramig, P. R. (1986). Acoustic measures of stutterers' and nonstutterers' fluency in two speech contexts. *Journal of Speech and Hearing Research, 29*, 325–331.

Hegde, M. N. (1978). Fluency and fluency disorders: Their definition, measurement, and modification. *Journal of Fluency Disorders, 3*, 51–71.

Hegde, M. N., & Brutten, G. J. (1977). Reinforcing fluency in stutterers: An experimental study. *Journal of Fluency Disorders, 2*, 315–328.

Hegde, M. N., & Hartman, D. E. (1979a). Factors affecting judgments of fluency. I: Interjections. *Journal of Fluency Disorders, 4*, 1–11.

Hegde, M. N., & Hartman, D. E. (1979b). Factors affecting judgments of fluency. II: Word repetitions. *Journal of Fluency Disorders, 4*, 13–22.

Hieke, A. E. (1985). A componential approach to oral fluency evaluation. *The Modern Language Journal, 69*, 135–142.

Hillman, R. E., & Gilbert, H. R. (1977). Voice onset time for voiceless stop consonants in the fluent reading of stutterers and nonstutterers. *Journal of the Acoustical Society of America, 61*, 610–611.

Horii, Y. (1984). Phonatory initiation, termination, and vocal frequency change reaction times of stutterers. *Journal of Fluency Disorders, 9*, 115–124.

Howell, P., & Vause, L. (1986). Acoustic analysis and perception of vowels in stuttered speech. *Journal of the Acoustical Society of America, 79*, 1571–1579.

Huffman, E., & Perkins, W. H. (1974). Dysfluency characteristics identified by listeners as "stuttering" and "stutterer." *Journal of Communication Disorders, 7*, 89–96.

Hutchinson, J., & Navarre, B. (1977). The effect of metronome pacing on selected aerodynamic patterns of stuttered speech: Some preliminary observations and interpretations. *Journal of Fluency Disorders, 2*, 189–204.

Iacono, T. A. (1984) The effect of pre-information on naive listeners' perceptual judgment of post treatment stutterers. *Australian Journal of Human Communication Disorders, 12*, 25–34.

Ingham, R. J. (1984). *Stuttering and behavior therapy: Current status and experimental foundations.* San Diego: College-Hill Press.

Ingham, R. J. (In press). Stuttering: Recent trends in research and therapy. In H. Winitiz (Ed.), *Human communication and its disorders.* Norwood, NJ: Ablex.

Ingham, R. J., & Carroll, P. J. (1977). Listener judgments of differences in stutterers' nonstuttered speech during chorus- and nonchorous-reading conditions. *Journal of Speech and Hearing Research, 20*, 293–302.

Ingham, R. J., Gow, M., & Costello, J. M. (1985). Stuttering and speech naturalness: Some additional data. *Journal of Speech and Hearing Disorders, 50*, 217–219.

Ingham, R. J., Martin, R. R., Haroldson, S. K., Onslow, M., & Leney, M. (1985). Modification of listener-judged naturalness in the speech of stutterers. *Journal of Speech and Hearing Research, 28*, 495–504.

Ingham, R. J., Montgomery, J., & Ulliana, L. (1983). The effect of manipulating phonation duration on stuttering. *Journal of Speech and Hearing Research, 26*, 579–587.

Ingham, R. J., & Packman, A. C. (1978). Perceptual assessment of normalcy of speech following stuttering therapy. *Journal of Speech and Hearing Research, 21*, 63–73.

Ingham, R. J., & Packman, A. (1979). A further evaluation of the speech of stutterers during chorus- and nonchorus-reading conditions. *Journal of Speech and Hearing Research, 22*, 784–793.

Ingham, R. J., Southwood, H., & Horsburgh, G. (1981). Some effects of the Edinburgh Masker on stuttering during oral reading and spontaneous speech. *Journal of Fluency Disorders, 6*, 135–154.

Janssen, P., Wienke, G., & Vaane, E. (1983). Variability in the initiation of articulatory movements in the speech of stutterers and normal speakers. *Journal of Fluency Disorders, 8*, 341–358.

Johnson, W., & Associates (1959). *The onset of stuttering.* Minneapolis: University of Minnesota Press.

Klich, R., & May G. (1982). Spectrographic study of vowels in stutterers' fluent speech. *Journal of Speech and Hearing Research, 25*, 364–370.

Krikorian, C., & Runyan, C. (1983). A perceptual comparison: Stuttering and nonstuttering children's nonstuttered speech. *Journal of Fluency Disorders, 8*, 283–290.

Leeson, R. (1975). *Fluency and language teaching.* London: Longman.

The living Webster encyclopedic dictionary of the English language. (1975). Chicago: North American Educational Guild.

Love, L. R., & Jeffress, L. A. (1971). Identification of brief pauses in the fluent speech of stutterers and nonstutterers. *Journal of Speech and Hearing Research, 14*, 229–240.

Luper, H. L. (1956). Consistency of stuttering in relation to the goal gradient hypothesis. *Journal of Speech and Hearing Disorders, 21*, 336–342.

MacDonald, J. D., & Martin, R. R. (1973). Stuttering and disfluency as two reliable and unambiguous response classes. *Journal of Speech and Hearing Research, 16*, 691–699.

Malecot, A. (1968). The force of articulation of American Stops and Fricatives as a function of position. *Phonetica, 18*, 95–102.

Mallard, A. R., & Westbrook, J. B. (1985). Vowel duration in stutterers participating in precision fluency shaping. *Journal of Fluency Disorders, 10*, 221–228.

Manning, W. H., Trutna, P. A., & Shaw, C. K. (1976). Verbal versus tangible reward for children who stutter. *Journal of Speech and Hearing Disorders, 41*, 52–62.

Martin, R. R., & Haroldson, S. K. (1981). Stuttering identification:

Standard definition and moment of stuttering. *Journal of Speech and Hearing Research, 46,* 59–63.

Martin, R. R., & Haroldson, S. (1986). Stuttering as involuntary loss of speech control: Barking up a new tree. *Journal of Speech and Hearing Disorders, 51,* 187–190.

Martin, R. R., Haroldson, S. K., & Triden, K. A. (1984). Stuttering and speech naturalness. *Journal of Speech and Hearing Research, 49,* 53–58.

Martin, R. R., & Siegel, G. M. (1966). The effects of simultaneously punishing stuttering and rewarding fluency. *Journal of Speech and Hearing Research, 9,* 466–475.

McClean, M. (1973). Forward coarticulation of velar movement at marked junctural boundaries. *Journal of Speech and Hearing Research, 16,* 286–296.

McFarlane, S. C., & Prins, D. (1978). Neural response time of stutterers and nonstutterers in selected oral motor tasks. *Journal of Speech and Hearing Research, 21,* 768–778.

McFarlane, S., & Shipley, K. (1981). Latency of vocalization onset for stutterers and nonstutterers under conditions of auditory and visual cueing. *Journal of Speech and Hearing Research, 46,* 307–311.

McKnight, R. C., & Cullinan, W. L. (1987). Subgroups of stuttering children: Speech and voice reaction times, segmental durations, and naming latencies. *Journal of Fluency Disorders, 12,* 217–233.

McMillan, M. O., & Pindzola, R. H. (1986). Temporal disruptions in the "accurate" speech of articulatory defective speakers and stutterers. *Journal of Motor Behavior, 18,* 279–286.

Metz, D. E., Conture, E. G., & Caruso, A. (1979). Voice onset time, frication, and aspiration during stutterers' fluent speech. *Journal of Speech and Hearing Research, 22,* 649–656.

Metz, D. E., Onufrak, J. A., & Ogburn, R. S. (1979). An acoustical analysis of stutterers' speech prior to and at termination of speech therapy. *Journal of Fluency Disorders, 4,* 249–254.

Metz, D. E., Samar, V. J., & Sacco, P. R. (1983). Acoustic analysis of stutterers' fluent speech before and after therapy. *Journal of Speech and Hearing Research, 26,* 531–536.

Meyers, S. C., & Freeman, F. J. (1985a). Interruptions as a variable in stuttering and disfluency. *Journal of Speech and Hearing Research, 28,* 428–435.

Meyers, S. C., & Freeman, F. J. (1985b). Mother and child speech rates as a variable in stuttering and disfluency. *Journal of Speech and Hearing Research, 28,* 436–444.

Moore, JR., W. H., & Ritterman, S. I. (1973). The effects of response contingent reinforcement and response contingent punishment upon the frequency of stuttered verbal behavior. *Behaviour Research and Therapy, 11,* 43–48.

Mowrer, D. (1975). An instructional program to increase fluent speech of stutterers. *Journal of Fluency Disorders, 1,* 25–35.

Mowrer, D. (1978). Effects of audience reaction upon fluency rates of six stutterers. *Journal of Fluency Disorders, 3,* 193–203.

Murphy, M., & Baumgartner, J. (1981). Voice initiation and termination time in stuttering and nonstuttering children. *Journal of Fluency Disorders, 6,* 257–264.

O'Connell, D. C., & Kowal, S. (1984). Comparisons of native and foreign language poetry readings: Fluency, expressiveness, and their evaluation. *Psychological Research, 46,* 301–313.

Oller, D. K. (1973). The effect of position in utterance on speech segment duration in English. *Journal of the Acoustical Society of America, 54,* 1235–1247.

Onslow, M., & Ingham, R. J. (1987). Speech quality measurement and the management of stuttering. *Journal of Speech and Hearing Disorders, 52,* 2–17.

Perkins, W. H. (1971). *Speech pathology: An applied behavioral science.* Saint Louis: C. V. Mosby.

Perkins, W. H. (1973). *Behavioral management of stuttering: Final report.* Washington, DC: Social & Rehabilitation Service Research Grant. Department of Health, Education, and Welfare.

Perkins, W. H. (1983). The problem of definition: Commentary on "stuttering." *Journal of Speech and Hearing Disorders, 48,* 247–249.

Perkins, W. H., Rudas, J., Johnson, L. Michael, W. B., & Curlee, R. F. (1974). Replacement of stuttering with normal speech. III: Clinical effectiveness. *Journal of Speech and Hearing Research, 39,* 416–428.

Peters, A. D. (1977). The effect of positive reinforcement on fluency: Two case studies. *Language, Speech, and Hearing Services in Schools, 8,* 15–22.

Pindzola, R. H. (1986). Acoustic evidence of aberrant velocities in stutterers' fluent speech. *Perceptual and Motor Skills, 62,* 399–405.

Pindzola, R. H. (1987). Durational characteristics of the fluent speech of stutterers and nonstutterers. *Folia Phoniatrica, 39,* 90–97.

Prosek, R. A., & House, A. S. (1975). Intraoral air pressure as a feedback cue in consonant production. *Journal of Speech and Hearing Research, 18,* 133–147.

Prosek, R. A., Montgomery, A. A., Walden, B. E., & Hawkins, D. B. (1987). Formant frequency of stuttered and fluent vowels. *Journal of Speech and Hearing Research, 30,* 301–305.

Prosek, R. A., Montgomery, A., Walden, B., & Schwartz, D. (1979). Reaction-time measures of stutterers and nonstutterers. *Journal of Fluency Disorders, 4,* 269–278.

Prosek, R. A., & Runyan, C. M. (1982). Temporal characteristics related to the discrimination of stutterers' and nonstutterers' speech samples. *Journal of Speech and Hearing Research, 25,* 29–33.

Prosek, R. A., & Runyan, C. M. (1983). Effects of segment and pause manipulation on the identification of treated stutterers. *Journal of Speech and Hearing Research, 26,* 510–516.

Ramig, P. R., & Adams, M. R. (1981). Vocal changes in stutterers and nonstutterers during high- and low-pitched speech. *Journal of Fluency Disorders, 6,* 15–33.

Ramig, P. R., Krieger, S. M., & Adams, M. R. (1982). Vocal changes in stutterers and nonstutterers when speaking to children. *Journal of Fluency Disorders, 7,* 369–384.

Rastatter, M. P., & Dell, C. (1987a). Simple visual versus lexical decision vocal reaction times of stuttering and normal subjects. *Journal of Fluency Disorders, 12,* 63–69.

Rastatter, M. P., & Dell, C. (1987b). Vocal reaction times of stuttering subjects to tachistoscopically presented concrete and abstract words: A closer look at cerebral dominance and language processing. *Journal of Speech and Hearing Research, 30,* 306–310.

Rastatter, M. P., Loren, C., & Colcord, R. (1987). Visual coding strategies and hemisphere dominance characteristics of stutterers, *Journal of Fluency Disorders, 12,* 305–315.

Reich, A., Till, J., & Goldsmith, H. (1981). Laryngeal and manual reaction times of stuttering and nonstuttering adults. *Journal of Speech and Hearing Research, 24,* 192–196.

Rieber R. W., Breskin, S., & Jaffe, J. (1972). Pause time and phonation time in stuttering and cluttering. *Journal of Psycholinguistic Research, 1*, 149–154.

Robb, M. P., Lybolt, J. T., & Price, H. A. (1985). Acoustic measures of stutterers' speech following an intensive therapy program. *Journal of Fluency Disorders, 10*, 269–280.

Runyan, C. M., & Adams, M. R. (1978). Perceptual study of the speech of "successfully therapeutized" stutterers. *Journal of Fluency Disorders, 3*, 25–39.

Runyan, C. M., & Adams, M. R. (1979). Unsophisticated judges' perceptual evaluations of the speech of "successfully treated" stutterers. *Journal of Fluency Disorders, 4*, 29–38.

Runyan, C. M., Hames, P. E., & Prosek, R. A. (1982). A perceptual comparison between paired stimulus and simple stimulus methods of presentation of the fluent utterances of stutterers. *Journal of Fluency Disorders, 7*, 71–77.

Russell, J. C., Clark, A. W., & Van Sommers, P. (1968). Treatment of stammering by reinforcement of fluent speech. *Behaviour Research and Therapy, 6*, 447–453.

Sacco, P. R., & Metz, D. E. (1987). Changes in stutterers' fundamental frequency contours following therapy. *Journal of Fluency Disorders, 12*, 1–8.

Samar, V., Metz, D., & Sacco, P. (1986). Changes in aerodynamic characteristics of stutterers' fluent speech associated with therapy. *Journal of Speech and Hearing Research, 29*, 106–113.

Seymour, C. M., Ruggerio, A., & McEneaney, J. (1983). The identification of stuttering: Can you look and tell? *Journal of Fluency Disorders, 8*, 215–220.

Shaffer, G. L. (1940). Measures of jaw movement and phonation in non-stuttered and stuttered production of voiced and voiceless plosives. *Speech Monographs, 7*, 85–92.

Shapiro, A. (1980). An electromyographic analysis of the fluent and dysfluent utterances of several types of stutterers. *Journal of Fluency Disorders, 5*, 203–231.

Shaw, C. K., & Shrum, W. F. (1972). The effects of response-contingent reward on the connected speech of children who stutter. *Journal of Speech and Hearing Disorders, 37*, 75–88.

Shenker, R. C., & Finn, P. (1985). An evaluation of the effects of supplemental "fluency" training during maintenance. *Journal of Fluency Disorders, 10*, 257–268.

Siegel, G. M. (1987). The limits of science in communication disorders. *Journal of Speech and Hearing Disorders, 52*, 306–312.

Starkweather, C. W. (1984). On fluency. *NSSLHA Journal, 12*, 30–37.

Starkweather, C. W. (1987). *Fluency and stuttering.* Englewood Cliffs, NJ: Prentice-Hall.

Starkweather, C. W., Franklin, S., & Smigo, T. (1984). Vocal and finger reaction times in stutterers and nonstutterers, Differences and correlations. *Journal of Speech and Hearing Research, 27*, 193–196.

Starkweather, C. W., Hirschman, P., & Tannenbaum, R. S. (1976). Latency of vocalization onset: Stutterers versus nonstutterers. *Journal of Speech and Hearing Research, 19*, 481–492.

Starkweather, C. W., & Myers, M. (1979). Duration of subsegments within the intervocalic interval in stutterers and nonstutterers. *Journal of Fluency Disorders, 4*, 205–214.

Stephenson-Opsal, D., & Bernstein Ratner, N. (1988). Maternal speech rate modification and childhood stuttering. *Journal of*

Fluency Disorders, 13, 49–56.

Subtelny, J. D., Worth, J. H., & Sakuda, M. (1966). Intraoral pressure and rate of flow during speech. *Journal of Speech and Hearing Research, 9*, 498–518.

Till, J., Reich, A., Dickey, S., & Seiber, J. (1983). Phonatory and manual reaction times of stuttering and nonstuttering children. *Journal of Speech and Hearing Research, 26*, 171–180.

Umeda, N. (1977). Consonant duration in American English. *Journal of the Acoustical Society of America, 61*, 846–858.

Venkatagiri, H. S. (1981). Reaction time for voiced and whispered /a/ in stutterers and nonstutterers. *Journal of Fluency Disorders, 6*, 265–271.

Venkatagiri, H. S. (1982). Reaction time for /s/ and /z/ in stutterers and nonstutterers: A test of discoordination hypothesis. *Journal of Communication Disorders, 15*, 55–62.

Watson, B. C., & Alfonso, P. J. (1982). A comparison of LRT and VOT values between stutterers and nonstutterers. *Journal of Fluency Disorders, 7*, 219–241.

Watson, B. C., & Alfonso, P. J. (1983). Foreperiod and stuttering severity effects on acoustic laryngeal reaction time. *Journal of Fluency Disorders, 8*, 183–205.

Watson, B. C., & Alfonso, P. J. (1987). Physiological bases of acoustic LRT in nonstutterers, mild stutterers, and severe stutterers. *Journal of Speech and Hearing Research, 30*, 434–447.

Weismer, G., & Ingrisano, D. (1979). Phrase-level timing patterns in English: Effects of emphatic stress location and speaking rate. *Journal of Speech and Hearing Research, 22*, 516–533.

Wendahl, R. W., & Cole, J. (1961). Identification of stuttering during relatively fluent speech. *Journal of Speech and Hearing Research, 4*, 281–286.

Williams, D. E. (1957). A point of view about stuttering. *Journal of Speech and Hearing Disorders, 22*, 390–397.

Wingate, M. E. (1964). A standard definition of stuttering. *Journal of Speech and Hearing Disorders, 29*, 484–489.

Wingate, M. E. (1984). Fluency, disfluency, dysfluency, and stuttering. *Journal of Speech Fluency Disorders, 9*, 163–168.

Wingate, M. E. (1987). Fluency and disfluency; Illusion and identification. *Journal of Fluency Disorders, 12*, 79–101.

Winkler, L. E., & Ramig, P. (1986). Temporal characteristic in the fluent speech of child stutterers and nonstutterers. *Journal of Fluency Disorders, 11*, 217–229.

Young, M. A. (1964). Identification of stutterers from recorded samples of their "fluent" speech. *Journal of Speech and Hearing Research, 7*, 302–303.

Young, M. A. (1984). Identification of stuttering and stutterers. In R. F. Curlee & W. H. Perkins (Eds.), *Nature and treatment of stuttering: New directions.* (pp. 13–30) San Diego: College-Hill Press.

Zebrowski, P., Conture, E., & Cudahy, E. (1985). Acoustic analyses of young stutterers' fluency: Preliminary observations. *Journal of Fluency Disorders, 10*, 173–192.

Zimmermann, G. (1980). Articulatory dynamics of fluent utterances of stutterers and nonstutterers. *Journal of Speech and Hearing Research, 23*, 95–107.

Zimmermann, G. N., & Hanley, J. M. (1983) A cinefluorographic investigation of repeated fluent productions of stutterers in an adaptation procedure. *Journal of Speech and Hearing Research, 26*, 35–42.

SUMMARY TABLE

These reports published in journals were selected on the basis that fluent speech of a stutterer was chosen by the experimenter as the dependent variable for analysis. The types of analyses included the following: acoustic measures, perceptual evaluations, measures of temporal characteristics of fluent speech, effects of novel stimulation and fluency-inducing conditions, and effects of treatment. The last study cited in this table was published in February 1988.

Both authors independently coded each study according to the criteria below. Any discrepancies in coding were either resolved by a subsequent rereading of the study or the category label was marked "not clear."

Coding procedures. Each study was examined and coded as follows:

1. Criteria for choosing a fluent utterance:
   A = Definition of stuttering or fluency was reported; where:
   bs = behavioral definition of stuttering
   ps = perceptual definition of stuttering
   bd = behavioral definition of disfluency
   pd = perceptual definition of disfluency
   b* = behavioral definition of dysfluency
   p* = perceptual definition of dysfluency
   bf = behavioral definition of fluency
   pf = perceptual definition of fluency
   A definition was coded as "behavioral" when speech characteristics were specifically stated (ie., sound repetitions , prolongations, etc.).
   A definition was coded as "perceptual" when specific speech characteristics were not stated. It was assumed that the sample of interest was identified on the basis of the listener's own criteria.
   B1 = Judgment based on auditory cues.
   B2 = Judgment based on visual cues.
   C = The surrounding context of the target utterance was inspected for the presence or absence of disfluency or stuttering.
   D = The stutterer's judgment of fluency or stuttering was included.
2. Reliability reported on observer judgments based on criteria for choosing a fluent utterance.
   Intrajudge: S1 = Intrajudge reliability of stuttering, or dysfluency judgments.
   F1 = Intrajudge reliability of fluency judgments.
   Interjudge: S2 = Interjudge reliability of stuttering, disfluency, or dysfluency judgments.
   F2 = Interjudge reliability of fluency judgments.

nc = not clear
— = not reported

Authors	1. Criteria for choosing a fluent sample					2. Reliability Intrajudge		Interjudge		3. Speech Sample Size
	A	B1	B2	C	D	S1	F1	S2	F2	
Adams (1987)	pf	x	—	—	—	—	—	—	—	syllable
Adams & Hayden (1976)	—	—	—	—	—	—	—	—	—	/a/
Adams & Ramig (1980)	bs bd	x	—	—	—	—	—	x	—	CVC
Adams, Runyan, & Mallard (1975)	pf ps	x	—	—	—	—	—	—	—	CVC
Adams, Sears, & Ramig (1982)	bs bd	x	—	—	—	—	—	x	—	nc
Andrews, Howie, Dozsa, & Guitar (1982)	bs	x	—	—	x	—	x	—	—	sentence

Authors	1. Criteria for choosing a fluent sample					2. Reliability Intrajudge		Interjudge		3. Speech Sample Size
	A	B1	B2	C	D	S1	F1	S2	F2	
Baken, McManus, & Cavello (1983)	bs	x	—	—	—	—	—	x	—	/a/
Bar (1971)	pf	nc	nc	—	—	—	—	—	—	nc
Borden (1983)	bs	x	x	—	—	—	—	—	—	syllable (counting)
Borden, Baer, & Kenney (1985)	ps b*	x	x	—	—	—	—	—	—	syllable (counting)
Borden, Kim, & Spiegler (1985)	ps b*	x	x	—	—	—	—	—	—	syllable (counting)
Brayton & Conture (1978)	bs	x	—	—	x	—	x	—	—	syllable
Howell & Vause (1986)	p*	x	—	—	—	—	—	—	—	syllable
Hutchinson & Navarre (1977)	p*	—	—	—	—	—	—	—	—	consonants
Iacono (1984)	bs	x	—	—	—	—	—	x	—	1 min.
Ingham & Carroll (1977)	ps	x	—	—	—	—	—	x	—	10 sec.
Ingham, Gow, & Costello (1985)	ps	x	—	—	—	—	—	x	—	1 min.
Ingham, Montgomery, & Ulliana (1983)	ps	x	—	—	—	—	—	x	—	151–176 syllables
Ingham & Packman (1978)	ps	x	—	—	—	—	—	x	—	15–20 words
Ingham & Packman (1979)	ps	x	—	—	—	—	—	x	—	1 min.
Ingham, Southwood, & Horsburgh (1981)	ps	x	—	—	—	—	—	x	—	10–15 words
Janssen, Wieneke, & Vaane (1983)	pf	x	x	—	—	—	—	—	x	CVC & CVCC
Klich & May (1982)	pd	x	x	—	—	—	—	x	—	vowels
Krikorian & Runyan (1983)	bs	x	—	—	—	—	—	x	—	nc
Love & Jeffress (1971)	—	—	—	—	—	—	—	—	—	367–469 words— reading
Mallard & Westbrook (1985)	bs	x	—	x	—	—	—	x	—	spontaneous speech
Manning, Trutna, & Shaw (1976)	bs pf	x	nc	—	—	x	x	—	—	monologue
Martin & Siegel (1966)	ps	x	x	—	—	—	—	x	—	reading passage
McFarlane & Prins (1978)	ps pd	x	—	—	—	—	—	—	—	CV
McFarlane & Shipley (1981)	pf bd	x	nc	—	x	—	—	x	—	nonsense syllables

(Continued on next page)

SUMMARY TABLE. *continued*

Authors	1. Criteria for choosing a fluent sample					2. Reliability Intra-judge		Inter-judge		3. Speech Sample Size
	A	B1	B2	C	D	S1	F1	S2	F2	
McKnight & Cullinan (1987)	—	—	—	—	—	—	—	—	—	1) words 2) nonsense syllables 3) digits
McMillan & Pindzola (1986)	pf	x	nc	—	—	—	—	—	—	VCV
Metz, Conture, & Caruso (1979)	bd	x	—	—	—	—	—	—	—	syllables
Metz, Onufrak, & Ogburn (1979)	bs	x	—	—	—	—	—	x	—	CVC
Metz, Samar, & Sacco (1983)	bs	x	—	—	—	x	—	x	—	CVC
Meyers & Freeman (1985a)	bs bd bf	x	x	—	—	—	—	x	x	conversation
Meyers & Freeman (1985b)	bd	x	x	—	—	—	—	x	—	conversation
Moore & Ritterman (1973)	bs	x	x	—	—	—	—	x	—	word reading
Mowrer (1975)	bs	x	x	—	—	—	—	—	—	word & continuous speech
Mowrer (1978)	bs	x	x	—	—	—	—	x	—	monologue
Murphy & Baumgartner (1981)	—	—	—	—	—	—	—	—	—	/a/
Peters (1977)	bs	x	x	—	—	—	—	x	—	monologue
Pindzola (1986)	pf ps	x	x	—	x	—	—	—	—	VCV
Pindzola (1987)	p*	x	nc	—	x	—	—	—	—	VCV
Prosek, Montgomery, Walden, & Hawkins (1987)	bs bd	x	—	—	—	—	—	—	—	vowels
Prosek, Montgomery, Walden, & Schwartz (1979)	—	—	—	—	—	—	—	—	—	VC
Prosek & Runyan (1982)	ps pd	x	—	x	—	—	—	x	—	same as Runyan & Adams (1978)
Ramig & Adams (1981)	bd	x	—	—	—	—	—	x	—	sentence
Ramig, Krieger, & Adams (1982)	bd	x	—	x	—	—	—	x	—	sentence
Rastatter & Dell (1987a)	—	—	—	—	—	—	—	—	—	/a/
Rastatter & Dell (1987b)	—	—	—	—	—	—	—	—	—	/a/
Rastatter, Loren, & Colcord (1987)	—	—	—	—	—	—	—	—	—	/a/
Reich, Till, & Goldsmith (1981)	pd	x	nc	—	x	—	—	—	—	vowel & word
Rieber, Breskin, & Jaffe (1972)	—	—	—	—	—	—	—	—	—	oral reading
Robb, Lybolt, & Price (1985)	pf	x	x	—	—	—	x	—	x	words
Runyan & Adams (1978)	ps pd	x	—	x	—	—	—	x	—	reading & conversation
Runyan & Adams (1979)	ps pd	x	—	x	—	—	—	x	—	same as above
Runyan, Hames, & Prosek (1982)	ps pd	x	—	x	—	—	—	—	—	same as above
Russell, Clark, & Van Sommers (1968)	bs	x	nc	—	—	—	—	—	—	reading
Brown & Colcord (1987)	bs bd	x	—	—	—	—	—	x	—	3-21 syl.
Ciambrone, Adams, & Berkowitz (1983)	bs	x	—	—	—	—	—	—	—	/a/
Colcord & Adams (1979)	bs bd	x	—	—	—	—	—	x	x	word
Colcord & Gregory (1987)	bd	x	—	—	—	—	—	x	—	sentence
Conture, Rothenberg, & Molitor (1986)	pf pd	x	—	—	—	—	—	—	x	syllable
Cross & Luper (1979)	ps	x	x	—	—	—	—	—	—	/a/
Cross & Olson (1987a)	ps pd	x	x	—	x	—	—	—	—	/a/
Cross & Olson (1987b)	ps	—	—	x	—	—	—	—	—	/a/
Cross, Shadden, & Luper (1979)	—	—	—	—	—	—	—	—	—	/a/
Cullinan & Springer (1980)	—	—	—	—	—	—	—	—	—	/a/
Di Simoni (1974)	bs pf	x	—	—	—	—	—	—	—	multi-syllable
Few & Lingwall (1972)	bs	x	—	—	—	—	—	x	—	10 sec.
Frayne, Coates, & Marriner (1977)	pf	x	—	—	—	—	—	—	—	10 sec.
Freeman & Ushijima (1975)	—	—	—	—	—	—	—	—	—	word
Goldsmith & Anderson (1984)	b*	x	x	—	—	—	—	x	—	nc
Gronhovd (1977)	bd	x	—	—	—	—	—	—	—	150 syl.
Halvorson (1971)	ps pf	x	—	x	—	—	—	nc	—	monologue

Authors	1. Criteria for choosing a fluent sample					2. Reliability Intra-judge		2. Reliability Inter-judge		3. Speech Sample Size
	A	B1	B2	C	D	S1	F1	S2	F2	
Harrold & Murdoch (1986)	bs	x	—	—	—	—	—	x	—	1 min.
Hayden, Adams, & Jordahl (1982)	—	—	—	—	—	—	—	—	—	/a/
Hayden, Jordahl, & Adams (1982)	—	—	—	—	—	—	—	—	—	/a/
Healey (1982)	bs	x	—	—	—	—	—	x	—	sentence
Healey & Adams (1981a)	pd	x	—	—	—	—	—	—	—	sentence
Healey & Adams (1981b)	pd	x	—	—	—	—	—	—	—	sentence
Healey & Gutkin (1984)	bd	x	x	—	—	—	—	—	—	syllable
Healey & Howe (1987)	bd	x	—	—	—	—	—	x	—	vowel & phrase
Healey & Ramig (1986)	bd pf	x	x	—	—	x	x	x	x	phrase
Hegde & Brutten (1977)	bd	x	x	—	—	x	—	x	—	reading passage
Hillman & Gilbert (1977)	pd	x	—	—	—	—	—	x	—	reading passage
Horii (1984)	—	—	—	—	—	—	—	—	—	/i/
Sacco & Metz (1987)	p*	x	—	—	—	—	—	x	—	words
Samar, Metz, & Sacco (1986)	bs	x	—	—	—	x	—	x	—	IVI
Shaffer (1940)	ps	x	—	—	x	—	—	—	—	words
Shapiro (1980)	pf b*	x	x	x	x	—	—	x*	x	words
Shaw & Shrum (1972)	bs	x	x	—	—	x	—	—	—	monologue
Shenker & Finn (1985)	pf	x	—	—	—	—	—	—	—	word
Starkweather, Franklin, & Smigo (1984)	bs	x	—	—	—	—	—	—	—	uh
Starkweather, Hirschman, & Tannenbaum (1976)	ps	x	—	—	—	—	—	—	—	nonsense syllable
Starkweather & Myers (1979)	ps	x	—	—	—	—	—	—	—	IVI
Stephenson-Opsal & Bernstein Ratner (1988)	pd	x	—	—	—	—	—	nc	—	conversation
Till, Reich, Dickey, & Sieber (1983)	pd	x	nc	—	x	—	—	nc	—	vowel & word
Venkatagiri (1981)	—	—	—	—	—	—	—	—	—	/a/
Venkatagiri (1982)	—	—	—	—	—	—	—	—	—	/s/ & /z/
Watson & Alfonso (1982)	p*	x	—	—	x	—	—	—	—	nonsense syllable
Watson & Alfonso (1983)	p*	x	—	—	x	—	—	—	—	/a/
Watson & Alfonso (1987)	pf	x	—	—	x	—	—	—	—	/a/
Wendahl & Cole (1961)	bd	x	—	x	—	—	—	—	—	5–22 words
Winkler & Ramig (1986)	pf	x	—	—	—	—	—	—	—	sentence
Young (1964)	bd	x	—	x	—	—	—	—	—	same as Wendahl & Cole (1961)
Zebrowski, Conture, & Cudahy (1985)	pf	x	—	—	—	—	—	—	—	words
Zimmermann (1980)	pf bd	x	nc	x	—	—	—	—	x	CVC
Zimmermann & Hanley (1983)	pf bd	x	nc	—	—	—	—	x	x	VC or CV

Coordination of Aerodynamic and Phonatory Processes in Fluent Speech Utterances of Stutterers

Herman F. M. Peters
Louis Boves

The production of fluent speech requires precise coordination of respiratory, phonatory, and articulatory movements. Further, abnormal laryngeal function is an important element in several theories of stuttering. Schwartz (1974) and Wyke (1974) described stuttering as a consequence of deviant reflex mechanisms that disrupt normal laryngeal muscle activity. A number of authors (Adams, 1974; Agnello, 1975; Wingate, 1976), have suggested that the failure to coordinate expiratory actions and adjustment of the laryngeal musculature in preparation for phonation is associated with stuttering disfluencies. Adams (1974) and Zimmermann (1980) pointed out that a disruption of coordinated muscle activity within the laryngeal system may be a central factor in stuttering. Others (Van Riper, 1982; Wingate, 1976) have drawn attention to the disruption of coordination between the laryngeal system and the respiratory and articulatory systems.

Physiological studies indicate that the initiation of voicing is particularly difficult for stutterers. A number of processes involved in starting phonation in fluent and disfluent speech utterances of stutterers were found to differ from control speakers. Aberrant muscle activity, including a lack of reciprocity between abductor and adductor muscle groups, was observed by Freeman and Ushijima (1978), Freeman (1979) and Shapiro (1980). Yoshioka and Löfqvist (1981) described a disruption of temporal control of the abductory and adductory gestures of the vocal folds in stuttering, particularly in relationship to supraglottal articulation and respiratory functions in speech. Conture, McCall, and Brewer (1977) and Conture, Schwartz and Brewer (1985) observed inappropriate vocal fold position and hypothesized that a complex interaction among the laryngeal, articulatory, and respiratory systems contributes to the occurrence of inappropriate abductory and/or adductory laryngeal behav-

ior. In a study of the programming and initiation of fluent speech utterances (Peters & Hulstijn, 1987a) it was shown that stutterers have longer latency times as well as longer initiation times in starting phonatory movements than nonstutterers. Recently, Peters and Boves (1984, 1987) observed that stutterers use unusual subglottal air pressure buildup patterns before starting phonation in perceptually fluent speech utterances more often than nonstuttering controls.

The initiation of phonation is a complex process, involving the adduction of the vocal folds, adjustment of numerous laryngeal muscles, and increase of subglottal pressure. All subprocesses must be coordinated with one another. Thus it is clear that to obtain a complete picture of the initiation of phonation, multiple physiological processes on several levels should be measured simultaneously. Most of the studies cited above, however, obtained data from a single process or a single level in speech production. Given the complexity of the relationships and the level of our understanding of their details, present knowledge is inadequate to characterize fully the dynamic principles underlying fluent and disfluent speech (Baer & Alfonso, 1982). Also, different measurement techniques have been used, which makes it difficult to compare results between studies. In general, important limitations in technical aspects of measurement have prevented a comprehensive description of speech motor dynamics. Research in the coordination of respiratory functions, the adjustment of the larynx, and the start of phonation seems to be especially limited (Ford & Luper, 1975). The present study is concerned with the relationship between several aerodynamic functions and the start of phonation in fluent speech utterances of stutterers. To this end, simultaneous recordings were made of the acoustic signal, or subglottal air pressure and of the electroglottograph.

Although all utterances to be included in the study were carefully judged perceptually for their fluency, so that differences between stutterers and nonstutterers on the acoustic level may seem to be unlikely, a detailed acoustic

Reprinted from *Journal of Speech and Hearing Research, 31*, no. 3, 352–361. Copyright © 1988, American Speech-Language-Hearing Association.

analysis of voice onset and speech rate, features that were not specifically judged in the fluency ratings, was still considered worthwhile. Subglottal pressure (henceforward Psg) is the power source for speech production. Although it might be argued that Psg is only a result of the action of the respiratory muscles that are the primary source of energy, the number of factors influencing Psg is quite large. Thus from a practical point of view it is advantageous to measure the one-dimensional result instead of the multidimensional underlying actuators, even if its measurement, by necessity, is invasive. For if measurement of Psg does not lead to the conclusion that stutterers manage Psg differently from nonstutterers, then there is no need to go through the tedious measurements of all muscles that might have caused the differences, had they been present.

To be able to give an unequivocal account of the onset of phonation, one should probably record glottal area (using a photoglottograph) to assess vocal fold adduction and EMG activity of several laryngeal muscles to obtain information regarding laryngeal adjustment. Such a setup would likely limit the number of subjects to one or two stutterers and controls, resulting in what is essentially a single subject per group study. We considered that at present, somewhat less complete measurements on larger groups would be more informative. Therefore, we decided to restrict our measurements of laryngeal activity to the completely noninvasive electroglottography (EGG). It is by now generally accepted that the EGG reflects time variations of the area of contact between the vocal folds (Childers & Krishnamurthy, 1985; Childers, Smith, & Moore, 1984; Fourcin, 1981; Gilbert, Potter, & Hoodin, 1984). When needed, some global information on the adjustment of the laryngeal muscles can be inferred from the EGG by means of models like the ones described by Titze (1984) and Childers, Hicks, Moore, and Alsaka (1986). Also, in many cases the EGG allows one to determine whether phonation started with the vocal folds adducted or abducted, because glottal closure in preparation for phonation usually results in an isolated pulse in the EGG preceding the onset of quasi-periodic oscillation.

This report is part of a more comprehensive investigation of the timing and coordination of the respiratory, phonatory, and articulatory subsystems in the fluent and nonfluent speech of stutterers. A previous report (Peters & Boves, 1984, 1987) focused on the process of prephonatory Psg buildup in the fluent speech of stutterers and controls, and on the manner in which patterns of Psg buildup were affected by conscious changes in voice onset and the reduction of articulatory effect. The present study goes further in that, in addition to Psg buildup, it also describes voice onset as measured from the EGG and from the acoustic signal. Finally, an analysis of the combination of Psg buildup and voice onset is carried out, to investigate the interdependence of these processes.

The major aim of this report is to provide descriptions of our observations of aerodynamic, laryngeal, and acoustic processes in two nonrandom groups of subjects. Some of our observations are stated in terms of differences between the group of stutterers and the group of nonstutterers. This way of formulating should not lead the reader to believe that it was our aim to enlarge the store of factors on which stutterers have been found to differ from nonstutterers with some additional items. The management of Psg and the abruptness of voice onset have not been investigated in any detail for any type of speech. Therefore, we need observations of nonstutterers as a reference against which we may interpret observations in the group of stutterers.

METHOD

Subjects

Fifteen adult male stutterers between 19 and 28 years of age and 15 nonstuttering men, matched for age, served as subjects. All subjects were native speakers of Dutch who reported normal hearing sensitivity and normal language proficiency and voice quality. None of the stutterers had been enrolled in any kind of stuttering therapy during the 2 years preceding the experiment. From five stutterers and eight controls no useful recordings could be obtained due to the failure to position the catheter for measuring Psg properly in the posterior commissure, where it does not interfere with phonation. These failures were caused by anatomic idiosyncracies of the subjects and the inability to control the movements of the tip of the catheter with great precision (Blok, personal communication, May 1985). Thus there were 10 stutterers and 7 controls from whom data were available for analysis.

The relevant characteristics of the subjects' stuttering are summarized in Table 1. The classification of stutterers as mild, moderate, or severe was based on measures of subjects' conversational speech and oral reading. These measures combine ratings of three aspects of speech behavior, namely, the proportion of nonfluent words (P), visible muscle tension (T), and body movements not directly related to speech production (M). The severity of muscle tension and nonspeech related body movements was rated on a three-point scale by an experienced speech-language pathologist. The number of nonfluent words was counted from audio-recordings of each subject's speech and converted to a proportion of the total number of words in the recording. It is our experience that the classification of stutterers from a weighted combination of these measures is a valid and useful indication of the severity of their speech problem and seems to be similar to the one used in the study of Borden, Baer, and Kenney (1985).

Criteria for Perceptual Fluency

Only those speech utterances that were judged to have been spoken fluently were analyzed. To be accepted as fluent, an utterance had to satisfy two criteria. First, there could not be

TABLE 1. Rating scale values on a 3-point scale for conversational speech and reading (P = proportion of non-fluent words; T = visible muscle tension and M = body movements) and stuttering severity classification.

Subject	Conversational speech			Reading test			Stuttering severity classification
	P	T	M	P	T	M	
1	3	3	3	3	3	3	severe
2	3	3	3	3	3	3	severe
3	2	2	2	1	2	2	moderate
4	1	2	1	1	2	1	mild
5	2	3	3	2	3	3	severe
6	3	3	3	3	3	3	severe
7	2	1	2	2	1	2	moderate
8	3	3	3	3	3	3	severe
9	2	2	2	2	2	2	moderate
10	2	2	2	1	2	1	moderate

any visible sign of struggle in a subject's face or body directly before or during the production of an utterance. The presence of visible signs of disfluency was judged by an experimenter during the recording session. Secondly, the utterance could not contain audible hesitations, prolongations, or repetitions. After the experiment an audio-recording of each subject's speech was independently judged by two trained raters to check for the presence of audible disfluencies. All utterances on which the judges disagreed were deferred to an additional rating session, in which the two judges were both present to discuss their original ratings. The purpose of this session was to reach a consensus on all utterances. Initial disagreement occurred on roughly 15 percent of the items. The large majority of the utterances on which the raters initially disagreed (approximately 95%) were readily recognized as containing stuttering disfluencies that had been missed for some reason by one of the raters during the individual rating. This procedure was used to ensure that virtually no perceptually disfluent utterance was erroneously categorized as fluent or vice versa.

Stimulus Words

The speech material used consisted of 80 words. Half of these were one-syllable words of the VC or CVC type, most of which are commonly used, meaningful words in Dutch. A small number of monosyllables were nonsense utterances. The rest were polysyllabic words containing three or four syllables, with stress on the first syllable. All polysyllabic utterances are meaningful Dutch words, although not equally common words. Some polysyllabic words contained clusters of up to three consonants. The initial sounds of all utterances consisted of two contrasted vowels /a/ and /o/ and two contrasted consonants /s/ and /p/. These four initial sounds were equally represented in the word list. The choice of these

sounds was motivated by the requirements of a more comprehensive study of speech motor behavior in stuttering (Peters & Hulstijn, 1987a). In the present study, these sounds allowed us to compare the initiation of phonation from closed (/a/ and /o/) and open vocal fold positions (/s/ and /p/).

Speech Task

At each experimental session an otorhinolaryngologist who inserted the catheter for measuring Psg and a technician were present, in addition to an experimenter and a subject. Subjects were seated in front of a TV monitor, coupled to an Apple II+ microcomputer that controlled the experiment. The words displayed on the TV screen were preceded by an auditory (100 Hz tone of 100 msec-duration) and a visual warning signal (a row of asterisks displayed on the screen). Subjects were instructed to say the word as soon as possible after an auditory response signal (a 1 kHz tone lasting 100 msec). The period between the warning and the response signals was chosen at random from the set |1, 2, 3| seconds to prevent subjects from anticipating a routine.

A complete experimental session consisted of two parts. In each part a subject produced 40 stimulus words after 5 practice words. In one part of the experiment a word was shown on the TV screen simultaneously with the warning signal. Thus subjects had an opportunity to prepare for the production of the utterance. In the second part of the experiment the word was not shown on the screen until the signal to respond was presented. In this condition, subjects were not given time to prepare their responses. Approximately half of the subjects did the preparation condition first, the rest did the immediate reading condition first. These different conditions were included in the design, because it has been hypothesized that prepared and unprepared speech production are dissimilar (Watson & Alfonso, 1987).

Instrumentation

A schematic diagram of the instrumentation used for the research is illustrated in Figure 1. Stimuli were presented by an Apple II+ microcomputer that controlled the experiment. All signals, including the warning and response signals, were recorded on an FM recorder (Philips Analog 14) running at a tape speed of 15 inches per second, which gives a frequency response that is flat within 3 dB from DC to 5 kHz. Speech was recorded using a condensor microphone (AKG type 451E) placed at a distance of approximately 30 cm in front of each subject. The electroglottograph (EGG) signal was picked up by a pair of gold plated circular electrodes placed on a subject's skin, one at each side of the neck at the level of the thyroid cartilage and recorded by a Laryngograph (Fourcin, 1981). The electrodes were held in place with an elastic band fixed around the subject's neck. The EGG signal was constantly monitored during the experiment on an oscilloscope.

Subglottal pressure was recorded by means of a Millar PC 350 Micro tip transducer, connected to a control unit of

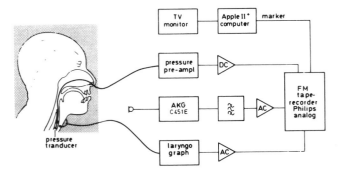

Figure 1. Schematic representation of the experimental set-up during the experiment.

our own design and construction (Koike, 1981; Boves, 1984). The catheter was inserted pernasally and positioned in the posterior commissure so as not to impede normal phonatory functions. The positioning of the catheter was checked by means of indirect laryngoscopy and by having the subject perform selected laryngeal maneuvers (cough, sustain a vowel) while monitoring the Psg trace on an oscilloscope.

Signal Analysis

Analysis of Subglottal Air Pressure Signals. Psg signals were classified according to the pattern of pressure change from the moment of its first rise to the onset of phonation. Analyses were made from paper recordings of Psg, EGG, and audio signals taken at a paper speed of 5 cm/sec. Seven different types of pressure buildup were distinguished. In the description and interpretation of some types, the identity of the word initial phoneme is of crucial importance. The eventual classification of buildup patterns was based on a consensus of both authors. Using our knowledge of the physiology of phonation and the subglottal pressure traces of the control subjects as a reference, we concluded that of the seven types, three could be designated as normal, whereas the remaining four should be considered as somewhat unnatural in completely fluent speech. Observations of the registrations of the control subjects and the fact that some of the buildup patterns do not comply with predictions from existing models of speech production support the decision to summarize Psg patterns under two general headings "normal" and "deviant." The categories and the categorization procedure are described in full detail in Peters and Boves (1987).

The seven types are illustrated in Figure 2. A short description of each type follows.

Normal types:

Type 1a. Monotonically increasing pressure with phonation starting shortly before pressure reaches its maximum. This type is seen both in VC and CVC words.

Type 1b. Monotonically increasing pressure with phonation starting just as pressure reaches its maximum

level (both in VC and CVC words) or, alternatively, some time after the maximum has been reached (only in CVC words).

Type 1c. Monotonically increasing pressure; but with a small pressure drop before phonation. This type is restricted to words starting with /p/.

Deviant types:

Type 2. Monotonically increasing pressure with phonation starting at least 100 msec after pressure has

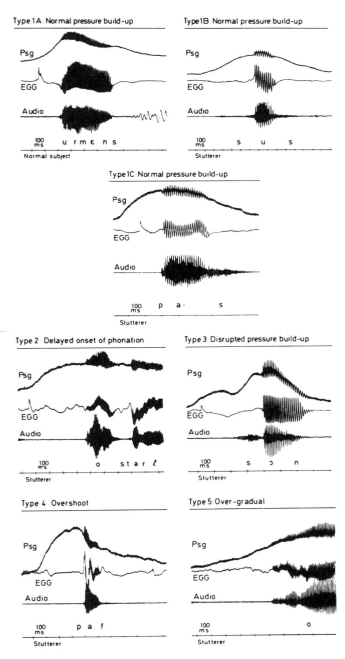

Figure 2. Recordings of normal (Type 1A, 1B and 1C) and deviant types (Type 2, 3, 4 and 5) of pressure build-up in fluent speech utterances. Signals: Audio = speech signal; Psg = subglottal pressure and EGG = electroglottogram.

reached maximum. Delayed start of phonation is only considered as deviant type 2 in words starting with a vowel.

Type 3. Nonmonotically increasing pressure before the start of phonation.

Type 4. Pressure overshoot: pressure increases—possibly in a monotonic way—to a level that is too high for comfortable phonation. Pressure is reduced to a lower level before phonation commences.

Type 5. Extremely slow build up of pressure: phonation begins at the lowest possible pressure level, well before the eventual maximum level is reached.

Analysis of the EGG Signals.   Analysis of EGG recordings was restricted to the first 10 pitch pulses of each word. The recordings were classified on the basis of two criteria: (a) the form of the amplitude envelope and (b) the presence or absence of major irregularities in period duration (jitter) and/or amplitude (shimmer) of individual EGG cycles.

Amplitude envelope was determined by measuring the height of the curves at the rising slope, from the moment when the vocal folds first touch to the moment where the contact area no longer increases (see Figure 3A,B). Some authors have established EGG amplitudes by measuring the distance between the lowest and the highest points in a cycle (Borden, Baer, & Kenney, 1985; Haji, Horiguchi, Baer, &

Gould, 1986). Because the rising slope of the EGG corresponds with an increase in vocal fold contact area, we believe our measures are more reliable.

These amplitude envelopes were classified as reflecting either abrupt or gradual voice onset. An envelope was categorized as gradual if it contained at least five consecutive pulses with amplitudes more than 10 percent larger than the preceding pulses (cf. Figure 3A). All others were classified as abrupt (cf. Figure 3B).

Gross amplitude irregularities were said to be present if one or more of the pulses was more than 15 percent higher or lower than neighboring pulses. In a similar way, gross irregularities in period duration were defined as individual periods with durations that differed by at least 15 percent from both of its neighbors (see Figure 3C, 1 and 2).

Analysis of the Speech Signals.   Only words beginning with a vowel were analyzed. Two kinds of measures were computed: abruptness of the onset of phonation and syllable duration. A schematic representation of these measures is shown in Figure 4.

The measure used for determining the abruptness of voice onset was the logarithm of the time it takes for the amplitude of the audio signal to increase from 10 percent to 90 percent of its eventual maximum value. This measure has

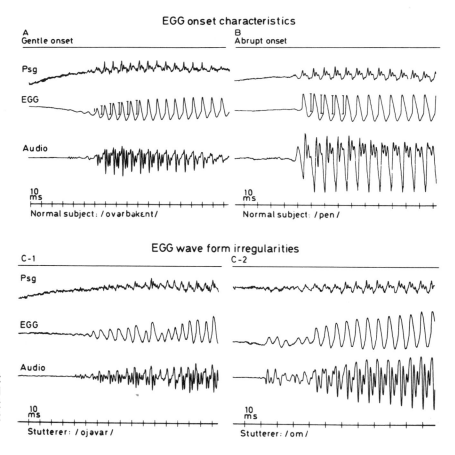

Figure 3. EGG Recordings of gentle and abrupt onset of phonation (A and B) and frequency and amplitude wave form irregularities in fluent speech utterances (C 1 and C 2). Only the first part of the utterance is shown in the figure.

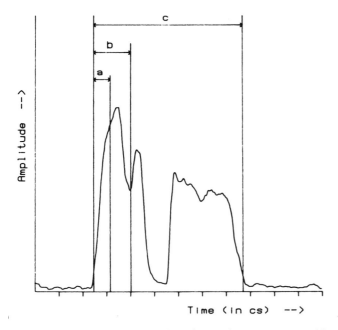

Figure 4. Schematic representation of acoustic measures: a = 10–90% rise time; b = duration first syllable and c = duration of the word, mean syllable duration is computed by dividing the duration by the phonological number of syllables.

been shown to be the best predictor of perceived abruptness of voice onset (Peters, Boves, & van Dielen, 1986).

The duration of the first syllable of words and the average duration of syllables was measured as follows. The average duration of the syllables was determined by searching for the start and the end of the words, and dividing that time difference by the number of phonological syllables in the word.

Data Processing

Although the present study is mainly descriptive in nature, the data were subjected to (post hoc) statistical tests to present results in a compact and insight lending way. A statistically significant difference between groups (mostly stutterers vs. nonstutterers, but also vowels vs. consonants as word initial sounds) should not be construed as demonstrating a causal relation between group membership and measurement result.

The relative frequency of occurrence of the types of Psg buildup and voice onset measured from the EGG were submitted to an analysis of variance. Similar analyses using absolute value data were carried out with the acoustic measurements (steepness of amplitude envelope, duration of the first syllable and average syllable duration). Relations between the levels of measurement (Psg, EGG, acoustics) were analyzed with chi-square tests of 2 × 2 and 2 × 3 contingency tables.

One of the stutterers produced only 21 words that were considered fluent. A second stutterer provided only 13 utterances that were considered fluent. Because much of the

data processing was based on proportional measures, which can be unreliable when based on a small number of observations, the data of these subjects were discarded, so that the number of stutterers in the final analysis was reduced to eight. Each of the remaining stutterers produced at least 50 fluent utterances.

Seven of the 560 utterances (7 subjects times 80 utterances) of the controls and 23 of the 640 (8 × 80) utterances of the stutterers were not used due to coughs or due to failures of the instrumentation. Slightly more than 12 percent of the utterances of the stutterers (74 of 613) were judged to be nonfluent. This leaves a data base of 539 fluent utterances of 8 stutterers and 553 utterances of 7 control subjects.

RESULTS AND DISCUSSION

Prepared Versus Unprepared Speech Production

The difference between prepared and unprepared reading is an experimental variable that has proven to be significant in several studies (Peters & Hulstijn, 1987a, 1987b; Watson & Alfonso, 1982). In the present study, however, this factor did not approach significance for any of the dependent variables. Thus, although an opportunity to preplan an utterance may influence various aspects of speech production (including reaction time and proportion of disfluencies) it did not affect the details of the physiological processes involved in the production of these utterances, nor the rise time of the amplitude envelope or syllable duration. This result may suggest that the opportunity to prepare the production of an utterance does not affect the execution of the motor program once it is started. In any case, the data from these two conditions were combined for presentation of the remaining results.

Subglottal Air Pressure Build-up

Because utterance initial sounds play a decisive role in classifying Psg buildup patterns, separate analyses of variance were carried out for the vowels, the plosive, and the fricative. The data are summarized in Table 2.

The Vowels /a/ and /o/. From Table 2 it can be seen that control subjects used a type 1a Psg buildup more often than stutterers [(F(1,13) = 5.26, p < .05]. The different proportions for types 1b and 1c are not significant. For the total proportions of normal pressure buildup, however, a fairly large, statistically significant difference between the groups can be seen [$F(1,13) = 6.87, p < .05$].

As might be expected, the difference between the summed proportions of occurrence of deviant pressure types (type 2 + 3 + 4 + 5), is also significant [$F(1,13) = 7.89, p < .01$]. For the individual deviant pressure build-up types only the data for type 3 are significant. The larger difference

TABLE 2. Mean relative frequency scores of Psg build-up in fluent utterances in vowels and consonants for normal speakers (N) and stutterers (ST).

| Types of pressure build-up | Vowels (/a/ + /o/) | | Consonants | | | |
| | | | /p/ | | /s/ | |
	N	ST	N	ST	N	ST
Normal pressure build-up						
Type 1a	89.06	68.89	29.62	18.10	41.43	37.95
Type 1b	6.27	12.74	4.78	7.21	48.57	45.27
Type 1c	1.07	0.00	61.21	37.60	4.46	0.00
Type 1a + 1b + 1c	96.41	81.61	95.61	62.91	94.46	83.23
Deviant pressure build-up						
Type 2	1.07	10.06	0.00	7.64	0.00	1.68
Type 3	1.45	5.94	2.81	7.72	1.43	11.04
Type 4	0.71	0.81	1.57	18.35	2.68	1.35
Type 5	0.00	0.68	0.00	0.00	0.00	0.00
Type 2 + 3 + 4 + 5	3.24	17.41	4.39	33.67	4.11	14.06

for type 2 is not significant, probably due to a large within group variance [$F(1,13) = 2.57, p = .13$].

The Plosive /p/. The only significant differences between the groups are for the total proportions of normal and deviant types of Psg buildup [respectively $F(1,13) = 10.48, p < .01$ and $F(1,13) = 7.69, p < .02$]. For /p/ there was a nonsignificant ($p = .07$) tendency for stutterers to use type 4, which suggests that stutterers may occasionally raise Psg to a level that is too high and has to be reduced before the eventual start of phonation.

The Fricative /s/. For /s/ between group differences are limited to type 3 [$F(1,13) = 7.06, p < .05$].

Subjects. Table 2 does not give data for individual subjects. As described in Peters and Boves (1987) there are no systematic patterns for individuals or any subgroups of stutterers that could be identified based on the proportions with which they use specific pressure build-up types. Finally, there is no relation between subjects' severity of stuttering (Table 1) and the proportion of deviant pressure buildup types used (Kendall's *tau* = .277, $z = -1.127$, $p = .13$).

Discussion. In general, there is a fairly clear distinction between the group of stutterers and the control group with respect to the proportion with which several types of Psg build-up were used. It is of some importance that such differences were found in a study in which the fluency criteria were strict. It appears that even in utterances that are perceptually fluent, stutterers quite often exhibit Psg buildup patterns that differ from the more prevalent patterns we classified as normal. It is not yet clear whether these deviant Psg buildup types should be considered as subclinical or physiological stutters. However, this finding, which corroborates previous observations of Freeman (1984) and Watson and Alfonso (1982), calls into question the outcomes of a

number of other experiments in which perceptually fluent utterances of stutterers were analyzed. This conclusion is consistent with those of Adams and Runyan (1981) and Starkweather (1982), which were based on their reviews of the pertinent literature. It may be that a considerable proportion of perceptually fluent utterances should be considered as physiological stutters and should be analyzed separately from other perceptually fluent utterances. Such reanalyses might lead to more homogeneous pictures of stuttering behavior.

Electrographic Measurements

The results of the EGG signal measurements and classifications are summarized in Table 3. The data for each type of EGG (i.e., abrupt onset, gentle onset, and presence of amplitude and/or frequency perturbations), were subjected to analyses of variance with two main factors: group (stutterers vs. controls) and word-initial sound (vowels /a,o/ vs. consonants /p,s/).

Onset Abruptness. The analysis of the abrupt vs. gentle onset showed that both factors are significant: groups $F(1,13) = 10.95$, $p < .01$ and word-initial sounds $F(1,13) = 8.0$, $p < .01$. As can be seen from Table 3 stutterers evidenced abrupt voice onsets significantly more often than control subjects. Also, abrupt onsets occurred significantly more often in words that start with a consonant than in those beginning with a vowel.

Jitter/Shimmer. Irregularities in amplitude and/or duration of individual periods in EGG tracings tended to occur more often in the utterances produced by the stutterers. Except in the case of jitter in words beginning with a vowel [$F(1,13) = 17.7, p < .001$] the differences are, however, not significant.

TABLE 3. Mean relative frequency scores of the onset of phonation and waveform deviations in EGG in vowels (/a/ and /o/), consonants (/p/ and /s/) and all sounds (/a/ + /o/ + /p/ + /s/) for normal speakers (N) and stutterers (ST).

	Vowels		Consonants		All sounds	
	N	ST	N	ST	N	ST
Onset of phonation						
abrupt	39.72	65.71	68.79	79.98	54.25	72.84
gentle	57.04	30.14	28.60	15.73	42.82	22.94
Waveform deviations						
amplitude	13.38	17.85	11.40	15.04	12.39	16.44
frequency	9.38	22.71	7.73	5.67	8.55	14.20
amplitude and/or frequency	18.11	31.66	13.19	16.20	15.65	23.93

Discussion. In a recent study, Borden et al. (1985) observed that amplitude envelopes of EGGs showed abrupt onsets, both in the productions of control subjects and in fluent utterances of stutterers. A gradual increase in EGG amplitude envelopes occurred in the fluent utterances of stutterers only after a number of unsuccessful attempts to produce an utterance. Borden et al.'s measurements were confined to the onset of voicing in vowels following the fricative /f/. Therefore, their results should be compared only with our measurements on words beginning with /p/ and /s/. Abrupt onsets were found more often in stutterers than in control subjects in the present study.

There are several explanations that may account for the discrepancy between the findings of Borden et al. (1985) and our results. One is that the discrepancy is due to differences in measurement and/or classification procedures. A second explanation, which we think is more probable, lies in the different character of the speech task. Our subjects had to produce 80 words once, and only the fluent productions were analyzed. In Borden's experiment, stutterers repeated words until the required number of fluent utterances was obtained. This task would likely encourage stutterers to use strategies to prevent disfluencies, and use of gradual voice onset may reduce the rate of disfluencies considerably (Webster, 1980). In fact, in a related experiment, Peters and Boves (1987) found that stutterers' deliberate use of very gradual voice onset reduced the number of stuttered utterances significantly, compared with a normal speaking condition.

Acoustic Measures of Voice Onset and Syllable Duration

The measurements obtained from acoustic speech signals are summarized in Table 4. Analyses of variance on the rise time data, the duration of the first syllable and average syllable duration showed that the differences between the group means all failed to reach statistical significance. This may not be surprising, given the strict criteria an utterance had to fulfill to be considered fluent.

The failure to find significant differences between the groups on these measures is not consistent with what has been reported for the physiological measures. The most notable discrepancy concerns the voice onset measure obtained from the EGG and its acoustic counterpart. There are several reasons why EGG amplitude does not necessarily correspond with the acoustic energy radiated at the lips.

First, amplitude of the EGG may not be a valid index of the strength of vocal tract excitation. The magnitude of the time derivative of the EGG at the moment of glottal closure, perhaps combined with the duty cycle, may be a more direct indicator of the rate of change of air flow that forms vocal tract excitation. Secondly, the amplitude of the acoustic pressure wave radiated from the lips is to some extent dependent on lip opening. It is possible that even small changes in the timing of voice onset and lip movements may cause considerable variations in the relation between amplitude envelopes of the voice source and the speech signal. Moreover, the time needed for the speech signal to build to its eventual amplitude may be affected by a number of different factors, like the damping of the vocal tract walls or the ratio between fundamental frequency and that of the first formant.

The failure to find significant group effects in acoustic measures precluded any attempt to analyze the interrelations between these measures and the patterns of Psg buildup.

Relationship Between Pressure Buildup and Onset of Phonation

To ascertain if deviant Psg buildup is related either to abrupt or gentle voice onset as determined from the EGG or to the presence of jitter and shimmer, chi-square tests were performed on 2 × 2 contingency tables, both for individual subjects (for whom absolute frequencies allowed for mean-

TABLE 4. Mean scores of rise time, duration first syllable and mean syllable time in ms in speech utterances with initial /a/ and /o/ for normal subjects (N) and stutterers (ST).

Acoustical measurements	N	ST
Rise time	70.1	71.2
Duration first syllable	284.5	303.6
Mean syllable duration	292.0	322.4

ingful tests) and for groups of subjects. None of these chi-square tests approached significance. This result strongly suggests that respiratory maneuvers involved in the generation and control of Psg and laryngeal maneuvers that initiate and maintain vocal fold vibration are, to a large extent, independent processes. There is, of course, some dependence. Phonation cannot start unless Psg has exceeded a minimum threshold and, in the absence of closure of the vocal tract, Psg cannot start to rise before the glottis begins closing. But apart from these boundary conditions, the processes seem independent. This finding suggests that it may be unwise to extrapolate or generalize results from one process to another.

One of the criteria for classifying Psg buildup patterns was the time span between the start of phonation and the moment when maximum pressure is reached. Three categories can, in fact, be discerned: type 1a, where phonation starts on the rising slope of the Psg curve; type 1b, where phonation commences at the moment when maximum pressure is reached; and type 2, where phonation starts well after the moment when maximum pressure is attained. Using these three categories and the two classes (abrupt vs. gentle) of voice onset obtained from the EGG, 3×2 contingency tables were constructed. A chi-square test showed stutterers' voice onset to become more abrupt if the start of phonation is delayed relative to the pressure maximum [χ^2 (2, $N = 28.22$), $p < .001$]. It seems sensible to hypothesize that this relationship is an effect of the coordination of respiratory maneuvers and laryngeal adjustment. The exact nature of this interdependence remains, however, to be determined. Model simulations, like those of Ishizaka and Flanagan (1972) and Titze and Talkin (1979), might lend considerable insight into the physiological limits of the interplay of subglottal pressure build-up and muscular adjustments of the larynx.

CONCLUSIONS

From the work reported in this paper several conclusions can be drawn. First, and probably most important, is that there is ample reason to doubt that the perceptually fluent utterances of stutterers are homogeneous. From the data on subglottal pressure buildup it is obvious that the stutterers differed significantly from the control group with respect to the occurrence of deviant buildup types, in spite of the strictness of the criteria for fluency.

Secondly, EGG analyses demonstrated that stutterers use an abrupt voice onset significantly more often than do nonstutterers. Again, this points toward differences between these groups with respect to the physiological processes underlying fluent speech utterances.

Lastly, our findings suggest that various levels of measurement of the process of speech production are, to a considerable extent, independent, at least in the sense that knowledge of one level is of little help in predicting or in inferring what happens at another level. This seems particu-

larly true if the speech production system is in its normal working condition. This conclusion is completely in line with an increasing number of experimental studies of the speech production system that seem to suggest that, at least superficially, the actions of many articulators may be relatively independent (Fujimura, 1987). One important consequence of this conclusion is that extreme caution has to be observed in generalizing conclusions from one specific set of measurements, unless this is done in the framework of a comprehensive model of the speech production mechanism.

ACKNOWLEDGMENTS

We should like to thank Philip Blok, M.D., for his able assistance with the measurements of subglottal pressure. Ine van Dielen ran most of the experiments, and she took care of much of the work associated with the analysis of the recordings. Martin Nicolasen and Hans Zondag managed to keep the instrumentation in working order, both during and between the recording sessions. Ron Frissen designed a preliminary scheme for classifying pressure buildup types; Eric Jan de Rijk did a similar job for the EGG signals. Comments of Drs. Martin R. Adams, John W. Folkins and C. Woodruff Starkweather on previous versions of this text helped to improve it considerably. Last but not least we appreciate the help of Wouter Hulstijn, Ph.D., in the statistical processing of the data.

REFERENCES

Adams, M. (1974). A physiologic and aerodynamic interpretation of fluent and stuttered speech. *Journal of Fluency Disorders, 1,* 35–47.

Adams, M., & Runyan, C.M. (1981). Stuttering and dysfluency: Exclusive events or points on a continuum? *Journal of Fluency Disorders, 6,* 197–218.

Agnello, J.C. (1975). Voice onset and termination features of stutterers. In L.M. Webster & L. Furst (Eds.), *Vocal tract dynamics and dysfluency* (pp. 40–70). New York: Speech and Hearing Institute.

Baer, T., & Alfonso, P.J. (1982). On simultaneous neuromuscular, movement and acoustic measures of speech articulation. New Haven: *Haskins Laboratories Status Report on Speech Research.* SR 71–72, 89–110.

Borden, G.J., Baer, T., & Kenney, M.K. (1985). Onset of voicing in stuttered and fluent utterance. *Journal of Speech and Hearing Research, 28,* 363–372.

Boves, L. (1984). *The phonetic basis of perceptual ratings of running speech.* Dordrecht: Foris Publications.

Childers, D.G., Hicks, D.M., Moore, G.P., & Alsaka, Y.A. (1986). A model for vocal fold vibratory motion, contact area, and the electroglottogram. *Journal of the Acoustical Society of America, 80,* 1309–1320.

Childers, D.G., & Krishnamurthy, A.K. (1985). A critical review of electroglottography. *CRC Critical Review in Bioengineering, 12,* 131–161.

Childers, D.G., Smith, A.M., & Moore, G.P. (1984). Relationships between electroglottograph, speech and vocal cord contact. *Folia Phoniatrica, 36,* 105–118.

Conture, E.A., McCall, G., & Brewer, D. (1977). Laryngeal behavior during stuttering. *Journal of Speech and Hearing Research, 20,* 661–668.

Conture, E.G., Schwartz, H.D., & Brewer, D.W. (1985). Laryngeal behavior during stuttering: A further study. *Journal of Speech and Hearing Research, 28,* 233–240.

Ford, S., & Luper, H. (1975). *Aerodynamic, phonatory and labial EMG patterns during fluent and stuttered speech.* Paper presented at the Annual Convention ASHA, Washington, DC.

Fourcin, A.J. (1981). Laryngographic assessment of phonatory function. In C. Ludlow & M. O'Connell, (Eds.), *Proceedings of the conference on assessment of vocal pathology. ASHA Reports (11)* 116–125.

Freeman, F. (1979). Phonation in stuttering: A review of current research. *Journal of Fluency Disorders, 4,* 79–89.

Freeman, F. (1984). Laryngeal muscle activity of stutterers. In R.F. Curlee & P.H. Perkins (Eds.), *Nature and treatment of stuttering: New directions* (pp. 104–114). San Diego: College-Hill Press.

Freeman, F.J., & Ushijima, T. (1978). Laryngeal muscle activity during stuttering. *Journal of Speech and Hearing Research, 21,* 538–562.

Fujimura, O. (1987). Fundamentals and applications in speech production research. *Proceedings 11th International Congress of Phonetics.* Tallinn, *Part 6,* 10–27.

Gilbert, H.R., Potter, C., & Hoodin, R. (1984). Laryngograph as a measure of vocal fold contact area. *Journal of Speech and Hearing Research, 25,* 178–182.

Haji, T., Horiguchi, S., Baer, T., & Gould, I. (1986). Frequency and amplitude perturbation analysis of electroglottograph during sustained phonation. *Journal of the Acoustical Society of America, 80* (1), 58–62.

Ishizaka, K., & Flanagan, J. (1972). Synthesis of voiced sounds from a two-mass model of the vocal folds. *Bell System Technical Journal, 51,* 1233–1268.

Koike, Y. (1981). Sub- and supraglottal pressure variation during phonation. In K.N. Stevens & M. Hirano (Eds.), *Vocal fold physiology* (pp. 181–192). Tokyo: University of Tokyo Press.

Peters, H.F.M., & Boves, L. (1984, November). *Timing of aerodynamics and laryngeal functions in stuttering.* Convention address, ASHA, San Francisco.

Peters, H.F.M., & Boves, L. (1987). Aerodynamic functions in fluent speech utterances of stutterers in different speech conditions. In H.F.M. Peters & W. Hulstijn (Eds.), *Speech motor dynamics in stuttering* (pp. 229–245). Wien: Springer-Verlag.

Peters, H.F.M., Boves, L., & van Dielen, I. (1986). Perceptual judgment of abruptness of voice onset in vowels as a function of the amplitude envelope. *Journal of Speech and Hearing Disorders, 51,* 299–308.

Peters, H.F.M., & Hulstijn, W. (1987a). Programming of speech utterances in stuttering. In H.F.M. Peters & W. Hulstijn (Eds.), *Speech motor dynamics in stuttering* (pp. 185–197). Wien: Springer-Verlag.

Peters, H.F.M., & Hulstijn, W. (Eds.). (1987b). *Speech motor dynamics in stuttering.* Wien: Springer-Verlag.

Schwartz, H.F. (1974). The core of the stuttering block. *Journal of Speech and Hearing Disorders, 39,* 169–178.

Shapiro, A.I. (1980). An electromyographic analysis of fluent and dysfluent utterances of several types of stutterers. *Journal of Fluency Disorders, 5,* 203–232.

Starkweather, C.W. (1982). *Stuttering and laryngeal behavior: A review. ASHA Monographs, 21.* Rockville, MD: American Speech-Language-Hearing Association.

Titze, I.R. (1984). Parameterization of the glottal area, glottal flow, and vocal fold contact area. *Journal of the Acoustical Society of America, 75,* 570–580.

Titze, I.R., & Talkin, D.T. (1979). A theoretical study of the effects of various laryngeal configurations on the acoustics of phonation. *Journal of the Acoustical Society of America, 66,* 60–79.

Van Riper, C. (1982). *The nature of stuttering.* Englewood Cliffs, NJ: Prentice-Hall.

Watson, B.C., & Alfonso, P.I. (1982). A comparison of LRT and VOT values between stutterers and nonstutterers. *Journal of Fluency Disorders, 7,* 219–241.

Watson, B.C., & Alfonso, P.I. (1987). Coordination of prephonatory events in mild and severe stutterers. In H.F.M. Peters & W. Hulstijn (Eds.), *Speech motor dynamics in stuttering* (pp. 197–209). Wien: Springer-Verlag.

Webster, R.L. (1980). Evolution of a target-based behavioral therapy for stuttering. *Journal of Fluency Disorders, 5,* 303–320.

Wingate, M. (1976). *Stuttering theory and treatment.* New York: Irvington.

Wyke, B. (1974). Phonatory reflex mechanisms and stammering. *Folia Phoniatrica, 26,* 321–338.

Yoshioka, H., & Löfqvist, A. (1981). Laryngeal involvement in stuttering: A glottographic observation using a reaction time paradigm. *Folia Phoniatrica, 33,* 348–357.

Zimmermann, G. (1980). Stuttering: A disorder of movement. *Journal of Speech and Hearing Research, 23,* 122–136.

Constancy of Relative Timing for Stutterers and Nonstutterers

Robert A. Prosek
Allen A. Montgomery
Brian E. Walden

Since Williams (1957) presented his point of view that stuttering is a continuous process to be considered in its entirety, evidence has accumulated that the fluent speech of stutterers is different from that of nonstutterers. Investigations of this aspect of the speech of stutterers and nonstutterers have shown that their speech is different perceptually (Krikorian & Runyan, 1983; Prosek & Runyan, 1983; Runyan & Adams, 1978, 1979; Wendahl & Cole, 1961; Young, 1984), physiologically (Baken, McManus, & Cavallo, 1983; Freeman & Ushijima, 1978; Shapiro, 1980; Zimmermann, 1980), and acoustically (Hillman & Gilbert, 1977; Horii & Ramig, 1987; Love & Jeffress, 1971; Pindzola, 1987; Prosek & Runyan, 1982; Starkweather & Myers, 1979). On the other hand, some properties of the fluent speech signal do not seem to be affected by stuttering, primarily fundamental vocal frequency (Healey, 1984; Horii & Ramig, 1987; Lechner, 1979; Schmitt & Cooper, 1978), vowel formant frequencies (Prosek, Montgomery, Walden, & Hawkins, 1987), and the duration of segments immediately following repetitions (Montgomery & Cooke, 1976). Although it appears that many aspects of speech can be affected within the stuttering moment, it also is evident that not all aspects of the speech signal are affected.

In addition to studies concerning the fluent speech of stutterers, considerable research has been done on relative timing in normal talkers. Relative timing, for purposes of this paper, refers to the temporal regularities among articulatory events associated with the specification of phonetic segments (Fowler, 1980). Relative articulatory timing typically is defined in terms of the phase relations among events in the acoustic, electromyographic (EMG), or kinematic data (Tuller & Kelso, 1984). This requires definition of (a) a period of articulatory activity, and (b) the latency of an articulatory event within that defined period. Typically, it has been found that the latency is a constant fraction of the period. Variations in linguistic stress and speaking rate will change the absolute durations of the latency and the period, but their ratio remains unchanged. That is, the intervals change in a proportionately related manner.

Tuller, Kelso, and Harris (1982, 1983) have demonstrated that in VCV sequences, the latency of the onset of the stop consonant (measured from the onset of the first vowel) is in a constant ratio to the articulatory period (defined by the onsets of the first and second vowels). This constancy was observed in both EMG and kinematic (lip and jaw) activity during syllable production. In spite of the changes in rate and stress that affected the absolute durations of sounds, the relative timing of these articulatory events remained constant. They interpreted their results as a possible explanation for the constancy of consonant perception in the face of radical duration changes.

Weismer and Fennell (1985) extended the work of Tuller et al. (1982, 1983) in an experiment that measured relative speech timing acoustically in the fluent utterances of normal and neurologically impaired subjects across rate and stress conditions. They expanded the measurements to include nonoverlapping latencies and periods, and complex, as well as simple, sequences. The overall results showed that relative timing tended to be statistically invariant across conditions for all subjects. The result is surprising because the absolute measures of speech duration for the dysarthrics and apraxics in the study typically were aberrant. Weismer and Fennell interpreted this result to be a function of fluency. They argued that the relative speech timing of the normal and neurologically disordered talkers was similarly restricted due to the fluent articulatory sequences. They concluded that ratio measures captured an important constraint associated with speech production.

For purposes of the present study, it is assumed that stuttering behavior not only includes disturbances in the temporal aspects of speech, but affects variables in the fluent speech signal as well. If fluency is critical to maintaining constant relative timing during speech production, then some insight can be gained into the motor control exerted by stutterers over their speech by examining the relative timing

Reprinted from *Journal of Speech and Hearing Research, 31*, no. 4, 654–658. Copyright © 1988, American Speech-Hearing-Language Association.

of their articulations. The purpose of this study was to examine the relative timing of stutterers' speech in two fluent utterances of the same phonetic content. In one utterance, the surrounding speech material included instances of stuttering; the second utterance was produced in a fluent environment and at a faster rate than the first one. In addition, a control group was used to compare the relative timing of the stutterers to that of normally fluent talkers.

METHOD

Subjects

The experimental subjects for this study were 13 men and 2 women who stuttered, ranging in age from 18 to 35 years (mean age = 24.7 years). None of the stutterers had participated in an experiment concerning stuttering prior to the current study, but all had received varying amounts and kinds of therapy in the past. None, however, had received treatment for stuttering for at least two years prior to participation in the current project. Nine of the subjects were moderate stutterers and 6 were severe, as judged by a certified speech pathologist who participated in the clinical evaluation of each subject. For each stutterer, a nonstuttering control subject was selected of the same sex and age, plus or minus 6 months (mean age = 24.5 years).

Speech Material

Speech samples were obtained from the subjects using an adaptation task in order to provide a fluent utterance produced in a stuttering and stutter-free environment. For this purpose, a 120-word passage appropriate for a sixth grade reading level was used. All of the readings were recorded on high-quality audio-cassette recording equipment. Each person was seated in a double-wall sound-treated room approximately 38 cm from the recording microphone. When signaled by the experimenter, the subject read the passage five times in succession without rehearsal.

Procedures

The nature of the current study required the stutterers to produce two fluent utterances that were different in reading rate. In addition, we sought utterances that were surrounded by stuttering in one instance, but surrounded by fluency in the second. Thus, when searching for samples to analyze, two criteria had to be met. First, it was necessary that the rate used to produce the utterance differ between the two readings, and second, the speech material surrounding one reading had to be disfluent, and that of the second reading had to be fluent.

Two speech-pathologists who were not familiar with the speech of any of the stutterers analyzed the tape recordings for instances of stuttering. For this study, stuttering was defined as the occurrence of repetitions or prolongations.

The judges indicated on typed transcripts of the passage where stuttering instances occurred. Agreement between the judges was 98 percent, and any sentence that contained stuttering instances was not selected for further analysis.

After reviewing all of the tapes, the second sentence of the reading passage "The pitcher sends a baseball whizzing toward him," was analyzed for 26 of the 30 subjects. Each of these subjects had produced this utterance fluently at least twice, once in the first reading and once in the fifth reading. For the first reading by the stutterers, the sentence surrounding the selected utterance contained disfluencies; for the fifth reading, the surrounding sentences were produced fluently. For the nonstutterers, however, the sound environment of both the first and the fifth reading was fluent.

For the remaining four subjects, the fourth sentence of the passage "Off into the wild blue yonder goes the ball" was selected for analysis. Again, these subjects produced this utterance fluently twice, once in the first reading and once in the fifth reading. As with the other stutterers, these subjects had moments of disfluency in the sentences surrounding the first reading of the passage, but the sound environment of the fifth reading was fluent. For the matched nonstutterers, the sound environment for both the first and the fifth readings was fluent.

Measurements

All of the ratios to be described were defined by measuring an acoustic period and an acoustic latency, and then dividing the period by the latency. The use of several different ratio types guarded against the possibility that the results were due to one type of measurement, such as VCV material only. Weismer and Fennell (1985) demonstrated that the constancy of relative timing could be observed in acoustic ratios formed in a variety of ways. The ratio types used in the current study are defined in the same way they were defined by Weismer and Fennell.

Figure 1 is a spectrogram of the second sentence of the passage; It illustrates the ratios that were computed for 26 of the 30 subjects. Ratio A is similar to that used by Tuller et al. (1982). The period was defined from the onset of the vowel / ə / to the onset of the vowel /ɪ/ in the phrase / ðəpɪt ʃɚ/. The latency was defined from the onset of the vowel / ə / to the onset of the consonant /p/. Ratio B is similar to Ratio A because the latency and period share a common left-hand boundary, the period ends with the onset of a vowel, and the latency ends with the onset of a stop consonant. Ratio B, however, contains 16 segments where Ratio A contains only three segments.

In Ratio C, the latency and period do not share any boundaries, but the period completely overlaps the latency. In this ratio, the period begins with the onset of /p/ in /pɪt ʃɚ/ and ends with the release of /t/ in /t ɔ ɚ d/. The latency begins with the onset of /ɪ/ in /pɪt ʃɚ/ and ends with the onset of /t/. As with Ratio B, the period and the latency contain a large number of phones.

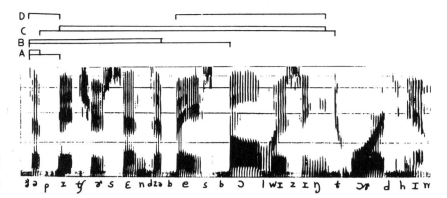

Figure 1. Spectrogram of the sentence "The pitcher sends a baseball whizzing toward him," illustrating the ratio types used in the present study for 26 subjects.

Ratio D may be contrasted with all of the other ratios because the latency and period share no boundaries and do not overlap. The period begins with the onset of /e/ and ends with the onset of /t/. The latency begins with the onset of the first / ə / and ends with the onset of the first /ɪ/. Note that the latency of Ratio D is the same as the period of Ratio A.

Figure 2 is a spectrogram of the fourth sentence of the reading passage; it was analyzed for four of the subjects. As can be seen, each of the ratio types defined for Figure 1 has an analogous ratio in Figure 2. The differences between Figures 1 and 2 are: (a) the sounds produced in the utterances are different, (b) the measurements for Figure 2 begin toward the end of the utterance, whereas those for Figure 1 are at the beginning of the sentence, and (c) the number of sounds involved in Ratios B, C, and D in Figure 2 is fewer than for Figure 1. Although these differences will influence some measurable parameters of the speech signal (absolute durations and fundamental vocal frequency, for example), they were not expected to influence unduly the ratios under investigation in the study.

Rate Differences

In order to determine that the reading rate had indeed changed between readings of the passage, the durations of the utterances produced by the stutterers in the first and fifth readings were measured using a digital sound spectrograph

(Voice Identification RT-1000). The durations were divided into the number of syllables in the utterance to form reading rate in syllables per second. These rates were compared with a t test for correlated measures and found to differ significantly [t (13) = 4.08, p = .001]. The first reading was always slower than the fifth reading. The same comparison was made using the data of the nonstutterers and again the result was significant [t (13) = 4.45, p = .006]. Once more, the rate used to produce the first reading was slower than that used to produce the fifth reading.

RESULTS

The ratio data were analyzed using a three factor analysis of variance with repeated measures on two factors. The first factor was group (stutterer or nonstutterer); the second factor was reading number (first or fifth); and the third factor was the ratio type (A, B, C, or D). Table 1 presents the mean and standard deviation for each factor in the analysis.

The results revealed no significant differences between the stutterers and the nonstutterers in terms of the ratios measured in this study [F (1,28) = 0.69, p = .41]. Also, no significant difference was found between the ratios measured in the first reading and those measured in the fifth reading [F (1,28) = 0.0002, p = .98]. Thus, the results indicate that the

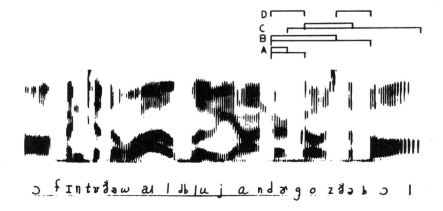

Figure 2. Spectrogram of the sentence "Off into the wild blue yonder goes the ball," which was used as the speech sample of 4 subjects. The ratio types shown are analogous to those in Figure 1.

TABLE 1. Means and standard deviations (in parentheses) for the factors investigated. Ratio types are defined in Figures 1 and 2.

Ratio type	First reading		Fifth reading	
	Stutterers	Nonstutterers	Stutterers	Nonstutterers
A	2.22 (0.56)	2.26 (0.43)	2.21 (0.69)	2.45 (0.84)
B	1.53 (0.4)	1.45 (0.18)	1.48 (0.47)	1.46 (0.2)
C	1.27 (0.4)	1.26 (0.42)	1.25 (0.39)	1.29 (0.53)
D	5.08 (2.17)	4.16 (1.52)	4.6 (1.73)	4.44 (1.62)

relative timing of articulatory events was not influenced by whether the talker was a stutterer or not, nor by the presence of fluency or disfluency in the environment in which the utterance occurred. If the talker produced a fluent utterance, the relative timing was quite consistent.

A significant difference was found among the various ratio types used in the study [F (3,84) = 78.71 p = .0001]. This result indicates that the ratio values obtained depended on the phonetic material in the utterance, the number of syllables spanned in the period and latency, and the boundaries defined for the ratio measurement. Note, however, that this result applies to the value of the ratios, not to the consistency of their production. Post hoc multiple comparisons using t tests were conducted between the first and fifth reading of each utterance separately for each ratio defined in Figures 1 and 2 and for each group. None of the tests reached significance. Thus, although the magnitudes of the ratios differed according to ratio type, this had no bearing on the consistency of the productions when the reading rate was altered.

Finally, it is worth noting that there were no significant interactions among the factors. Accordingly, relative timing was not influenced by any combination of the levels of each factor.

DISCUSSION

The results are consistent with the statement by Weismer and Fennell (1985) that relative timing characteristics are highly constrained by the requirements of fluency. In this study, articulatory control, as exemplified by relative timing, was not demonstrably different for stutterers and nonstutterers when the former were fluent. The support is indirect, however, because relative timing has not been measured in disfluent utterances and, in fact, it would be extremely difficult to obtain such measures in a meaningful way. Nonetheless, the important issue for the present is that fluently produced passages maintained their relative timing across changes in speaking rate even when the surrounding material was disfluent.

Williams (1957) proposed a manner of viewing stuttering that considered more than just the disfluent event itself. He preferred a conceptualization in which stuttering is a continuous process that affects psychological and physical aspects of an individual, as well as the individual's attitude toward speech and speaking situations. The most popular interpretation of this viewpoint is that stuttering is not an isolated event that is imposed on an otherwise normal speech signal. Indeed, evidence mentioned earlier does indicate that the fluent speech of stutterers is different from that of nonstutterers. On the other hand, the data of this study and of studies on fundamental frequency seem to indicate that not all aspects of the speech signal are affected. Because mild and moderate stutterers produce fluency for a large percentage of their utterances, many aspects of their speech are likely to be normal. Apparently, relative timing is a candidate for one of the parameters of speech that is "normal" when a stutterer is fluent. Other candidates appear to be fundamental vocal frequency and vowel formant frequencies (Healey, 1984; Horii & Ramig, 1987; Lechner, 1979; Prosek et al., 1987; Schmitt & Cooper, 1978).

This is not to say that stuttering is an isolated event that occurs only on occasion. Some points of view concerning "tenuous fluency" (Adams & Runyan, 1981), attitude (Guitar, 1976; Helps & Dalton, 1979), and anticipation (Martin & Haroldson, 1967) indicate that certain aspects of speech may be continuous and may require constant monitoring by the stutterer. This does not imply that every aspect of a stutterer's speech requires constant attention, because some will be within expected limits. Such selective attention may explain why a stutterer's fluent speech can be perceptually different from that of a nonstutterer's. That is, the durations of segments may have changed, thus providing the listener with information that a stutterer was speaking, even though the stutterer has maintained the articulator phasing required of an elegantly controlled normal mechanism.

Finally, it should be pointed out that relative timing should be measured at other levels of the speech signal in addition to the acoustic. EMG and kinematic data may reveal subtle mistimings that the acoustic signal does not reflect. Such information, combined with acoustic and perceptual data, should provide a clearer understanding of the motor control that stutterers can, and apparently do, exert over their speech production.

ACKNOWLEDGMENTS

This study was supported by the Department of Clinical Investigation, Walter Reed Army Medical Center, under Work Unit Number 2576, and approved by the Center's

Human Use Committee. All subjects provided written consent prior to their participation. The opinions and assertions contained herein are those of the authors and are not to be construed as official or as reflecting the views of the Department of the Army or the Department of Defense.

REFERENCES

Adams, M. R., & Runyan, C. M. (1981). Stuttering and fluency: Exclusive events or points on a continuum? *Journal of Fluency Disorders, 6,* 197–218.

Baken, R. J., McManus, D. A., & Cavallo, S. A. (1983). Prephonatory chest wall posturing in stutterers. *Journal of Speech and Hearing Research, 26,* 444–450.

Fowler, C. A. (1980). Coarticulation and theories of extrinsic timing. *Journal of Phonetics, 8,* 113–133.

Freeman, F. J. & Ushijima, T. (1978). Laryngeal muscle activity during stuttering. *Journal of Speech and Hearing Research, 21,* 538–562.

Guitar, B. (1976). Pretreatment factors associated with the outcome of stuttering therapy. *Journal of Speech and Hearing Research, 19,* 590–600.

Healey, E. C. (1984). Fundamental frequency contours of stutterer's vowels following fluent stop consonant productions. *Folia Phoniatrica, 36,* 145–151.

Helps, R., & Dalton, P. (1979). The effectiveness of an intensive group speech therapy programme for adult stammerers. *British Journal of Disorders of Communication, 14,* 17–30.

Hillman, R. E., & Gilbert, H. R. (1977). Voice onset time for voiceless stop consonants in the fluent reading of stutterers and nonstutterers. *Journal of the Acoustical Society of America, 61,* 610–611.

Horii, Y., & Ramig, P. R. (1987). Pause and utterance durations and fundamental frequency characteristics of repeated oral readings by stutterers and nonstutterers. *Journal of Fluency Disorders, 12,* 257–270.

Krikorian, C. M., & Runyan, C. M. (1983). A perceptual comparison: Stuttering and nonstuttering children's nonstuttered speech. *Journal of Fluency Disorders, 8,* 283–290.

Lechner, B. K. (1979). The effects of delayed auditory feedback and masking on the fundamental frequency of stutterers and nonstutterers. *Journal of Speech and Hearing Research, 22,* 343–353.

Love, L. R., & Jeffress, L. A. (1971). Identification of brief pauses in the fluent speech of stutterers and nonstutterers. *Journal of Speech and Hearing Research, 14,* 229–240.

Martin, R. R., & Haroldson, S. K. (1967). The relationship between anticipation and consistency of stuttered words. *Journal of Speech and Hearing Research, 10,* 323–327.

Montgomery, A. A., & Cooke, P. A. (1976). Perceptual and acoustic analysis of repetitions in stuttered speech. *Journal of Communication Disorders, 9,* 317–330.

Pindzola, R. H. (1987). Durational characteristics of the fluent speech of stutterers and nonstutterers. *Folia Phoniatrica, 39,* 90–97.

Prosek, R. A., Montgomery, A. A., Walden, B. E., & Hawkins, D. B. (1987). Formant frequencies of stuttered and fluent vowels. *Journal of Speech and Hearing Research, 30,* 301–305.

Prosek, R. A., & Runyan, C. M. (1982). Temporal characteristics related to the discrimination of stutterers' and nonstutterers' speech samples. *Journal of Speech and Hearing Research, 25,* 29–33.

Prosek, R. A., & Runyan, C. M. (1983). Effects of segment and pause manipulation on the identification of treated stutterers. *Journal of Speech and Hearing Research, 26,* 510–516.

Runyan, C. M., & Adams, M. R. (1978). Perceptual study of the speech "successfully therapeutized" stutterers. *Journal of Fluency Disorders, 3,* 25–39.

Runyan, C. M., & Adams, M. R. (1979). Unsophisticated judges' perceptual evaluations of the speech of "successfully treated" stutterers. *Journal of Fluency Disorders, 4,* 29–38.

Schmitt, L. S., & Cooper, E. B. (1978). Fundamental frequencies in the oral reading behavior of stuttering and nonstuttering male children. *Journal of Communication Disorders, 11,* 17–23.

Shapiro, A. I. (1980). An electromyographic analysis of the fluent and dysfluent utterances of several types of stutterers. *Journal of Fluency Disorders, 5,* 203–231.

Starkweather, C. W., & Myers, M. (1979). Duration of subsegments within the intervocalic interval in stutterers and nonstutterers. *Journal of Fluency Disorders, 4,* 205–214.

Tuller, B., & Kelso, J. A. S. (1984). The timing of articulatory gestures: Evidence for relational invariants. *Journal of Acoustical Society of America, 76,* 1030–1036.

Tuller, B., Kelso, J. A. S., & Harris, K. S. (1982). Interarticulator phasing as an index of temporal regularity in speech. *Journal of Experimental Psychology: Human Perception and Performance, 8,* 460–472.

Tuller, B., Kelso, J. A. S., & Harris, K. S. (1983). Converging evidence for the role of relative timing in speech. *Journal of Experimental Psychology: Human Perception and Performance, 9,* 829–833.

Weismer, G., & Fennell, A. M. (1985). Constance of (acoustic) relative timing measures in phrase-level utterances. *Journal of the Acoustical Society of America, 78,* 49–57.

Wendahl, R. W., & Cole, J. (1961). Identification of stuttering during relatively fluent speech. *Journal of Speech and Hearing Research, 4,* 281–286.

Williams, D. E. (1957). A point of view about "stuttering." *Journal of Speech and Hearing Disorders, 22,* 390–397.

Young, M. A. (1984). Identification of stuttering and stutterers. In R. F. Curlee & W. H. Perkins (Eds.), *Nature and treatment of stuttering: New directions* (pp. 13–30). San Diego: College-Hill Press.

Zimmerman, G. (1980). Articulatory dynamics of fluent utterances of stutterers and nonstutterers. *Journal of Speech and Hearing Research, 23,* 95–107.

Reaction Times of Moderate and Severe Stutterers to Monaural Verbal Stimuli: Some Implications for Neurolinguistic Organization

Michael P. Rastatter
Carl W. Dell

A number of investigations have shown that neurolinguistic organization in stutterers is different from that of nonstutterers (Andrews, Quinn, & Sorby, 1972; Curry & Gregory, 1969; Hand & Haynes, 1983; Jones, 1966; Moore, 1976; Moore & Haynes, 1980; Moore & Lang, 1977; Rosenfield & Goodglass, 1980; Sommers, Brady, & Moore, 1975; Sussman & MacNeilage, 1975; Travis & Malamud, 1937; Zimmermann & Knott, 1974). The findings of these studies indicate that stutterers appear to be more efficient in processing language in the right hemisphere than in the left. This is in contrast to the well-documented left hemisphere advantage of normal (fluent) speakers (Bryden, 1982). A series of other studies, however, has provided data that are contrary to the right-hemisphere processing theory (Cerf & Prins, 1980; Dell & Rastatter, 1985; Dorman & Porter, 1975; Fox, 1966; Pinsky & McAdam, 1980). These studies suggest that stutterers have linguistic processing capacities similar to those of nonstutterers.

It is not clear why these findings are inconsistent. Hand and Haynes (1983) suggested that many of the studies showing that stutterers' response patterns were similar to those of nonstutterers used "nonlinguistic" stimuli. There appear, however, to be other variables contributing to these discrepant findings. Specifically, the methods used to study perceptual asymmetries in stutterers may have influenced the magnitude and direction of the laterality effect (Bryden, 1982). For example, many of the studies showing no difference between stutterers and nonstutterers used dichotic listening and tachistoscopic viewing. These methods have been shown to introduce attentional biases that influence performance toward or away from a given sensory field (Bryden,

1982; Moscovitch, 1983). A number of reaction time procedures exist, however, that circumvent these performance biases yet still provide a measure of the "absolute" level of linguistic function of each hemisphere (Cousino & Rastatter, 1985; Day, 1977, 1979; Dell & Rastatter, 1984; Gallaher & Rastatter, 1985; McGuire, Loren, & Rastatter, 1986; Moscovitch, 1973, 1983; Rastatter, Dell, McGuire, & Loren, in press; Rastatter & Gallaher, 1982, 1983). One technique that has been widely used involves analyzing the manner in which reaction time differences between monaural, left-, and right-ear stimulations vary as a function of the hand responding. Although the hand used to respond in reaction time tasks has not always influenced performance in laterality studies (Moscovitch, 1973, 1983), Rastatter and Gallaher (1982) and Cousino and Rastatter (1985) provided evidence showing that reaction-time latencies are significantly different for the two hands when monaural, left-, and right-ear stimulations are compared.

When a significant ear effect is obtained regardless of the hand responding one may infer that the auditory information has been analyzed solely by the contralateral hemisphere. We will refer to this as the strict model of language processing. The neurodynamics of the response modes rendering this effect are as follows: When the right hand is used to react, the difference in reaction time between left- and right-ear stimulation represents T, the interhemispheric transfer time.[1] In this model, the pathway from right-ear stimulation requires no interhemispheric communication before a response is made with the right hand, given that the individual is left-hemisphere dominant for language processing. Conversely, the pathway from left-ear stimulation to the right-hand response mode differs from right-ear input only by the time required for interhemispheric communication to occur. Thus when right-ear, right-hand reaction times are subtracted from left-ear, right-hand ones, the remainder equals T. Similarly, reaction times with the left hand following right- and left-ear stimulation vary only by interhemi-

Reprinted from *Journal of Speech and Hearing Research, 30*, no. 1, 21–27.

spheric transfer time as well. That is, right-ear stimulation will arrive in the left hemisphere, undergo analysis and then transfer to the right hemisphere for a left-hand response to occur. Left ear stimulations will arrive in the right hemisphere, be transferred to the left hemisphere for processing and finally be returned to the right hemisphere for a left-hand response. Again when right-ear, left-hand responses are subtracted from left-ear, left-hand responses the remainder must equal T. Thus, in this situation, the T obtained for the right hand should be very similar to or equal the T obtained for the left hand.

An alternative, which we will refer to as the efficiency model, occurs when a significant interaction is found between the ear receiving the stimulation and the hand responding. Specifically, the right-ear, right-hand response configuration provides the fastest reaction times when language processing occurs in both the right and left hemispheres, but right hemisphere processing takes more time (Y) because of reduced efficiency. Again, this model has been shown to exist in the normal, intact brain (Cousino & Rastatter, 1985; Day, 1977; Rastatter & Gallaher, 1982) and appears to be consistent with the split-brain literature suggesting that the right hemisphere maintains varied linguistic abilities (Gazzaniga & Hillyard, 1971; Gazzaniga & Sperry, 1967; Levy, Nebes, & Sperry, 1971; Moscovitch, 1981; Zaidel, 1978a, 1978b). Nevertheless, the neurodynamics of the efficiency model are as follows: Right-ear stimulations are channeled directly to the left hemisphere, where linguistic processing occurs, followed by interhemispheric processing to the motor centers in the same hemisphere. Left-ear input is directed to the right hemisphere where less efficient language analysis takes place. The information is then directed to the left hemisphere for a right-hand response via a transcallosal route. As such, differences in reaction times between left-versus right-ear inputs for right-hand responses becomes $Y + T$. Alternately, for the hand controlled by the right hemisphere the differences in reaction times between left- and right-ear stimulations becomes $Y - T$. That is, right-ear stimulations are received in the left hemisphere, subjected to analysis, and then are shuttled across the corpus callosum to the reaction mechanism in the right hemisphere. However, reactions made with the left hand following left-ear stimulations need not transfer to the left hemisphere for analysis because of the reduced processing capacity (Y) of the minor hemisphere.

Because studies of hemispheric processing in stutterers are not in total agreement, and because absolute levels of hemispheric language processing have not been obtained for stutterers, an attempt was made to explore further the linguistic processing capacities of the left versus right hemispheres of stutterers. Specifically, the purpose of the present study was to measure the reaction times of the left and right hands while stimulating the left and right hemispheres in a group of stutterers in an effort to develop a clear picture of neurolinguistic organization in these subjects.

METHOD

Subjects

Stuttering Subjects. The experimental procedures were administered to 14 subjects (7 men and 7 women, aged 20–44 years) with a self-reported, life-long history of stuttering. Six of the stutterers (3 men and 3 women) were rated as being very severe while the remaining subjects were rated as moderate during reading and conversation on the Stuttering Severity Instrument (Riley, 1972). All subjects had normal hearing bilaterally; pure-tone, air-conduction levels were 10 dB HL for the octave frequencies 250 to 8000 Hz. They were native speakers of English and had no history of neurological damage. All subjects indicated right-handed preferences for all items on the Classification of Hand Preferences by Association Analysis (Annette, 1970).

Normal-speaking Subjects. Fourteen normal-speaking subjects (7 men and 7 women) matched with the experimental subjects for age (within 2 months) and educational level (ranging from undergraduate to doctoral students) were administered the experimental procedures. None of the subjects had a history of speech, hearing, or neurological anomalies. All were right-handed and evidenced normal hearing at the time of testing as determined by the procedures described above.

Stimuli

Auditory Stimuli. The verbal stimuli were 24 monosyllabic words, composing 12 word pairs, each pair representing a minimal phonemic contrast. Each word was either a consonant-vowel (CV) or a consonant-vowel-consonant (CVC) syllable. Holding manner and voice constant, these stimulus pair contrasted place of articulation. Plosive contrasts were employed to maximize the laterality effect (Studdert-Kennedy & Shankweiler, 1970). Half of the word-pairs contrasted prevocalic place of articulation (e.g., tea-key); the other half contrasted postvocalic place of articulation (e.g., soup-suit). The length of each verbal segment was approximately the same, but segment length was not a variable because an identical word was presented to both ears.

Picture Stimuli. All stimulus pictures were hand sketched in color by a professionally trained artist on a 1 inch (2.5 cm) × 1½ inch (3.8 cm) piece of construction paper. To assure that each stimulus picture was readily identifiable, each picture was briefly shown to 30 college students who were instructed to write down the name of each item. The students correctly identified the picture items with at least 96 percent accuracy (29/30) in all cases. Additionally, subjects participating in the study were required to name each picture prior to the experiment to ensure recognition. If a picture was misnamed the experimenter provided the subject with the correct name.

Stimulus Tapes. Master recordings of verbal stimuli were prepared using both channels of a dual channel tape deck (Sony, Model TC-105). The 24 stimulus words were spoken by a male speaker of General American English having no speech anomalies. Stimulus tapes were created on a two-channel cassette tape recorder (AIWA, Model 6650); however, the stimulus tapes employed only one channel at a time, thus creating monaural stimulation of individual ears when replayed through stereo headphones. Stimuli were recorded in a random block design. Random time intervals from 3 to 6 sec were left between verbal items.

Instrumentation

Each subject viewed three response plates in a row mounted on a BCI Programmer (Model SR 400) situated directly in front of them. The middle plate was specified for the subjects as a handrest; the plates on the left and right were used to present stimulus pictures. The center plate measured 2¾ (6.5 cm) × 3½ (8.5 cm) while the response plates each were 2¾ (6.5 cm) × 1¾ (4.0 cm). The two response plates were located immediately adjacent to the hand rest. The distance from the center line of the hand rest to the corresponding center point of response plates was 2¾ inches (6.5 cm). The stimulus tape was replayed on a two-channel cassette tape recorder (AIWA, Model 6650). Auditory stimuli were presented to both the subject and the experimenter via headphones at 90 dB SPL. In addition, the auditory signal was sent to a voice-operated relay (Grason-Stadler, Model E7300-1), which in turn activated a digital timer (CMC, Model 7078) capable of reading 1 msec. Prior to being sent to the voice-operated relay, however, the acoustic waves were low-pass filtered at 1000 Hz by a DKI bandpass filter. The timer was stopped by a signal from either response plate after a subject touched it. The examiner, situated behind the subject out of view, stopped the tape recorder at will, recorded responses, changed the stimulus pictures, and reset the timer.

Procedures

Initially, each subject received a training procedure. In this procedure, subjects were instructed to keep the left or right hand on the center plate and to move as rapidly as possible to the correct picture (on the right or left response plate) after hearing a word (presented to only one ear). Subjects were instructed further that once the pictures were set in place they were to reposition their responding hand on the hand rest plate. They were told that once their hand was in position the next word would be presented and to ready themselves for a response. All 24 vocabulary items were presented in the

training session; the picture choices did not pose minimal phonemic contrasts. Once the training procedure was completed successfully (no subject erred), the experimental task was presented immediately. The two pictures presented with each auditory stimuli now posed a minimal phonemic contrast. Each subject made 96 responses with each hand. The stimulus words, ear stimulated, and direction of hand movement were presented an equal number of times in a random block design. To prevent equipment biases, the headset was reversed on each subject half the time.

RESULTS

Table 1 presents the means, standard deviations, and ranges for each of the independent variables for the stuttering and normal subjects.

Figures 1 and 2 present the mean reaction times for the various ear-hand response conditions for the stuttering and normal-speaking subjects, respectively.

For the stutterers, the difference in reaction times for the right hand equalled 1 msec while the corresponding differ-

TABLE 1. Means, standard deviations, and ranges reported in ms for stutterers' and normal-speaking subjects' reaction times as a function of sex, hand of response, ear, direction of hand movement, and stuttering severity for the stutterers.

Variable	M	SD	Range
Stutterers*			
Sex			
Male	561	133	127–875
Female	556	127	136–922
Hand of response			
Right	556	115	127–842
Left	542	122	134–922
Ear stimulated			
Right	548	144	127–900
Left	549	140	139–922
Direction of hand movement			
Right	549	125	140–922
Left	558	130	127–900
Severity			
Moderate	551	130	127–922
Severe	554	144	130–910
Normal speakers			
Sex			
Male	460	101	116–925
Female	458	105	128–970
Ear stimulated**			
Right	408	126	116–930
Left	508	122	131–970
Direction of hand movement			
Right	462	125	116–957
Left	454	126	135–970

*All means non-significant at $p > .05$.
**Significantly different at $p < .01$.

ence obtained for the left hand also equalled 1 msec. The corresponding differences for the normal subjects proved to be 120 msec for the right hand and 78 msec for the left hand.

Analysis of Variance

Stuttering Subjects.   To test the significance of main effects and interactions among variables, the data were submitted to an analysis of variance with repeated measures design. Results showed that the main effects of sex [$F(1,12) = 0.32$, $p > .05$], hand of response [$F(1,12) = 0.98, p > .05$], ear stimulated [$F(1,12) = 0.06$, $p > .05$], direction of hand movement [$F(1,12) = 1.04, p > .04$], and stuttering severity [$F(1,12) = 0.82, p > .05$] proved nonsignificant. Additionally, all tests of two-, three-, four-, and five-way interactions were nonsignificant.

Normal-speaking Subjects.   Again, the analysis of variance with repeated measures procedure was applied to the data to test the significance of the main effects and interactions among variables. Results showed that the main effect for ear proved significant [$F(1,12) = 64.01, p < .01$], but the main effects for sex [$F(1,12) = 0.33, p > .05$], hand of response [$F(1,12) = 0.84, p > .05$], and direction of hand movement [$F(1,12) = 0.92, p > .05$] were not significant.

The interaction between ear stimulated and hand of response proved significant [$F(1,12) = 22.10, p < .01$]. Bonferroni post-hoc tests were used to determine the source of the significant interaction. The results showed that the right-ear, right-hand response condition was significantly faster than the remaining response conditions. The right-ear, left-hand condition was significantly faster than the two left-ear conditions while the left-ear, right-hand and the

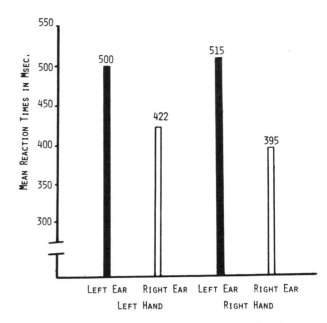

Figure 2. Mean reaction-times for the various ear-hand response configurations for the normal-speaking subjects.

left-ear, left-hand responses were not significantly different from one another.

The remaining interactions proved nonsignificant.

Error Data

Analysis of Errors.   Normal subjects erred 1 percent of the time during the experiment, while stuttering subjects erred approximately 2 percent of the time. When a subject chose the wrong picture, the reaction-time value was not submitted along with correct response values to statistical analysis. Wilcoxon matched-pairs signed-rank tests were performed on the number of errors dichotimized by independent variables: ear stimulated, hand used to respond, direction of hand movement, group responding, and severity level for the stutterers. None of these tests proved significant at the .05 level.

DISCUSSION

The results of the present study showed that both the normal-speaking and stuttering subjects evidenced left and right hemispheric auditory-verbal processing capacities. However, major differences were found to exist between the two groups regarding the extent to which each hemisphere participated in the analysis of the verbal information.

The results obtained for the normal-speaking subjects are consistent with the efficiency model of linguistic organization. The interaction that occurred between the ear stimulated and the hand used to respond suggests that the left

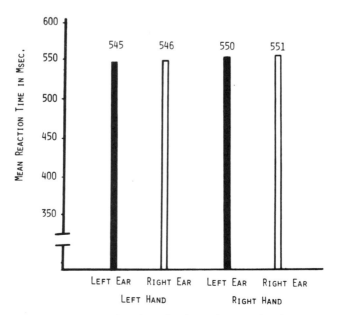

Figure 1. Mean reaction times for the various ear-hand response configurations for the stuttering subjects.

hemisphere is dominant for processing language, while the right hemisphere maintains some reduced, inefficient capacity to process auditory-verbal information (Cousino & Rastatter, 1985; Moscovitch, 1973; Rastatter & Gallaher, 1982). Additionally, when the data in Figure 2 are applied to the formula that test for the strict model, clearly the values of T (interhemispheric transfer time) generated for the right versus left hands are not equal. That is, the T value for the right hand equals 120 msec while the value of T for the left hand equals 78 msec. As stated earlier, in the strict model these T values should be equal. Alternately, the formula for the efficiency model provides a more realistic value of T while an absolute measure of right hemisphere processing time (Y) is derived. It must be kept in mind that in the efficiency model the difference between reaction times with the right hand equals $Y + T$, the processing time in the right hemisphere plus the interhemispheric transfer time of that processing to the reaction mechanism in the left hemisphere. Therefore, when Y (derived by subtracting the mean right ear score from the mean left ear score shown in Table 1) is subtracted from the T value for the right hand (Figure 2), the remainder equals transcallosal time. For the present data, when Y (100 msec) is subtracted from the right-hand T value (120 msec) a transfer time of 20 msec is obtained. Even though this value is based on behavioral estimates, it parallels other physiological measures of transcallosal time, which are on the order of 10 to 35 msec (Teitelbaum, Shipless, & Byck, 1968). These findings are very similar to those posited earlier by Rastatter and Gallaher (1982) and Cousino and Rastatter (1985).

The results obtained for the stuttering subjects showed that neither a significant ear effect or interaction of any order occurred, findings which can be described best by a bilateral model of neurolinguistic organization, wherein both hemispheres must participate simultaneously in the auditory-verbal decoding process. Support for the bilateral processing theory proposed in this paper can be marshalled from the null effects in laterality, and also from the values of T derived from the stutterers which proved to be 1 msec for both the right and left hand (see Figure 1). These values are far below the electrophysical estimates of transcallosal time noted above. Furthermore, they are not in concert with other values of interhemispheric transfer based on complex manual reac-

tion times (Bashore, 1981; Cousino & Rastatter, 1985; Rastatter & Gallaher, 1982). Therefore, T values obtained for the stutterers cannot be considered to reflect the time it took the information to transfer across the corpus callosum immediately prior to the occurrence of a crossed response (right-ear stimulation followed by a right-hand response). Alternately, we would suggest that the auditory information was present in each hemisphere before a motor response occurred. Figure 3 presents a schematic of the simultaneous, bilateral processing model; only contralateral pathways that transmit more rapidly than ipsilateral pathways are shown. Under the right-ear, right-hand response condition (Figure 3A) the auditory stimuli is received in the left hemisphere and is partially analyzed. In order for decoding to occur completely, however, the stimuli is sent across the corpus callosum to the right hemisphere. Once analysis is completed (this occurs when both hemispheres are engaged and simultaneously analyze the stimuli) a signal is sent to the motor centers of the left hemisphere via an interhemispheric pathway where a response is initiated with the right hand. The neurodynamics of left-ear, right-hand responses (Figure 3B) are similar. Left ear input is channeled to the right hemisphere and is partially analyzed. Again, complete processing and subsequent motor response occurs following interhemispheric communication. Therefore, differences between left- and right-ear stimulation for the right hand are nearly nonexistent. Figures 3C and 3D illustrate the schematics for a left-hand response following right- and left-ear stimulations. As these figures illustrate, the processing model is identical to the one described above for the right hand. Because of simultaneous hemispheric processing, interhemispheric transfer-time becomes impossible to parcel out of the present data and, by extension, may be considered to be a component of the decoding process. Such a theory may well help explain, at least in part, the increased latencies in reaction time observed in stutterers. It is felt that bilateral processing accounts for only a portion of the slower responses noted for our stuttering subjects since our earlier work showed that at least two neurophysiological factors serve to influence stutterers' reaction time latencies (Rastatter & Dell, 1985). These include aberrancies in both motor control and auditory processing capacity. Perhaps similar factors may be held

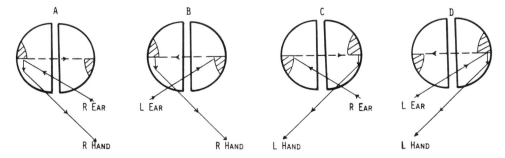

Figure 3. Schematic of the simultaneous, bilateral stimulus-processing model.

accountable for the increases in reaction time found in other stuttering subjects (Adams & Hayden, 1976; McFarlane & Prins, 1978; Reich, Till, & Goldsmith, 1981; Starkweather, Hirschman, & Tannenbaum, 1976).

If a bilateral model of language processing where each hemisphere maintained equal and individual capacities to process the stimuli was supported, reaction-time values would have been influenced differently.

Figure 4 presents the schematic for this model; again only contralateral pathways are shown. Left-ear input (Figure 4A) is sent directly to the right hemisphere where complete processing takes place. For a response to occur, the signal is sent across the corpus callosum to the motor centers in the left hemisphere.

Right-ear input (Figure 4B) would be analyzed solely in the left hemisphere followed by intrahemispheric processing to the motor centers in the same hemisphere. Based on this model differences in reaction times between the left and right ears for the right hand would favor the right ear by a factor of T, interhemispheric transfer time. Figures 4C and 4D present a schematic for left-hand responses. An identical processing model is derived in this situation, except reaction times would favor left-ear stimulation. Because of these response configurations tests of significance would have yielded an interaction between ear stimulated and hand of response. Obviously such was not the case, and the independent, bilateral processing model is not supported.

A Theoretical Framework

Moscovitch (1973) asserts that the right hemisphere in right-handed people maintains some limited underlying "verbal competence." Our normal-speaking subjects' data, and those posited by Day (1977), Rastatter and Gallaher (1982), and Cousino and Rastatter (1985) support such a claim. According to Moscovitch, however, the limit of this verbal competence "depends on the degree to which the dominant hemisphere can control the verbal behavior of the minor hemisphere via midline commissures and other pathways" (1973, p. 114). Geschwind (cited in Moscovitch, 1973) contends that access to minor, right-hemisphere verbal functions may be inhibited by the left hemisphere, resulting in a "masking" effect on nondominant verbal output. There is considerable evidence supporting Geschwind's thesis based on the verbal behavior of commissurotomized patients (Gazzaniga & Sperry, 1967). Once disconnected from the dominant hemisphere, the right hemisphere is released from the inhibiting effects of a superior neurostructure.

Based on our data, and the concepts proposed by Moscovitch (1973) and Geschwind (cited in Moscovitch, 1973), it seems reasonable to assert that the left hemisphere in the stuttering population relies on certain linguistic functions of the right hemisphere. In effect, the left hemisphere does not assume total control, which appears to hold true regardless of the severity of stuttering. The main effect for stuttering severity was nonsignificant. As a result of the left hemisphere's inability to totally integrate the right, it remains possible that the speech-motor programmer in stuttering populations may receive conflicting information from each hemisphere, or at a more fundamental level, similar information that is temporally out of phase. Zimmermann, Smith, and Hanley (1981) maintain that a disturbance in coordination may occur among muscle groups when input to motor neuron pools is aberrant. They indicate that stuttering behavior (e.g., tension prior to speech, stuttering on initial sounds) "indicate that the period before movement may be a time in which aberrant inputs to motor neuron pools are likely to occur in stutterers" (p. 27). Theoretically, dissimilar or out of phase signals from both the left and right hemispheres to the motor neuron pools possibly may be the source (at least in part) of the aberrant input referred to by Zimmermann et al. (1981).

This study does not answer, unequivocally, whether the left and right hemispheres in stutterers are in competition for verbal function; however, our data, although based on a decoding model, seem to point in that direction. Currently, investigations are being undertaken that examine the encoding capacities of the left and right hemispheres in stutterers in order to further test the theories proposed in this paper.

NOTES

1. It should be noted that the interhemispheric transfer times referred to under the present experimental conditions are

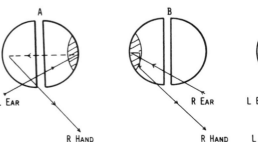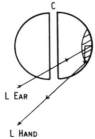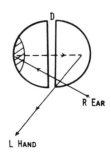

Figure 4. Schematic of the individual, bilateral stimulus-processing model.

behavioral estimates based on reactions to complex information. They are not considered to reflect callosal transfer time solely (see Bashore, 1981, for a review of these issues). Rather, the "*T*" times are used as a relative measure of interhemispheric communication that serve to delineate right versus left hemisphere processing capacities.

REFERENCES

Adams, M.R., & Hayden, P. (1976). The ability of stutterers and nonstutterers to imitate and terminate phonation during production of an isolated vowel. *Journal of Speech and Hearing Research, 19,* 290–296.

Andrews, G., Quinn, P.T., & Sorby, W.A. (1972). Stuttering: An investigation into cerebral dominance for speech. *Journal of Neurology, Neurosurgery and Psychiatry, 35,* 414–418.

Annette, M. (1970). A classification of hand preference by association analysis. *British Journal of Psychology, 61,* 303–321.

Bashore, T.R. (1981). Vocal and manual reaction-time estimates of interhemispheric transmission time. *Psychological Bulletin, 89,* 352–368.

Bryden, M.P. (1982). *Laterality: Functional asymmetry in the intact brain.* New York: Academic Press.

Cerf, A., & Prins, D. (1980, November). *Stutterers' ear preference for dichotic syllables.* Paper presented at the Annual Convention of the American Speech-Language-Hearing Association, Detroit, MI.

Cousino, M., & Rastatter, M.P. (1985). Reaction times of four year old children to monaurally presented verbal stimuli: Some evidence for right hemispheric linguistic function. *Cortex, 21,* 445–452.

Curry, F.K.W., & Gregory, H.H. (1969). The performance of stutterers and dichotic listening tasks thought to reflect cerebral dominance. *Journal of Speech and Hearing Research, 12,* 73–82.

Day, J. (1977). Right-hemispheric language processing in normal right-handers. *Journal of Experimental Psychology: Human Perception and Performance, 3,* 518–528.

Day, J. (1979). Visual half-field word recognition as a function of syntactic class and imageability. *Neuropsychologia, 17,* 515–520.

Dell, C.W., & Rastatter, M.P. (1984). *Reaction times of stutterers to monaural, verbal information.* Paper presented at the Annual Convention of the American Speech-Language-Hearing Association, San Francisco.

Dell, C.W., & Rastatter, M.P. (1985). *Reading reaction times of stutterers to tachistoscopically presented words.* Paper presented at the Annual Convention of the American Speech-Language-Hearing Association, Washington, DC.

Dorman, M.F., & Porter, R.J. (1975). Hemispheric lateralization for speech perception in stutterers. *Cortex, 11,* 181–185.

Fox, D.R. (1966). Electroencephalographic analysis during stuttering and nonstuttering. *Journal of Speech and Hearing Research, 9,* 488–497.

Gallaher, A.J., & Rastatter, M.P. (1985). Reaction times of severe Broca's aphasics to monaural verbal stimuli. *Brain and Language, 25,* 134–143.

Gazzaniga, M.S., & Hillyard, S.A. (1971). Language and speech capacity of the right hemisphere. *Neuropsychologia, 9,* 273–280.

Gazzaniga, M., & Sperry, R. (1967). Language after section of the cerebral commissure. *Brain, 90,* 131–148.

Hand, C.R., & Haynes, W.O. (1983). Linguistic processing and reaction time differences in stutterers and nonstutterers. *Journal of Speech and Hearing Research, 26,* 181–185.

Jones, R.K. (1966). Observations on stammering after localized cerebral injury. *Journal of Neurology, Neurosurgery, and Psychiatry, 29,* 192–195.

Levy, J., Nebes, R.D., & Sperry, R.W. (1971). Expressive language in the surgically separated minor hemisphere. *Cortex, 7,* 49–59.

McFarlane, S.C., & Prins, D. (1978). Neural response time of stutterers and nonstutterers in selected oral motor tasks. *Journal of Speech and Hearing Research, 21,* 768–778.

McGuire, R.A., Loren, C., & Rastatter, M.P. (1986). Naming reaction times to tachistoscopically presented pictures: Some evidence for right hemispheric encoding capacity. *Perceptual and Motor Skills, 62,* 303–306.

Moore, W.H. (1976). Bilateral tachistoscopic work perception of stutterers and normal subjects. *Brain and Language, 3,* 434–442.

Moore, W.H., & Haynes, W.O. (1980). Alpha hemispheric asymmetry and stuttering: Some support for a segmentation dysfunction hypothesis. *Journal of Speech and Hearing Research, 23,* 229–247.

Moore, W.H., & Lang, M.K. (1977). Alpha asymmetry over the right and left hemisphere of stutterers and control subjects preceding massed oral reading: A preliminary investigation. *Perceptual and Motor Skills, 44,* 223–230.

Moscovitch, M. (1973). Language and the cerebral hemispheres: Reaction-time studies and their implications for models of cerebral dominance. In P. Pliner, L. Kramer, & T. Alloway (Eds.), *Communication and affect: Language and thought* (pp. 89–126). New York: Academic Press.

Moscovitch, M. (1981). Right-hemisphere language. *Topics in Language Disorders, 1,* 41–66.

Moscovitch, M. (1983). The linguistic and emotional functions of the normal right hemisphere. In E. Perecman (Ed.), *Cognitive processing in the right hemisphere* (pp. 57–82). New York: Academic Press.

Pinsky, S.D., & McAdam, D.W. (1980). Electroencephalographic and dichotic indices of cerebral laterality in stutterers. *Brain and Language, 11,* 374–397.

Rastatter, M.P., & Dell, C.W. (1985). Simple motor and phonemic processing reaction times of stutterers. *Perceptual and Motor Skills, 61,* 463–466.

Rastatter, M.P., Dell, C.W., McGuire, R.A., & Loren, C. (in press). Vocal reaction times to unilaterally presented concrete and abstract words: Towards a theory of differential minor hemispheric semantic processing. *Cortex.*

Rastatter, M.P., & Gallaher, A.J. (1982). Reaction times of normal subjects to monaurally presented verbal and tonal stimuli. *Neuropsychologia, 20,* 465–473.

Rastatter, M.P., & Gallaher, A.J. (1983). Cerebral asymmetry for verbal information in severe aphasia. *The Journal of Auditory Research, 23,* 271–279.

Reich, A., Till, J., & Goldsmith, H. (1981). Laryngeal and manual reaction times of stuttering and nonstuttering adults. *Journal of Speech and Hearing Research, 24,* 192–196.

Riley, G.D. (1972). A stuttering severity instrument for children and adults. *Journal of Speech and Hearing Disorders, 37,* 314–321.

Rosenfield, D.B., & Goodglass, H. (1980). Dichotic testing for cerebral dominance in stutterers. *Brain and Language, 11,* 170–180.

Sommers, R.K., Brady, W.A., & Moore, W.H. (1975). Dichotic ear preferences of stuttering children and adults. *Perceptual and Motor Skills, 41,* 931–938.

Starkweather, C.W., Hirschman, P., & Tannenbaum, R.S. (1976). Latency of vocalization onset: Stutterers versus nonstutterers. *Journal of Hearing Research, 19,* 481–492.

Studdert-Kennedy, M., & Shankweiler, D. (1970). Hemispheric specialization for speech perception. *Journal of the Acoustical Society of America, 48,* 576–594.

Sussman, H.M., & MacNeilage, P.F. (1975). Hemispheric specialization for speech production and perception in stutterers. *Neuropsychologia, 13,* 19–26.

Teitelbaum, H., Shipless, S.K., & Byck, R. (1968). Role of somatosensory cortex in interhemispheric transfer of tactile habits. *Journal of Comparative Psychology, 66,* 623–632.

Travis, L.E., & Malamud, W. (1937). Brain potentials from normal subjects, stutterers and schizophrenic patients. *American Journal of Psychiatry, 93,* 929–936.

Zaidel, E. (1978a). Lexical organization in the right hemisphere. In P.A. Buser & A. Rougel-Buser (Eds.), *Cerebral correlates of conscious experience* (pp. 177–198). Amsterdam: Elsevier/North-Holland.

Zaidel, E. (1978b). Concepts of cerebral dominance in the split brain. In P.A. Buser & A. Rougel-Buser (Eds.), *Cerebral correlates and conscious experience* (pp. 263–284). Amsterdam: Elsevier/North-Holland.

Zimmermann, G.N., & Knott, J.L. (1974). Slow potentials of the brain related to speech processing in normal speakers and stutterers. *Electroencephalography and Clinical Neurophysiology, 37,* 599–607.

Zimmermann, G., Smith, A., & Hanley, J. (1981). Stuttering: In need of a unifying conceptual framework. *Journal of Speech and Hearing Research, 24,* 25–31.

CHAPTER 3 ADDITIONAL READINGS

Adams, M.R. (1981). The speech production abilities of stutterers: Recent, ongoing, and future research. *Journal of Fluency Disorders, 6,* 311–326.

Adams, M.R. (1985). The speech physiology of stutterers: Present status. *Seminars in Speech and Language, 6,* 177–189.

Adams, M.R., & Runyan, C.M. (1981). Stuttering and fluency: Exclusive events or points on a continuum? *Journal of Fluency Disorders, 6,* 197–218.

Bakker, K., & Brutten, G.J. (1989). A comparative investigation of the laryngeal premotor, adjustment, and reaction times of stutterers and nonstutterers. *Journal of Speech and Hearing Research, 32,* 239–244.

Bergmann, G. (1986). Studies in stuttering as a prosodic disturbance. *Journal of Speech and Hearing Research, 29,* 290–300.

Blood, G.W., & Blood, I.M. (1987). Laterality preferences in adult female and male stutterers. *Journal of Fluency Disorders, 14,* 1–10.

Blood, G.W., & Blood, I.M. (1989). Multiple data analyses of dichotic listening advantages of stutterers. *Journal of Fluency Disorders, 14,* 97–108.

Blood, I.M., & Blood, G.W. (1984). Relationship between stuttering severity and brainstem-evoked response testing. *Perceptual and Motor Skills, 59,* 935–938.

Boberg, E., Yeudall, L.T., & Schopflocher, D. (1983). The effect of an intensive behavioral program on the distribution of EEG alpha power in stuttering during the processing of verbal and visuospatial information. *Journal of Fluency Disorders, 8,* 245–263.

Borden, G.J., Kim, D.H., & Spiegler, K. (1987). Acoustics of stop consonant-vowel relationships during fluent and stuttered utterances. *Journal of Fluency Disorders, 12,* 175–184.

Carpenter, M., & Sommers, R.K. (1987). Unisensory and bisensory perceptual and memory processing in stuttering adults and normal speakers. *Journal of Fluency Disorders, 12,* 291–304.

Caruso, A.J., Abbs, J.H., & Gracco, V.L. (1988). Kinematic analysis of multiple movement coordination during speech in stutterers. *Brain, 111,* 439–456.

Code, C. (1979). Genuine and artificial stammering: An EMG comparison. *British Journal of Disorders of Communication, 14,* 5–16.

Cox, M.D. (1982). The stutterer and stuttering: Neuropsychological correlates. *Journal of Fluency Disorders, 7,* 129–140.

Cross, D.E. (1987). Comparison of reaction time and accuracy measures of laterality for stutterers and normal speakers. *Journal of Fluency Disorders, 12,* 271–286.

Cross, D.E., & Olson, P. (1987). Interaction between jaw kinematics and voice onset for stutterers and nonstutterers in a VRT task. *Journal of Fluency Disorders, 12,* 367–380.

Cross, D.E., & Olson, P.L. (1987). Articulatory-laryngeal interaction in stutterers and normal speakers: Effects of a bite-block on rapid voice initiation. *Journal of Fluency Disorders, 12,* 407–418.

Decker, T.N., Healey, E.C., & Howe, S.W. (1982). Brainstem auditory electrical response characteristics of stutterers and nonstutterers: A preliminary report. *Journal of Fluency Disorders, 7,* 385–402.

Doslak, M., Healey, E.C., & Riese, K. (1986). Eye movements of stutterers. *Investigative Ophthalmology and Visual Science, 27,* 1410–1414.

Finn, P., & Ingham, R.J. (1989). The selection of "fluent" samples in research on stuttering: Conceptual and methodological considerations. *Journal of Speech and Hearing Research, 32,* 401–418.

Guitar, B., Guitar, C., Neilson, P., O'Dwyer, N., & Andrews, G. (1988). Onset sequencing of selected lip muscles in stutterers and nonstutterers. *Journal of Speech and Hearing Research, 31,* 28–35.

Hayden, P.A., Jordahl, N., & Adams, M.R. (1982). Stutterers' voice initiation times during conditions of novel stimulation. *Journal of Fluency Disorders, 7,* 1–7.

Healey, E.C., & Adams, M.R. (1981). Speech timing skills of normally fluent and stuttering children and adults. *Journal of Fluency Disorders, 6,* 233–246.

Healey, E.C., & Ramig, P.R. (1986). Acoustic measures of stutterers' and nonstutterers' fluency in two speech contexts. *Journal of Speech and Hearing Research, 29,* 325–331.

Horii, Y., & Ramig, P.R. (1987). Pause and utterance durations and fundamental frequency characteristics of repeated oral reading by stutterers and nonstutterers. *Journal of Fluency Disorders, 12,* 257–270.

Janssen, P., Wieneke, G., & Vaane, E. (1983). Variability in the initiation of articulatory movements in the speech of stutterers and normal speakers. *Journal of Fluency Disorders, 8,* 341–358.

Kelly, E.M., & Conture, E.G. (1988). Acoustic and perceptual correlates of adult stutterers' typical and imitated stutterings. *Journal of Fluency Disorders, 13,* 233–252.

Liebetrau, R.M., & Daly, D.A. (1981). Auditory processing and perceptual abilities of "organic" and "functional" stutterers. *Journal of Fluency Disorders, 6,* 219–232.

McClean, M.D. (1987). Surface EMG recording of the perioral reflexes: Preliminary observations on stutterers and nonstutterers. *Journal of Speech and Hearing Research, 30,* 283–287.

McClean-Muse, A., Larson, C.R., & Gregory, H.H. (1988). Stutterers' and nonstutterers' voice fundamental frequency changes in response to auditory stimuli. *Journal of Speech and Hearing Research, 31,* 549–555.

Meyers, S.C., Hughes, L.F., & Shoney, Z.G. (1989). Temporal-phonemic processing skills in adult stutterers and nonstutterers. *Journal of Speech and Hearing Research, 32,* 274–280.

Moore, W.H. (1984). Hemispheric alpha asymmetries during an electromyographic biofeedback procedure for stuttering: A single-subject experimental design. *Journal of Fluency Disorders, 9,* 143–162.

Moore, W.H. (1986). Hemispheric alpha asymmetries of stutterers and nonstutterers for the recall and recognition of words and connected reading passages: Some relationships to severity of stuttering. *Journal of Fluency Disorders, 11,* 71–89.

Moore, W.H., Craven, D., & Faber, M. (1982). Hemispheric alpha asymmetries of words with positive, negative, and neutral arousal values preceding tasks of recall and recognition: Electrophysiological and behavioral results from stuttering males and nonstuttering males and females. *Brain and Language, 17,* 211–224.

Moore, W.H., Flowers, P., & Chunko, C. (1981). Some relationships between adaptation and electromyographic activity at laryngeal and masseter sites in stutterers. *Journal of Fluency Disorders, 6,* 81–94.

Neilson, P.D., Andrews, G., Guitar, B.E., & Quinn, P.T. (1979). Tonic stretch reflexes in lip, tongue, and jaw muscles. *Brain Research, 178,* 311–327.

Newman, P.W., Channell, R., & Palmer, M.L. (1986). A comparative study of the independence of unilateral ocular motor control in stutterers and nonstutterers. *Journal of Fluency Disorders, 11,* 105–116.

Newman, P.W., Harris, R.W., & Hilton, L.M. (1987). Vocal jitter and shimmer in stuttering. *Journal of Fluency Disorders, 14,* 87–96.

Nowack, W.J., & Stone, R.E. (1987). Acquired stuttering and bilateralcerebral disease. *Journal of Fluency Disorders, 12,* 141–146.

Peters, H.F., & Hulstijn, W. (1984). Stuttering and anxiety: The difference between stutterers and nonstutterers in verbal apprehension and physiologic arousal during the anticipation of speech and non-speech tasks. *Journal of Fluency Disorders, 9,* 67–84.

Pinsky, S.D., & McAdam, D.W. (1980). Electroencephalographic and dichotic indices of cerebral laterality in stutterers. *Brain and Language, 11,* 374–397.

Prosek, R.A., Montgomery, A.A., Walden, B.E., & Hawkins, D.B. (1987). Formant frequencies of stuttered and fluent vowels. *Journal of Speech and Hearing Research, 30,* 301–305.

Rastatter, M.P., & Dell, C.W. (1987a). Simple visual versus lexical decision vocal reaction times of stuttering and normal subjects. *Journal of Fluency Disorders, 12,* 63–69.

Rastatter, M.P., & Dell, C.W. (1987b). Vocal reaction times of stuttering subjects to tachistoscopically presented concrete and abstract words: A closer look at cerebral dominance and language processing. *Journal of Speech and Hearing Research, 30,* 306–310.

Rastatter, M.P., & Dell, C.W. (1988). Reading reaction times of stuttering and nonstuttering subjects to unilaterally presented concrete and abstract words. *Journal of Fluency Disorders, 13,* 319–329.

Rastatter, M.P., & Loren, C.A. (1987). Visual coding dominance in stuttering: Some evidence from central tachistoscopic stimulation (tachistoscopic viewing and stuttering). *Journal of Fluency Disorders, 13,* 89–96.

Rastatter, M.P., Loren, C., & Colcord, R. (1987). Visual coding strategies and hemisphere dominance characteristics of stutterers. *Journal of Fluency Disorders, 12,* 304–316.

Rastatter, M.P., McGuire, R.A., & Loren, C. (1987). Linguistic encoding dominance in stuttering: Some evidence for temporal and qualitative hemispheric processing differences. *Journal of Fluency Disorders, 13,* 215–224.

Rosenfield, D.B. (1980). Cerebral dominance and stuttering. *Journal of Fluency Disorders, 5,* 171–186.

Rosenfield, D.B. (1982). The brain and the stutterer. *Journal of Fluency Disorders, 7,* 81–92.

Rosenfield, D.B., & Goodglass, H. (1980). Dichotic testing of cerebral dominance in stutterers. *Brain and Language, 11,* 170–180.

Sacco, P.R., & Metz, D.E. (1987). Changes in stutterers' fundamental frequency contours following therapy. *Journal of Fluency Disorders, 12,* 1–8.

Sacco, P.R., & Metz, D.E. (1989). Comparison of period-by-period fundamental frequency of stutterers and nonstutterers over repeated utterances. *Journal of Speech and Hearing Research, 32,* 439–444.

Shapiro, A.I. (1980). An electromyographic analysis of the fluent and dysfluent utterances of several types of stutterers. *Journal of Fluency Disorders, 5,* 203–232.

Smith, A. (1989). Neural drive to muscles in stuttering. *Journal of Speech and Hearing Research, 32,* 252–264.

Starkweather, C.W. (1982). Stuttering and laryngeal behavior: A review. *ASHA Monographs, 21,* 1–45.

Starkweather, C.W. (1984). On fluency. *Journal of the National Student Speech-Language-Hearing Association, 12,* 30–37.

Starkweather, C.W., Franklin, S., & Smigo, T.M. (1984). Vocal and finger reaction times in stutterers and nonstutterers: Differences and correlations. *Journal of Speech and Hearing Research, 27,* 193–196.

Strub, R.L., Black, F.W., & Naeser, M.A. (1987). Anomalous dominance in sibling stutterers: Evidence from CT scan asymmetries, dichotic listening, neuropsychological testing, and handedness. *Brain and Language, 30,* 338–350.

Sussman, H.M. (1982). Contrastive patterns of intrahemispheric interference to verbal and spatial concurrent tasks in right-handed, left-handed and stuttering populations. *Neuropsychologia, 20,* 675–684.

Timmons, B.A. (1982). Physiological factors related to delayed auditory feedback and stuttering: A review. *Perceptual and Motor Skills, 55,* 1179–1189.

Venkatagiri, H.S. (1982). Reaction time for /s/ and /z/ in stutterers and nonstutterers: A test of the discoordination hypothesis. *Journal of Communication Disorders, 15,* 55–68.

Watson, B.C., & Alfonso, P.J. (1982). A comparison of LRT and VOT values between stutterers and nonstutterers. *Journal of Fluency Disorders, 7,* 219–242.

Watson, B.C., & Alfonso, P.J. (1983). Foreperiod and stuttering severity effects on acoustic laryngeal reaction time. *Journal of Fluency Disorders, 8,* 183–205.

Watson, B.C., & Alfonso, P.J. (1987). Physiological bases of acoustic LRT in nonstutterers, mild stutterers, and severe stutterers. *Journal of Speech and Hearing Research, 30,* 434–447.

Webster, W.G. (1986). Neuropsychological models of stuttering. II: Interhemispheric interference. *Neuropsychologia, 24,* 737–741.

Weiner, A.E. (1984). Patterns of vocal fold movement during stuttering. *Journal of Fluency Disorders, 9,* 31–50.

Wilkins, C., Webster, R.L., & Morgan, B.T. (1984). Cerebral lateralization of visual stimulus recognition in stutterers and fluent speakers. *Journal of Fluency Disorders, 9,* 131–142.

Wood, F., Stump, D., McKeehan, A., Sheldon, S., & Proctor, J. (1980). Patterns of regional cerebral blood flow during attempted reading aloud by stutterers both on and off haloperidol medication: Evidence for inadequate left frontal activation during stuttering. *Brain and Language, 9,* 141–144.

Wynne, M.K., & Boehmler, R.M. (1982). Central auditory function in fluent and disfluent speakers. *Journal of Speech and Hearing Research, 25,* 54–57.

Yoshioka, H., & Lofqvist, A. (1981). Laryngeal involvement in stuttering. A glottographic observation using a reaction time paradigm. *Folia Phoniatrica, 33,* 348–357.

Zimmermann, G. (1980). Articulatory behaviors associated with stuttering: A cinefluorographic analysis. *Journal of Speech and Hearing Research, 23,* 108–121.

CHAPTER FOUR

Diagnosis of Stuttering

The evaluation of stuttering in children and adults involves the careful observation and documentation of a number of behaviors and factors related to the disorder. The process of evaluation involves the determination of the nature of the problem as well as psychosocial, psycholinguistic, and physiologic factors that may accompany the disorder. Our primary concern as speech-language pathologists is to determine if a stuttering problem exists in individuals ranging in age from very young children (i.e., preschoolers) to adults who have been stuttering for several years. If a fluency problem is discovered, then the diagnostic information that is obtained will assist a clinician both in planning an appropriate treatment program and remedial procedures and in making a judgment regarding the prognosis.

In a typical stuttering evaluation, basic diagnostic information—such as the frequency, type, and duration of the stuttering in a variety of linguistically complex speaking situations (i.e., reading, monologues, telephone conversations)—is usually videotaped and audiotaped for analysis. Analyses of the stuttering with a number of speaking partners and situations outside of the clinic are also obtained. In addition to analyzing the stuttering in a number of contexts, a detailed history of the problem is acquired. From the case history we may find that there is a familial pattern to the disorder, a delay in articulation and language development, and/or some type of interpersonal behavior disorder or attention deficit. Moreover, a speech-language pathologist will want to describe the characteristics of the fluency problem; identify the primary environmental factors that contribute to the problem; identify verbal and nonverbal secondary coping behaviors associated with the stuttering; discover any negative attitudes or feelings that a stutterer has about the stuttering; and determine the overall severity of the stuttering. An interesting article by Martin, Haroldson, and Woessner concerning the perceptual scaling of stuttering severity leads off this chapter.

Before we discuss some aspects of the differential diagnosis of children and adults who stutter, an important issue related to the identification of stuttering needs to be addressed. The issue is concerned with the exact nature of the nonfluent problem we are evaluating. For instance, the term *stuttering* can refer to a number of different types of behaviors such as the repetition of sounds, words, or phrases and/or the hesitations, pauses, and interjections that occur in everyone's conversational speech. To date, no one has been able to develop a universally accepted definition of stuttering. Consequently, there is a great deal of confusion as to what stuttering is and how it differs from the nonfluencies that a normally fluent individual produces. Perhaps some of the disagreement about what stuttering reflects is related to the fact that stuttering and fluency can be considered a continuum of speech behavior that does not have well-specified boundaries (Adams & Runyan, 1981).

An interesting paradox about the identification of stuttering is that clinicians and researchers are confident that they can differentiate stutterers from nonstutterers but cannot agree on the specific types of behaviors that are used to separate the two sets of speakers. The types of disfluencies that lead to the identification of stuttering is still a source of much controversy and debate.

The profession's inability to resolve this issue has led to confusion and disagreement regarding the definition of stuttering and, in turn, its use in the perceptual evaluation of stuttering (Ingham, 1984). Some experts suggest that we should define stuttering in terms of specific speech behaviors that differentiate stutterers from nonstutterers. The definition of stuttering provided by Wingate (1964) has proved to be the most frequently used in the last 20 years. Wingate (1964) stated that stuttering is the "disruption in the fluency of verbal expression, which is characterized by involuntary, audible or silent, repetitions, or prolongations in the utterance of short speech elements, namely: sounds, syllables, and words of one syllable. These disruptions usually occur frequently or are marked in character and are not readily controllable" (p. 488). Although some believe that this definition is too narrow in scope and contains vague terminology, it continues to be the most referenced definition of stuttering.

In contrast to Wingate's definition of stuttering is the notion that stuttering is a perceptual event and should be defined in a broad sense as a "moment of stuttering." This refers to instances in the forward flow of speech in which a listener perceives some variation from a normal, fluent utterance. Although evaluating stuttering from the perspective of moments of stuttering seems easier than using a standard definition, it may not be as reliable as a definition that contains specific behaviors to identify. In 1981, Martin and Haroldson conducted a study to determine if listeners were more reliable in identifying stuttering when using a standard definition or moments of stuttering. They found that listeners who used the standard definition were not as reliable as those who were simply told to identify stuttering and given no further instructions. This article is included in this chapter so that readers can evaluate the Martin and Haroldson findings more closely.

Readers are also referred to the professional exchange that took place about this issue among Martin and Haroldson (1986), Wingate (1984), and Perkins (1984, 1986). The correspondence between Martin and Haroldson and Perkins in 1986 is reprinted in this chapter. The information in these letters is important because Perkins proposed a new perspective on how we should define stuttering.

Rather than use listener judgments, Perkins suggested that stuttering represented a temporary, overt, and covert involuntary loss of the ability to move forward through an utterance fluently. Thus, according to Perkins, the best way to know whether a stuttering moment occurred is to ask the stutterer. From this perspective, listener judgments become meaningless. Perkins' position is noteworthy because it shifts the identification of stuttering from the listener to the stutterer, the person who is experiencing the real or expected involuntary loss of control of speaking.

Given the lack of consensus about how to define stuttering, it is interesting that speech-language pathologists appear to do reasonably well in determining whether someone is a stutterer or a normally fluent individual. This is particularly true if the stuttering is frequent enough to call attention to itself and/or the person has been stuttering for several years. However, one age group that is sometimes difficult to evaluate is preschoolers, the age range when stuttering is known to begin. In evaluating young children who are disfluent, attention is focused on differentiating between a normally fluent child and a child showing signs of beginning to stutter. Many times, the normal hesitations and repetitions produced by young children can be confused with stuttering behavior. The article by Pindzola and White in this chapter provides us with specific guidelines that can assist the clinician in making the best possible judgment as to whether or not a child is exhibiting a fluency disorder. Although the guidelines are clear and well defined, the ultimate decision about whether a fluency problem exists resides with the clinician.

In addition to the guidelines mentioned above, a clinician might also want to assess a child's overall speech and language abilities. Articulation skills, expressive and receptive language abilities, and pragmatic language use are other important areas to evaluate in addition to the stuttering (Blood and Seider, 1981). Moreover, a clinician might want to assess the parent's speech rate and the level of the language complexity used during conversational interaction with their disfluent child. It is thought that the frequency of a child's stuttering could increase if the parents speak consistently with a rapid rate and an adult linguistic pattern.

When evaluating upper-elementary-grade children and adolescent stutterers, the stuttering pattern will be well established and somewhat more predictable than seen in young children. Typically, these children are referred to a speech-language pathologist for evaluation by a parent or teacher who has expressed some concern about the child's fluency. The assessment process in these cases involves the clarification and verification of a stuttering problem. Evaluations of the frequency and types of stuttering behaviors, attitudes about the problem, as well as language, learning, and other motor speech skill tests are conducted. If necessary, a psychological evaluation is recommended in order to determine if a stuttering child exhibits any inappropriate interpersonal behaviors that result from being a stutterer.

The diagnosis of adult stutterers typically involves having clients describe the present status of their fluency problem and discuss any changes in the stuttering that have occurred in the last few years. The evaluation process is focused on both the specification of the disfluent speech behavior and the client's attitudes about stuttering and motivation for enrolling in a treatment program. Stutterers with a long history of stuttering will have, most likely, adopted some negative feelings and reactions to the stuttering as a function of being a stutterer. These inner feelings and communication attitudes of a stutterer might be difficult to assess, but they can be evaluated indirectly through the use of the Erickson Scale (S24), which is a series of true/false questions that pertain to stutterers' reactions to their stuttering. The Erickson S24 scale was adapted from the original 39-item scale (Erickson, 1969) by Andrews and Cutler (1974) who found the S24 scale to be more valid and reliable than the original Erickson scale. The Erickson S24 scale can be found at the end of the Andrews and Cutler article cited in the references.

Other self-analysis and rating scales such as the self-efficacy scale constructed by Ornstein and Manning (1985) and the locus of control scale for stuttering developed by Craig, Franklin, and Andrews (1984) might also be used. Most recently, Watson, examined the difference between stutterers' and nonstutterers' communication attitudes through an inventory of affective, cognitive, and behavioral self-reports. Detailed information about the communication inventory and the results of this study can be found in the final reading contained in this chapter.

REFERENCES

Adams, M. R., & Runyan, C. M. (1981). Stuttering and fluency: Exclusive events or points on a continuum? *Journal of Fluency Disorders, 6,* 197–216.

Andrews, G., & Cutler, J. (1974). Stuttering therapy: The relation between changes in symptom level and attitude. *Journal of Speech and Hearing Disorders, 39,* 309–311.

Blood, G. and Seider, R. (1981). The concomitant problems of young stutterers. *Journal of Speech and Hearing Disorders, 46,* 31–33.

Craig, A. R., Franklin, J. A., & Andrews, G. (1984). A scale to measure locus of control of behaviour. *British Journal of Medical Psychology, 57,* 173–180.

Erickson, R. L. (1969). Assessing communication attitudes among stutterers. *Journal of Speech and Hearing Research, 1,* 12–22.

Ingham, R. J. (1984). *Stuttering and behavior therapy.* San Diego: College-Hill Press.

Martin, R., & Haroldson, S. K. (1986). Stuttering as involuntary loss of speech control: Barking up a new tree. *Journal of Speech and Hearing Disorders, 51,* 187–190.

Ornstein, A. F., & Manning, W. H. (1985). Self-efficacy scaling by adult stutterers. *Journal of Communication Disorders, 18,* 313–320.

Perkins, W. H. (1984). Stuttering as a categorical event: Barking up the wrong tree: Reply to Wingate. *Journal of Speech and Hearing Disorders, 49,* 431–434.

Perkins, W. H. (1986). More bite for a bark: Epilogue to Martin and Haroldson's letter. *Journal of Speech and Hearing Disorders, 51,* 190–191.

Wingate, M. E. (1964). A standard definition of stuttering. *Journal of Speech and Hearing Disorders, 29,* 484–489.

Wingate, M. E. (1984). Definition is the problem. *Journal of Speech and Hearing Disorders, 49,* 429–431.

Perceptual Scaling
of Stuttering Severity

Richard R. Martin
Samuel K. Haroldson
Garry L. Woessner

Measuring the severity of stuttering is an important consideration for professional workers interested in the area of stuttering. At first glance, identifying and assessing the severity of stuttering does not appear to pose a substantial problem. Upon closer inspection, however, determining the severity of stuttering is not always a straightforward activity. Statements such as "He stutters only occasionally," or "She stutters so severely that at times she simply can't talk," or "His stuttering gets worse when he's excited" do not carry sufficient accuracy to support meaningful clinical or laboratory research. It is not surprising, therefore, that a sizable body of experimental and clinical literature relating to stuttering severity has accumulated. It also probably is not surprising that professional workers have differing views on the preferred method for assessing and expressing the severity of stuttering. Ingham (1984), for example, believes that identifying and counting the number of stutterings or disfluencies is the most common and preferable dependent variable in the stuttering clinic or laboratory. Ingham (1984) indicates that the reasons stuttering counts are preferable is because they are "easy to administer, relatively precise, and may make a direct contribution to treatment" (p. 25). Cooper and Cooper (1985), on the other hand, express the notion that listener judgment is the most advantageous procedure for determining stuttering severity. These authors state that

> These instruments are based on the assumption that stuttering frequency may be the single *least* reliable and valid measure of stuttering severity, and that informed severity judgments are the single *most* reliable and valid measure of stuttering severity. For too long, too many clinicians have judged client progress in therapy on the basis of what might best be termed the *frequency fallacy*. . . . In an overzealous attempt to arrive at numbers on which to base clinical decisions, clinicians and researchers overlook the unreliability and the meaningless-

ness of stuttering frequency counts obtained in clinical situations. Therapy program creators go so far as to design progressions of therapeutic activities based on stuttering frequency counts obtained solely in the clinical situation. Is it any wonder that clients experience transfer problems from the clinic to the home, school, or office? (p. 37).

Historically, stuttering severity has been assessed and reported using one of three general procedures. The first of these involves statements or judgments about the overall severity of an individual stutterer's problem. Such a statement typically includes a consideration of the stutterer's speech behaviors, associated "secondary" behaviors, avoidance behaviors, and attitudinal behaviors. It is common for such global severity assessments to involve both objective and subjective measuring procedures. The Stuttering Severity (SS) Scale (Lanyon, 1967) and the Clinicians Perceptions of Stuttering Severity Scale (Cooper and Cooper, 1985) are two frequently employed overall stuttering severity scales.

A second procedure for assessing and reporting stuttering severity involves statements about the severity of stuttering derived from more or less objective measures of disfluency (disfluency type, disfluency frequency, disfluency duration, and speaking rate). Frequently, such assessments involve objective counts of specific struggle behaviors involving the speech musculature and/or associated "secondary" musculature. The Iowa Scale for Rating Severity of Stuttering (Johnson et al., 1963) is a widely used stuttering severity scale of the type discussed here. Another more recently developed severity instrument of this type is the Stuttering Severity Instrument (SSI) for Children and Adults (Riley, 1984).

A third procedure often used to assess stuttering severity involves statements derived from subjective observer judgments about the stuttering severity of words or specified speech samples. Typically, observers use psychophysical procedures such as equal-appearing-intervals or direct magnitude-estimation to scale their perceptions about the stuttering severity of a particular sample of speech. This paper reviews the available information about the perceptual scaling of stuttering severity and reports the results of two experiments designed to yield additional data about the subjective scaling of stuttering severity.

SCALING STUTTERING SEVERITY

Much of the early work concerning the psychophysical scaling of stuttering severity was conducted by Sherman and her colleagues at the University of Iowa. Initially, Lewis and Sherman (1951) conducted a study in which they had judges scale stuttering severity of 9-sec speech samples on a nine-point equal-appearing-intervals scale. These investigators found that reliable judgments of stuttering severity could be obtained from groups of observers. The experimenters also constructed training tapes containing 33 samples of stuttering representing a wide range of scaled severity. Publication in 1951 of the Lewis and Sherman equal-appearing-intervals procedures for scaling stuttering severity spawned much subsequent research relative to the psychological scaling of stuttering severity. This research has yielded a good deal of information about a number of variables that affect the scaling of stuttering severity.

Type of Scale

As indicated above, Sherman and her colleagues and students developed the nine-point equal-appearing-intervals scale of stuttering severity in the early 1950s, and this scale was employed in the majority of early studies involved with scaling stuttering severity (Aron, 1967; Hoops & Wilkinson, 1973; Lewis & Sherman, 1951; Naylor, 1953; Schiavetti, 1975; Sherman, 1952, 1955; Sherman & McDermott, 1958; Sherman & Trotter, 1956; Trotter, 1955, 1956; Trotter & Kools, 1955; Williams et al., 1963; Young, 1961, 1969a, 1969b, 1970; Young & Prather, 1962). In a widely cited and informative study, Cullinan, Prather, and Williams (1963) found only very small differences in either mean scale values or reliability among equal-interval scales with five, seven, or nine points. Consistent with the Cullinan et al. results, numerous experiments have been reported in which scales with other than nine points were employed: Curran and Hood (1977a, 1977b), 15 points; Rousey (1958), 7 points; Myers (1978), 6 points; and Manning, Emal, and Jamison (1975), 5 points.

In addition to the number of scale points utilized, data have been obtained about the amount of description associated with the scale points. In general, the experimental data indicate that reliability is not enhanced and scale values are not systematically different when scale points are accompanied by detailed or elaborated descriptions (Cullinan et al., 1963). Closely related to the description of scale points are the anchoring and sequencing effects reported by Young (1970). Relative to the anchoring effect, Young found that, when observers were allowed to hear samples representing the most and least severe stuttering, "maximum discrimina-

tion" among the samples being rated occurred when the anchors were "just slightly beyond" the severity range of the stimulus samples. Concerning the sequence effect, Young found that the scale value assigned to a given sample tended to influence the value assigned to the subsequent sample.

Berry and Silverman (1972) reported experimental results that cast doubt on the assumption that the nine-point equal-appearing-intervals scale indeed possesses equal intervals. Berry and Silverman asked observers to judge the size of the nine-point scale intervals relative to the standard (width of interval from scale value "4" to "5"). The judges rated the lower intervals ("1" to "2," "2" to "3," "3" to "4") to be approximately one-half as wide as the standard. These authors concluded that the original Lewis and Sherman nine-point equal-appearing-intervals scale for rating stuttering severity probably is an ordinal, rather than interval, scale.

Although equal-appearing-intervals scaling has been the most frequently used procedure for scaling stuttering severity, the method of direct magnitude-estimation also has been employed. Cullinan et al. (1963) compared the results of observers rating stuttering severity on a direct magnitude-estimation scale with observers rating stuttering severity on a five-, seven-, or nine-point interval scale. The authors reported no significant differences in group intrajudge reliability between the scales but reported that the group inter-judge reliability for the magnitude-estimation procedure was significantly lower than for any of the interval scales. In a later study, however, Martin (1965) found intraclass reliability coefficients of .90 or higher for each of 15 speech samples rated for stuttering severity using the direct magnitude-estimation scaling procedure.

Type of Speech Sample

A number of different kinds of speech samples have been scaled for stuttering severity. As part of their original experiment, Lewis and Sherman (1951) found that observers could rate reliably 9-sec samples of oral reading. Similar results have been reported by Cullinan et al. (1963), using 20-sec samples; Martin (1965), using 15-sec samples; and Young (1970), using 200-word samples. A number of studies have been reported in which observers scaled stuttering severity for longer speech samples. For example, Rousey (1958) utilized 4-min speech samples. Aron (1967) obtained nine-point severity ratings after five readings of the Rainbow Passage, and Naylor (1953) had stutterers make nine-point severity ratings of their own stuttering during the past "several months." Sherman (1955) extended the usefulness of scaling speech samples by demonstrating that observers could scale reliably the severity of stuttering for successive 10-sec periods during longer readings. In a number of experiments, observers have made reliable ratings of stuttering severity of individual words or instances of stuttering (Sherman & McDermott, 1958; Sherman & Trotter, 1956; Trotter, 1955, 1956). Not only has the severity of individual instances of stuttering been scaled but these instances have been scaled and analyzed differently in terms of such characteristics as disfluency type (Curran & Hood, 1977a, 1977b; Manning et al., 1975; Schiavetti, 1975), disfluency locus (Schiavetti, 1975), and word "conspicuousness" (Trotter, 1956).

Whether observers are presented audible, visible, or audible-visible portions of the speech sample is at least partially related to the magnitude and reliability of scaled stuttering severity. Williams, Wark, and Minifie (1963) found that the mean scale values of stuttering severity did not differ significantly among audible, visible, and combined samples but that observer reliability was lower in the visible condition. Martin (1965) found that audible-visible samples were rated significantly more severe than audible only samples. Aron (1967) reported that the addition of visual cues apparently had little effect on observers' severity of stuttering ratings.

Finally, although it has not been studied systematically, there is no evidence in the experimental literature to suggest that either the assigned scale values or observer reliability differ depending on whether the speech sample consists of oral reading or spontaneous speech.

Rater Characteristics

A consistent finding in studies relative to the scaling of stuttering severity is that the background experience of the rater is not a crucial variable. Groups of laymen unsophisticated about stuttering, undergraduate and graduate college students, undergraduate speech-language pathology students, graduate speech-language pathology students, experienced speech-language clinicians, elementary teachers, parents of stuttering children, and parents of nonstuttering children have not generated significantly different mean scale values of stuttering severity (Aron, 1967; Cullinan et al., 1963; Curran & Hood, 1977a, 1977b; Lewis & Sherman, 1951; Martin, 1965; Schiavetti, 1975; Trotter & Kools, 1955). Even groups of stutterers have not assigned significantly different severity scale values to speech samples of other stutterers than have groups of sophisticated or unsophisticated observers (Martin, 1965; Young, 1961). An interesting, and as yet unexplained, experimental result that seems to be an exception is the finding of Hoops and Wilkinson (1973) that a group of "advanced" speech-pathology students consistently assigned lower scale values of stuttering severity than either freshmen college students or elementary teachers.

The extent to which training of observers or practice by observers influences subsequent stuttering severity scaling has been the subject of a number of experiments. In their early experiments with the nine-point equal-appearing-intervals procedure, Sherman and her colleagues subjected observers to a rather extensive training procedure complete with recorded training tapes and practice rating sessions (Lewis & Sherman, 1951; Sherman, 1952, 1955; Sherman &

McDermott, 1958; Trotter, 1955). It is interesting that, beginning in the 1960s, the experimental convention of training observers to judge stuttering severity simply ceased. Few, if any, studies have been reported since 1960 in which raters received extensive training prior to scaling stuttering severity. The effects of rater practice on the assignment of subsequent scale values, however, has been explored experimentally. Lewis and Sherman (1951), Sherman (1955), and Young (1969a) found that experience with the scaling task alone was not sufficient to change the mean scale values or rater agreement. In an informative study, Young (1969b) provided raters with the group mean rating immediately following their severity ratings on each 20-sec sample. Young found that receiving feedback on the group mean ratings did not change interrater agreement.

The empirical observation that various types of observers can scale stuttering severity reliably without elaborate training or practice and without knowledge of results suggests that individual observers have a relatively stable perception about the various degrees of stuttering severity. This stability was evident in results of a study by Curran and Hood (1977b). These investigators had one group of observers rate severity with essentially no instructions, one group rate the same samples but with the instructions that the children were stutterers in therapy having "a great deal of difficulty talking," and a third group rate the same sample but with the instruction that the children had just been released from therapy and were "now doing a good job with their talking and fluency." Curran and Hood found no significant difference in mean severity ratings among the three groups.

Rater Reliability

In their initial experiment, Lewis and Sherman (1951) assessed rater reliability. They had 106 students judge 96 speech samples on a nine-point scale of stuttering severity on two separate occasions. The Pearson correlation coefficient between the first and second ratings across all observers and all samples was .96. In addition, the difference in mean scale values between the first and second rating was not statistically significant. Lewis and Sherman also correlated the scale values for 52 raters with those of 54 different raters. The correlation was .97, and once again the difference between mean scale values was not significant. On the basis of these results, Lewis and Sherman concluded that the nine-point equal-appearing-intervals technique for scaling stuttering severity produced satisfactory inter- and intraobserver reliability. In 1955, Sherman again assessed both intra- and interobserver agreement using correlational procedures and concluded that both groups of observers and individual observers could reliably place samples in relative positions along the severity dimension. Sherman pointed out, however, that observers did not necessarily agree on the absolute scale value for any sample. Sherman and McDermott (1958) reported high intraclass correlations between observers' ratings of the first 5 sec, the first 10 sec, the first

15 sec, and the entire 20 sec of a 20-sec speech sample. The authors also reported high correlations for the severity ratings of each of six raters with a group of raters.

In 1963, Cullinan et al. reported what has become an almost definitive study relative to observer reliability for scaling stuttering severity. Cullinan et al. found that intraobserver reliability was low for both the equal-intervals and magnitude-estimation procedures. These authors calculated that, if three or four independent ratings could be made of the same sample by the same judge, reliable mean scale values could be obtained using either magnitude-estimation or equal-intervals procedures. In terms of interrater reliability, Cullinan et al. found group reliability high for both rating procedures, but average individual reliability was unsatisfactory.

In a series of experiments designed to study the effects of certain procedural variables on scaling stuttering severity, Young (1969a, 1969b, 1970) assessed both intra- and interobserver reliability. In general, the results of Young's studies were in agreement with those reported by Cullinan et al. (1963). Groups of observers could reliably assign samples along a stuttering severity dimension, but individual raters differed considerably in terms of the absolute scale value assigned to any sample. These results pose a serious question about the confidence that can be placed in the results of case studies or single-subject studies in which one observer, often the clinician or experimenter, makes judgments about stuttering severity across times and treatments. There has been one study reported, however, in which a single observer has demonstrated the ability to scale stuttering severity reliably over time and across treatments. Aron (1967), as part of a larger study, had 46 stutterers read a passage five times in succession on three separate occasions. The experimenter rated stuttering severity of the entire five readings on a nine-point scale. Correlations between mean scale values of the first, second, and third reading occasions were from .95 to .97. A month after the subjects completed the study, five "qualified speech therapists" independently judged stuttering severity from tape recordings of the second and third reading occasions. Correlations between the experimenter's ratings and each judge's rating ranged from .85 to .92 for the first reading and from .86 to .93 for the second reading.

Some information has been reported about rater reliability for scaling stuttering severity when scaling procedures other than a nine-point equal-appearing-intervals scale were utilized. Martin (1965) had different groups of observers make stuttering severity ratings using a direct magnitude-estimation procedure. He reported that intraclass reliability coefficients were satisfactory for both the group and the average individual rater. Also, the rate-rerate correlations for each of the 15 samples were all .90 or higher. Curran and Hood (1977a) had observers rate severity of stuttering or disfluency types on a 15-point scale on two occasions. They found a rate-rerate correlation of .90. Rousey (1958), using a seven-point scale, had observers rate 4-min speech samples of stutterers and rerate 20 of the samples at a later time. Rousey obtained a rate-rerate correlation of .97.

EXPERIMENT I

The purpose of this experiment was to investigate two heretofore unstudied aspects of perceptually scaling stuttering severity. The first question concerned the relationship between judged severity of a speech sample and judged severity of individual instances of stuttering within that speech sample; the second concerned the relationship between identification and judged severity of individual instances of stuttering.

Method

Speech Samples. Ten-minute tape recordings were obtained from 30 adult stutterers speaking spontaneously. The experimenter selected one 15-sec sample from each tape recording. The samples were selected to represent a wide range of stuttering frequency and severity. Each sample contained at least one instance of stuttering in the judgment of the experimenter. The number of words in the sample ranged from 16 to 50. Each of the thirty 15-sec samples was dubbed six times in succession onto a master tape. A 7-sec silent interval separated all samples. The master stimulus tape was approximately 66 min in length.

Protocols. Verbatim lexical transcripts were prepared for each speech sample. Disfluencies such as repetitions, prolongations, and interjections were omitted from the transcripts. Transcripts of five samples were typed on a single page. At the top of each page a horizontal line of approximately 4 inches was drawn and divided evenly by nine short, vertical lines labeled "1" through "9." Above the left line ("1") was typed the word "mild" and above the right line ("9") was typed "severe." At the lower right of each sample on the transcript sheet was typed a short, blank line preceded by the words OVERALL SEVERITY.

Raters. Thirty graduate students in communication disorders served as raters. The raters were divided evenly into two groups (Groups A and B).

Procedure. A maximum of four raters were seated in student armchairs approximately 6 feet in front of a high-quality loudspeaker. The speaker was connected to an Ampex 440 audiotape recorder in an adjoining control room. Raters in Group A were given a packet of transcripts and the following instructions.

> In the packet are transcripts of a number of speech samples. The samples will be played over the speaker in the order they appear on your protocol.
> You will hear each sample six times in succession. For each playing of a sample, you are to do one of the following tasks in order.
> Playing 1 and 2. IDENTIFY EACH STUTTERED WORD. The first time the sample is played, draw a line under each word you consider to be stuttered. Use the second playing to verify or change your initial identifications of stuttered words.

Playing 3 and 4. RATE THE SEVERITY OF EACH INDIVIDUAL STUTTERED WORD. The third time the sample is played, use the 9-point scale at the top of the page to rate the stuttering severity of each underlined word. Write the appropriate scale number just above each underlined word. Use the fourth playing to verify or change the individual severity ratings you made during the third playing.

Playing 5 and 6. RATE THE OVERALL STUTTERING SEVERITY OF THE ENTIRE SAMPLE. The fifth time the sample is played, use the same scale to rate the stuttering severity of the entire sample. Enter this rating in the OVERALL SEVERITY blank following each sample. Use the sixth playing to verify or change the overall severity ratings made after the fifth playing.

Raters in Group B followed the same procedures and instructions except that they rated stuttering severity of the overall speech sample in readings 3 and 4 and individual stuttered words in readings 5 and 6. After all questions were resolved, the experimenter went into the control room and activated the tape recorder. The experimenter monitored the raters visually (one-way mirror) and auditorily (intercom) to ensure that the raters did not become lost or confused.

Results

Table 1 contains a summary of the experimental data for Group A, for Group B, and for the groups combined. Under Groups A and B, the $N = 450$ (15 raters $\times$ 30 samples); under combined, the $N = 900$ (30 raters $\times$ 30 samples). The first row in Table 1 gives the means and ranges of percent words identified as stuttered (underlined) per sample. The second row gives the means and ranges of stuttering severity scale values assigned to individual stuttered (underlined) words per sample. The third row gives the means and ranges of stuttering severity scale values assigned to overall speech samples.

Stuttering Severity Ratings. As indicated in Table 1, for both Group A and Group B raters, the mean stuttering severity scale value for individual stuttered words was lower than the mean stuttering severity scale value for the overall sample. To test the significance of the difference between these means, the data were submitted to a two-way analysis of variance in which the rating task (individual words versus overall sample) was a within factor and the task order (Group A versus Group B) was a between factor. The task by order interaction was not significant ($F = 3.58$; $df = 1, 28$; $p > 0.05$); the main effect for order was significant at the .05 but not at the .01 level ($F = 5.18$; $df = 1, 28$), and the main effect for task was significant ($F = 273.71$; $df = 1, 28$; $p < .01$). The finding that the task by order interaction was not significant but that the main effect for order was significant at the .05 level is problematic. To obtain additional information, t tests were calculated for the significance of the difference between task means in Group A and in Group B. Both t values (Group A: $t = 10.18$; $df = 14$; Group B: $t = 13.24$; $df = 14$) were significant beyond the .01 level. It seems reasonable to conclude, therefore, that in the present study raters in both Group A and Group B assigned significantly higher mean stuttering severity scale values to the overall speech sample than to the average individual stuttered word within the sample.

To investigate further the relationship between stuttering severity ratings for individual words and overall speech samples, a Pearson correlation coefficient was computed between the mean severity scale values assigned to individual stuttered words across raters and the mean severity values assigned to overall speech samples across raters. The resultant r of .78 indicated that raters who assigned high stuttering severity scale values to individual words also assigned high stuttering severity scale values to the overall speech sample. It is possible, of course, that the correlation between stuttering severity ratings of individual stuttered words and overall speech samples is spuriously high due to the influence of stuttering frequency. Accordingly, a partial correlation was calculated between mean severity ratings of individual stuttered words and overall speech samples with the effects of the number of stuttered words partialed out. The resulting r of .77 indicated that even when the variability due to the number of stuttered words in the different samples was removed, the relationship between severity ratings for individual stuttered words and overall speech samples remained high and positive.

Interrater Agreement. Interrater agreement for identifying stuttered words was computed in the following manner. The percent of raters who identified a specified word as stuttered was determined for each word. These percents were summed and divided by the total number of words identified as

TABLE 1. Means and ranges (in parentheses) of percent words identified as stuttered, stuttering severity scale values for words, and stuttering severity scale values for overall samples assigned by raters in Group A and Group B and the combined groups.

	Group A	Group B	Combined
Percent words identified as stuttered/sample	27.89	29.89	28.89
	(18.0–55.6)	(23.7–38.1)	(18.0–55.6)
Stuttering severity scale value for individual stuttered words/sample	3.73	4.04	3.88
	(2.32–5.77)	(3.59–4.77)	(2.32–5.77)
Stuttering severity scale value for overall speech sample/sample	4.77	5.35	5.06
	(3.77–6.33)	(4.32–6.07)	(3.77–6.33)

stuttered by at least one rater. The mean percent of interrater agreement on stuttered words was 44.5; that is, on the average, 44.5 percent of the raters agreed on the identification of a given stuttered moment.

Interrater agreement for scaling the severity of individual stuttered words was computed as follows. The modal stuttering severity scale value assigned by the raters to each stuttered word was determined. The interrater agreement for each stuttered word was expressed as the percent of raters who assigned a stuttering severity scale value at, or within plus or minus one scale value of, the modal scale value for the word. The percents for each individual word were summed and divided by the total number of words rated for stuttering severity. The mean percent agreement for assigning stuttering severity scale values to stuttered words was 79.8 percent; that is, 79.8 percent of the time a rater assigned a stuttering severity scale value to a given stuttered word, the scale value fell within plus or minus one of the modal scale value assigned by all raters to that word.

A similar analysis was performed to determine the interrater agreement for assigning stuttering severity scale values to overall speech samples. The resulting mean percent agreement was 74.1 percent, meaning that, 74.1 percent of the time a rater assigned a stuttering severity scale value to a given speech sample, the scale value fell within plus or minus one of the modal scale value assigned to that sample by all raters.

Identification and Scaled Severity of Stuttered Words.

In the present study, there were 52 words that all 30 raters identified as stuttered, and these were considered high-agreement words. A group of 52 words that only one rater identified as stuttered was selected randomly from all such words, and these were considered low-agreement words. The mean stuttering severity scale value for the 52 high-agreement words was 5.66; the mean for the low-agreement words was 2.83. A t test was computed on the difference between the two means and the t value of 9.76 was statistically significant ($df = 102$; $p < .001$). A Pearson correlation coefficient was computed between the percent interrater agreement for identification and the mean stuttering severity scale value across all 353 words identified by at least one rater as stuttered. The correlation was .91, indicating that, the higher the percent of raters who identified a word as stuttered, the higher the mean stuttering severity scale values assigned to that word.

EXPERIMENT II

The second study was designed to investigate the extent to which an individual observer can reliably rate the severity of individual instances of stuttering during "on-line" spontaneous speech.

Method

Subjects.   Twelve adult stutterers served as subjects for the present study.

Instrumentation.   Each subject was seated alone at a table in an experimental room. On the table were located a pair of earphones (TDH-39, housed in MX41-AR cushions), a microphone (Plantronics MS40-5), and a stack of 3×5 cards. On each card was typed a single noun.

The experimental room was connected to a control room by means of a one-way mirror and an intercom system. The earphones and microphone in the experimental room were patched through the wall and connected to an Artik delayed auditory feedback recorder. The recorder was adjusted so that the signal at the earphone was delayed approximately 250 msec from the signal at the microphone and was at a "comfortable loudness level."[1] Also housed in the control room were an Ampex 440 audiotape recorder, a panel of Grason-Stadler 1200 logic equipment, a Moduprint printing counter, and a panel containing seven pushbutton switches numbered "1" through "7." The button panel, logic system, and printing counter were connected and programmed so that, when a button on the panel was depressed, a "1" was registered in the left column of the printer and the button value ("1" through "7") was registered in the right column of the printer. All switch pulses were held in memory and automatically printed in chronological order at the end of each minute.

Procedure.   Subjects were seated in the experimental room and instructed to talk for about 40 min. They were told to talk about any topic and that they could use word cards if necessary to generate speaking topics. The headset, with microphone and earphones, was positioned. The microphone was adjusted so that it was 1.5 cm from the speaker's mouth and out of the direct breath stream. The subjects were advised that, at some point during the experiment, they would experience delayed auditory feedback but that they should continue talking.

In the control room, the experimenter listened to the subject and rated the severity of each perceived stuttering by pressing the appropriate button on the panel. The experimenter considered the button panel to be a seven-point equal-appearing-intervals scale, with "1" as least severe stuttering and "7" as most severe stuttering. During the first 10 min (pre), the subject spoke without DAF, and the experimenter judged severity. After 10 min, the DAF unit was activated automatically and remained active for the next 20 min (DAF 1, 10 min; DAF 2, 10 min). The DAF unit was switched off for the final 10 min (post). All sessions were audiotape recorded.

Reliability.   A 10-min portion of each subject's audiotape was selected randomly and dubbed onto a master reliability tape. The reliability tape contained twelve 10-min samples.

Two independent observers were asked to listen to the tape and rate the severity of each perceived stuttering using the same procedures and seven-button panel employed during the experiment. One observer was a graduate student in speech-language pathology (SO); the other was a college student with no courses or experience in speech-language pathology (UO). Approximately 2 months after the experimental sessions were completed, the experimenter rated stuttering severity on the reliability tape.

RESULTS

The means, ranges, and standard deviations of percent words stuttered, stuttering severity ratings, and words spoken per minute are given in Table 2. A one-way repeated measures analysis of variance was computed to determine if the percent words stuttered means differed significantly in the pre, DAF 1, DAF 2, and post periods. The resulting F value of 6.91 is significant beyond the .01 level. A Newman-Keuls analysis revealed that the mean percent of words stuttered was significantly less in DAF 1 than in pre and in DAF 2 than in pre. Percent words stuttered in post was significantly higher than in DAF 2. None of the other comparisons between means was significant.

Mean stuttering severity scale values in Table 2 also were subjected to a repeated-measures analyses of variance, and the F value of 5.61 was significant beyond the .01 level ($df = 3, 33$). Subsequent Newman-Keuls analyses revealed that mean stuttering severity in DAF 2 was significantly lower than in pre and that mean severity in post was significantly higher than in DAF 2. None of the other comparisons between means was significant.

Table 2 gives the means, standard deviations, and ranges of words spoken per minute by subjects in the various treatment periods. As indicated in the table, word output dropped slightly during the two DAF periods as compared with the pre period. A one-way repeated-measures analysis

of variance on these means, however, failed to reach statistical significance at the .05 level ($F = 2.68$; $df = 3, 33$).

Although studying the effects of DAF on the speech of stutterers was not the main purpose of the present experiment, the results are consistent with those reported in a number of previous studies; namely, in terms of group means, stutterers stutter less, speak louder, and speak somewhat slower under DAF than when speaking with normal auditory feedback.[2] In the present experiment, it was observed that rated stuttering severity, as well as stuttering frequency, were reduced substantially when the stutterers spoke under DAF. Of interest in the present study was the relationship between stuttering frequency and rated severity. For the pre, DAF 1, DAF 2, and post periods separately, a Pearson correlation coefficient was computed between subjects' mean stuttering frequency and mean stuttering severity scores. The correlations were .58, .74, .72, and .55 for the pre, DAF 1, DAF 2, and post periods, respectively.

Reliability. One major purpose of the present study was to explore the extent to which an observer can reliably assign stuttering severity scale values to individual instances of stuttering during continuous, spontaneous speech. As indicated earlier, reliability was assessed by having one sophisticated (SO) and one unsophisticated (UO) observer rate the severity of each instance of stuttering, and count the total words for each sample, on the reliability master tape. Comparable severity ratings and word counts were obtained from the experimenter's initial "on-line" ratings (OE) of the samples chosen for the reliability master tape and from the experimenter's subsequent rerating (RE) of the reliability master tape.

Pearson correlation coefficients were computed between all possible observer pairs for mean percent words stuttered, mean stuttering severity scale values, and mean words per minute on the reliability master tape. The correlations are given in Table 3. The correlations between OE and RE were calculated as dependent correlations and reflect

TABLE 2. Means, standard deviations, and ranges of percent words stuttered, mean stuttering severity scale value, and words per minute by 12 stutterers in the pre, DAF 1, DAF 2, and post periods.

	Pre	DAF 1	DAF 2	Post
Percent words stuttered				
Mean	15.7	10.0	8.8	12.9
S.D.	12.2	11.7	11.3	9.4
Range	4.0–48.8	0.7–47.0	0.4–45.2	5.0–39.7
Mean severity scale value				
Mean	−2.3	2.2	1.9	2.3
S.D.	0.6	0.7	0.7	0.7
Range	1.4–3.4	1.1–3.7	1.0–3.4	1.4–3.6
Words per minute				
Mean	81.9	66.9	68.3	78.2
S.D.	31.3	27.4	27.1	31.0
Range	25.6–131.3	15.1–107.6	19.7–115.3	20.9–129.2

TABLE 3. Correlation coefficients between all pairs of raters across 12 reliability speech samples.[a]

	RE	SO	UO
Mean percent words stuttered			
OE	.99	.88	.91
RE		.89	.91
SO			.98
Mean stuttering severity scale values			
OE	.99	.73	.75
RE		.74	.75
SO			.99
Mean words per minute			
OE	.99	.99	.99
RE		.99	.99
SO			.99

[a]OE, experimenter in original session; RE, experimenter rerate; SO, sophisticated observer; UO, unsophisticated observer.

intraobserver reliability. All other correlations in Table 3 were calculated as independent correlations and reflect interobserver reliability.

It is apparent from Table 3 that the various observers agreed closely with each other in terms of the mean words spoken per minute in the 12 reliability tape samples. With respect to mean percent words stuttered, all correlation coefficients were high and positive. The correlations for mean stuttering severity scale values also are high and positive. It is of interest to note that, for both mean percent words stuttered and mean stuttering severity scale values, the correlations between the two independent observers (SO and UO) are very high (.98 and .99), but these same correlations between each of the independent observers and the experimenter (OE) are somewhat lower (.88, .91, .73, and .75). In any event, results of the present study were that both intraobserver reliability (experimenter rate-rerate) and interobserver reliability (experimenter-sophisticated observer-unsophisticated observer) for scaling stuttering severity were satisfactory.

DISCUSSION

The data obtained in experiments I and II provide an addition to the available information about the perceptual scaling of stuttering severity reviewed and summarized in the Introduction. Perhaps the most significant results of the two studies reported above are those pertaining to observer reliability. There is considerable agreement in the literature that groups of observers can assign stuttering severity scale values in a reliable manner. There is considerable disagreement in the same literature, however, on whether individual observers can agree with themselves or other observers relative to the assignment of absolute scale values to a single speaker or a group of speakers. The results of experiment II indicate that the experimenter agreed with himself and with two different

independent observers in terms of the mean stuttering severity scale values he assigned to 12 stutterers across four 10-min periods. It is possible, of course, that the experimenter and the independent observers differed markedly in terms of the absolute stuttering severity scale values assigned to a given speaker in a given condition. It is unlikely that this occurred with any frequency, however, in view of the high correlations and lack of significant mean differences among the three observers in any of the four 10-min periods. The available experimental data, including those from the two present studies, suggest that individual clinicians and researchers can reliably scale the stuttering severity of clients or subjects. Such reliability should not be assumed, however, but should be determined empirically for any given situation.

The results of experiment II indicate not only that observers can scale reliably the severity of individual instances of stuttering but also that these individual moments of stuttering can be scaled for severity during ongoing spontaneous speech. This suggests that it may be possible for clinicians or researchers or independent observers to obtain information about a speaker's stuttering severity in pre and post "real-life" situations without the necessity of obtaining high-quality tape recordings in these difficult environments.

The results of experiments I and II suggest that the absolute scale value magnitudes of perceived stuttering severity can be influenced in part by the scaling procedures utilized. In experiment I, for the same speech sample, observers assigned significantly higher mean stuttering severity scale values to the overall speech samples than to the average individual stuttered words within a sample. Interestingly, in experiment II, where the experimenter assigned stuttering severity scale values to individual stutterings during ongoing spontaneous speech, the mean severity scale value assigned across speakers was lower than in either severity rating procedure in experiment II. Obviously, this difference in perceived severity may have been due entirely to the fact that different stutterers served as subjects in the two studies. Nevertheless, results of the present study and previous studies indicate that, if comparisons of stuttering severity scale values are to be made between speakers, or within the same speaker over time, the same scaling procedures should be utilized.

Finally, results of the experiments reported in this paper suggest that the perceptual scaling of stuttering severity is a complex process. An example of this complexity is the relationship between stuttering frequency and judged severity. In experiment II, the correlation coefficients between mean frequency of stuttering and mean severity scale values in the pre and post periods were .58 and .55, respectively. In the two DAF treatment periods, however, the comparable correlations were .74 and .72.[3] Both the percent words stuttered and the mean stuttering severity scale values decreased in the DAF periods relative to the pre and post periods. It is not immediately apparent why the significant reduction in both frequency and judged severity of stuttering occasioned by the DAF treatment increased the relationship between these two measures. It seems quite probable that the DAF procedure produced numerous changes in the stutterers' speech patterns—speech rate, vocal intensity, vowel duration, inflection. It seems reasonable to speculate that an observer's perceptions about the severity of instances of stuttering, and hence the relationship between stuttering frequency and severity, change as other features of the speech signal change.

The information available from the considerable experimental literature, including results of the two studies reported in this paper, suggests that the argument regarding whether frequency or severity is the preferred measure of stuttering may be unproductive. It is quite clear that both reliably identifying the frequency of stuttering and reliably scaling the perceived severity of stuttering are complex activities. Whether the effects of a particular experimental or clinical treatment should be assessed by measuring changes in stuttering frequency, stuttering severity, or both depends on the particular needs and purposes of the investigation. If the purpose of a particular treatment is to produce "zero stutterings" or "stutter-free speech," then quite obviously the efficacy of such a treatment should be assessed in terms of stuttering frequency. If, however, the purpose of a treatment is to produce "controlled" or "easy" stuttering, then severity of the "residual" stuttering should be assessed.

The complex manner in which various characteristics of the speech signal influence perceptions of stuttering severity were demonstrated quite dramatically in a multidimensional scaling of stuttering severity experiment reported by Prosek, Walden, Montgomery, and Schwartz (1979), and in a factor-analysis study of multiple audible and visible characteristics of stuttering reported by Prins and Lohr (1972). In both experiments, sophisticated statistical procedures revealed that the relationships among objective and perceptual characteristics of stuttered speech vary a great deal from speech sample to speech sample and from observer to observer.

Results of several recently reported experiments concerning speech naturalness appear quite relevant to the present discussion. An important finding of these studies is that observers can scale speech naturalness reliably (Ingham et al., 1985a, 1985b; Ingham & Onslow, 1985; Martin et al., 1984). In general, these naturalness experiments have demonstrated the existence of a complex relationship between the frequency of stuttering and judged speech naturalness. In the Martin et al. (1984) study, for example, observers scaled the speech naturalness of three groups of speakers: stutterers, stutterers speaking under DAF and "stutter-free," and nonstutterers. The mean naturalness ratings for the stutterers and the "stutter-free" stutterers under DAF were similar, but both these means were significantly higher (more unnatural) than that of the nonstutterers. To date, no attempts have been made to study systematically the relationships between perceptual ratings of stuttering severity, perceptual ratings of speech naturalness, and counts of stuttering frequency. Information from such experiments might help answer some

important questions, such as (1) Is it possible for a stutterer's speech to be perceived by listeners as highly natural even though that same stutterer's speech contains reliably identified instances of stuttering? (2) Is it possible for a stutterer's speech to be perceived by listeners as highly natural even though that same stutterer's speech contains one or more instances of stuttering perceived by observers as severe? (3) Is frequency of instances of stuttering or mean severity of instances of stuttering the better predictor of perceived speech naturalness? (4) Is mean severity of individual instances of stuttering or judged severity of an overall speech sample the better predictor of perceived speech naturalness?

ACKNOWLEDGMENTS

This research was supported in part by the Bryng Bryngelson Communication Disorders Research Fund, University of Minnesota.

NOTES

1. The volume (loudness) of the DAF unit was the same for all subjects. Prior to the study, 10 normal speakers spoke under DAF, with the volume adjusted to a "comfortable loudness." The "comfortable loudness" volume dial values for the 10 speakers were averaged, and this average value was increased by one dial unit. The result was the volume dial setting used with all experimental subjects.
2. For an excellent review of research relative to DAF and stuttering, the reader is directed to Ingham (1984).
3. These correlations are only slightly lower than the .85 correlation between rated severity and total disfluency frequency reported by Young (1961).

REFERENCES

Aron, M.L. (1967). The relationships between measurements of stuttering behavior. *Journal of the South African Logopedic Society, 14*, 15–34.

Berry, R.C., & Silverman, F.H. (1972). Equality of intervals on the Lewis-Sherman Scale of Stuttering Severity. *Journal of Speech and Hearing Research, 15*, 185–188.

Cooper, E.B., & Cooper, C.S. (1985). *Cooper personalized fluency control therapy: Revised.* Allen, TX: DLM Teaching Resources.

Cullinan, W.L., Prather, E.M., & Williams, D.E. (1963). Comparison of procedures for scaling severity of stuttering. *Journal of Speech and Hearing Research, 6*, 187–194.

Curran, M.F., & Hood, S.B. (1977a). The effect of instructional bias on listener ratings of specific disfluency types in children. *Journal of Fluency Disorders, 2*, 99–107.

Curran, M.F., & Hood, S.B. (1977b). Listener ratings of severity for specific disfluency types in children. *Journal of Fluency Disorders, 2*, 87–98.

Hoops, R., & Wilkinson, P. (1973). Group ratings of stuttering severity. In Y. LeBrun & R. Hoops (Eds.), *Neurolinguistic approaches to stuttering*. The Hague: Mouton.

Ingham, R.J. (1984). *Stuttering and behavior therapy: Current status and experimental foundations*. San Diego: College Hill Press.

Ingham, R.J., Gow, M., & Costello, J.M. (1985a). Stuttering and speech naturalness: Some additional data. *Journal of Speech and Hearing Disorders, 50*, 217–219.

Ingham, R.J., Martin, R.R., Haroldson, S.K., Onslow, M., & Leney, M. (1985b). Modification of listener-judged speech naturalness in the speech of stutterers. *Journal of Speech and Hearing Research, 28*, 495–504.

Ingham, R.J., & Onslow, M. (1985). Measurement and modification of speech naturalness during stuttering therapy. *Journal of Speech and Hearing Disorders, 50*, 261–281.

Johnson, W., Darley, F.L., & Spriestersbach, D.C. (1963). *Diagnostic manual in speech pathology*. New York: Harper.

Lanyon, R.I. (1967). The measurement of stuttering severity. *Journal of Speech and Hearing Research, 10*, 836–843.

Lewis, D., & Sherman, D. (1951). Measuring the severity of stuttering. *Journal of Speech and Hearing Disorders, 16*, 320–326.

Manning, W.H., Emal, K.C., & Jamison, W.J. (1975). Listener judgments of fluency: The effect of part-word CV repetitions and neutral vowel substitutions. *Journal of Fluency Disorders, 1*, 18–22.

Martin, R.R. (1965). Direct magnitude-estimation judgments of stuttering severity using audible and audible-visible speech samples. *Speech Monographs, 32*, 169–177.

Martin, R.R., Haroldson, S.K., & Triden, K. (1984). Stuttering and speech naturalness. *Journal of Speech and Hearing Disorders, 49*, 53–58.

Myers, F.L. (1978). Relationship between eight physiological variables and severity of stuttering. *Journal of Fluency Disorders, 3*, 181–191.

Naylor, R.V. (1953). A comparative study of methods of estimating the severity of stuttering. *Journal of Speech and Hearing Disorders, 18*, 30–37.

Prins, D., & Lohr, F. (1972). Behavioral dimensions of stuttered speech. *Journal of Speech and Hearing Research, 15*, 61–71.

Prosek, R.A., Walden, B., Montgomery, A., & Schwartz, D.M. (1979). Some correlates of stuttering severity judgments. *Journal of Fluency Disorders, 4*, 215–222.

Riley, G. (1984). *Stuttering Severity Instrument for Children and Adults*. Portland, OR: C.C. Publications.

Rousey, C.L. (1958). Stuttering severity during prolonged spontaneous speech. *Journal of Speech and Hearing Research, 1*, 40–47.

Schiavetti, N. (1975). Judgments of stuttering severity as a function of type and locus of disfluency. *Folia Phoniatrica, 27*, 26–37.

Sherman, D. (1952). Clinical and experimental use of the Iowa Scale of Severity of Stuttering. *Journal of Speech and Hearing Disorders, 17*, 316–320.

Sherman, D. (1955). Reliability and utility of individual ratings of severity of audible characteristics of stuttering. *Journal of Speech and Hearing Disorders, 20*, 11–16.

Sherman, D., & McDermott, R. (1958). Individual ratings of severity of moments of stuttering. *Journal of Speech and Hearing Research 1*, 61–67.

Sherman, D., & Trotter, W. (1956). Correlation between two measures of the severity of stuttering. *Journal of Speech and Hearing Research, 21*, 426–429.

Trotter, W.D. (1955). The severity of stuttering during successive readings of the same material. *Journal of Speech and Hearing Disorders, 20*, 17–25.

Trotter, W.D. (1956). Relationship between severity of stuttering and word conspicuousness. *Journal of Speech and Hearing Disorders, 21*, 198–201.

Trotter, W.D., & Kools, J.A. (1955). Listener adaptation to the severity of stuttering. *Journal of Speech and Hearing Disorders, 20*, 385–387.

Williams, D.E., Wark, M., & Minifie, F.D. (1963). Ratings of stuttering by audio, visual and audiovisual cues. *Journal of Speech and Hearing Research, 6*, 91–100.

Young, M.A. (1961). Predicting ratings of severity of stuttering. *Journal of Speech and Hearing Disorders, Monograph Supplement 7*, 31–54.

Young, M.A. (1969a). Observer agreement: Cumulative effects of rating many samples. *Journal of Speech and Hearing Research, 12*, 135–143.

Young, M.A. (1969b). Observer agreement: Cumulative effects of repeated ratings of the same samples and of knowledge of group results. *Journal of Speech and Hearing Research, 12*, 144–155.

Young, M.A. (1970). Anchoring and sequencing effects for the category scaling of severity of stuttering. *Journal of Speech and Hearing Research, 13*, 360–368.

Young, M.A., & Prather, E.M. (1962). Measuring severity of stuttering using short segments of speech. *Journal of Speech and Hearing Research, 5*, 256–262.

Stuttering as Involuntary Loss of Speech Control: Barking up a New Tree

Richard Martin
Samuel Haroldson

In a recent *JSHD* [*Journal of Speech and Hearing Disorders*] article (Perkins, 1983) and in a subsequent *JSHD* letter to the editor (Perkins, 1984), William Perkins offered the professional community a thoughtful, intriguing, and probably controversial view of stuttering. Specifically, Perkins proposed that stuttering be defined as "temporary overt and covert loss of control of the ability to move forward fluently in the execution of linguistically formulated speech" (Perkins, 1984, p. 431). In Perkin's view, loss of the ability to move forward fluently is involuntary and is a private experience available only to the stutterer. Obviously, such a conception of stuttering is markedly different from the two prevailing definitions: namely, that stuttering is defined by the presence of certain specific speech disruptions (repetitions and prolongations) or that stuttering is a perceptual phenomenon defined by observer agreement.

For the past almost 20 years, clinicians and researchers have been laboring with the definitional problem relative to stuttering. Those speech-language pathologists who employ a perceptual "moment of stuttering" definition are aware of and concerned about the fact that such a definition depends upon the notions, however idiosyncratic, a particular listener harbors as to what constitutes a stuttering. On the other hand, those professional workers who employ a "standard definition" of stuttering in terms of specific speech disfluencies recognize that such a definition results in a situation whereby the specific speech disfluencies that define stuttering also are present in the speech of nonstuttering speakers. Unfortunately, it seems that little progress has been made in recent years relative to the important definitional problem. To the extent that this is true, the appearance of Perkins's involuntary loss of control definition is most timely. The definition is relatively specific and straightforward. Both theoretically and procedurally the definition provides a refreshing alternative to the standard definition or perceptual phenomenon approach. For this, the profession is indebted to Professor Perkins.

Ultimately, of course, the utility of Perkins's definition will not depend upon whether it is right or wrong, that is, on whether stuttering is really an involuntary loss of speech control. In the final analysis, the usefulness of the Perkins definition will be determined primarily by the quality of the clinical and experimental questions it generates. The purpose of this letter is to discuss two features of the Perkins definition relative to its ability to generate meaningful, testable, and interesting questions.

One feature of the involuntary loss of control definition that will partially determine the nature and scope of its utility is the extent to which this definition differs from other definitions empirically. Does it make any difference in the clinic or the experimental laboratory whether the involuntary loss of control or a different definition of stuttering is utilized? For example, does the amount of reduction in stuttering frequency produced by a specific experimental treatment depend upon the definition of stuttering utilized? It is perhaps informative to note in this regard that differences between the standard definition and the moment of stuttering definition are primarily theoretical rather than empirical. A review of the many experimental research reports reveals quite clearly, for example, that stutterers experience reduced stuttering when speaking under noise or delayed auditory feedback (DAF), or when speaking rhythmically, or when reading the same passage aloud several times in succession. Interestingly, in all of the conditions just enumerated, plus many others, the effects of the experimental treatment procedures were observed in studies where stuttering was defined in terms of the standard definition and in studies where stuttering was defined in terms of perceptual agreement. Given this situation, much of the discussion about the relative advantages of one definition over the other centers around theoretical considerations.

At the present time, it simply is not known whether stuttering defined as involuntary loss of control differs empirically from stuttering defined as either specific speech

Reprinted from *Journal of Speech and Hearing Disorders*, 51, no. 2, 187–189. Copyright © 1986 American Speech-Language-Hearing Association.

disfluencies or perceptual moments. As Perkins indicated, no information is available from studies in which stutterers were requested to indicate when they experienced (or feared) a loss of control of speech. It is the case, however, that at least a few studies have been conducted in which stutterers reported in some way when they stuttered. At least two of these studies seem germane to the present discussion. In his early work with DAF, Goldiamond (1965) asked stutterers during baserate and during DAF treatment to depress a switch each time they stuttered. Goldiamond reported that stutterers experienced markedly reduced stuttering during treatment. Many studies have been reported subsequent to Goldiamond's work indicating that stutterers also experience reduced stuttering while speaking under DAF when the experimenter identifies and counts stutterings either as specific disfluencies or as moments of stuttering. Apparently, DAF results in reduced stuttering by many stutterers regardless of the definition of stuttering employed. Interestingly, with a few subjects prior to their exposure to DAF Goldiamond actually compared stuttering frequencies when stutterers identified and counted their own stutterings with stuttering frequencies when stuttering was identified and counted by the experimenter. Goldiamond concluded that "self-definition produced either no discernable effect or a transient change" in stuttering frequency (Goldiamond, 1965, p. 116). Although there is some indication in Goldiamond's early work that DAF effects a change in stuttering when either an observer or the stutterer identifies the stutterings, it is the case that the stutterers were not instructed specifically to identify stuttering as the loss of speech control.

The experimenter-administered and subject-administered time-out study reported by Martin and Haroldson (1982) also provides some data relevant to the experimental manipulation of stuttering when subjects' self-reports of stuttering are used as the dependent variable. In this study, stutterers spoke in a baserate, a time-out, and an extinction period. During the time-out period, 10 subjects were administered a time-out by the experimenter (EATO), and 10 subjects administered their own time-out (SATO) by pushing a hand switch each time they stuttered. The result of this study that is particularly relevant to the present discussion is that EATO and SATO subjects experienced similar reductions in stuttering during the first time-out session and similar increments in stuttering during the following extinction session.

Several other studies have been reported in which stutterers either recorded their own stutterings or delivered their own stimulation contingent upon stuttering (cf. Ingham, Adams, & Reynolds, 1978; James, 1981). Results of all of these experiments indicate quite clearly that when stutterers identify and consequate their own stutterings, this often results in a reduction in stuttering not unlike the reduction in stuttering observed when an experimenter or clinician identifies and consequates the stutterings. As was the case with Goldiamond's work with DAF, however, in none of those studies was the stutterer instructed explicitly to consider stuttering as the involuntary loss of speech control.

In order to obtain some information about the involuntary loss of control procedure, 10 adult stutterers were asked to read aloud "Arthur the Young Rat" (Johnson, Darley, & Spriestersbach, 1963) five times in succession. The subjects were given a hand switch and instructed to push this switch each time they experienced a loss of speech control. Each depression of the hand switch caused a brief 1000-Hz tone to be recorded on the second channel of an Ampex 440 audio recorder. At a later time, an observer unfamiliar with the project listened to the subject's speech on the first channel of the recorder but was unable to hear the tones on the second channel. The observer was instructed to push a hand switch "each time the subject stutters" (a "perceptual" definition). A computerized logic system was programmed so that if the observer's hand switch depression occurred between 1 sec before and 1 sec after a subject's tone (stuttering) on Channel 2, an agreement was indicated on a counter. At the end of each reading of a passage for each stutterer, the counter printed on tape the number of tones (subject switch depressions), the number of observer switch depressions, and the number of agreements.

With these data, a determination was made as to the amount of adaptation in stuttering that occurred when the observer identified stuttering and the amount of adaptation when the stutterer identified his or her own stutterings. These data appear in Figure 1. The figure shows the mean number of stutterings for each of the five readings when the subjects identified their own stutterings, when the observer identified the stutterings, and when the stutterer and observer agreed on a stuttering. All three curves in Figure 1 are similar to the classic adaptation curve reported in the literature. The percentages of reduction in stuttering from the first to the fifth reading are 60.2, 70.9, and 68.3 for the subject identification, observer identification, and agreed identification, respectively. It appears that even though stutterers and independent observers do not always agree as to the total number of stutterings or as to the precise location of individual occurrences of stuttering, they agree closely on the magnitude of the reduction in stuttering that accompanies each successive oral reading of a passage. The stutterers and independent observer even agreed relative to the slight increase in stuttering from the fourth to the fifth reading. Interestingly, the adaptation effect for only those occurrences of stuttering upon which the subject and observer agreed was not appreciably different from the amount of adaptation that resulted when only the subject or only the observer identifications were used.

The agreement data generated in the study just described are relevant to the definitional question. The mean numbers of stuttering identified by the 10 subjects in each of the five readings are shown in Figure 1. Of all the switch pushes by all subjects in Reading 1, 69 percent also occasioned a switch depression by the observer within the plus or

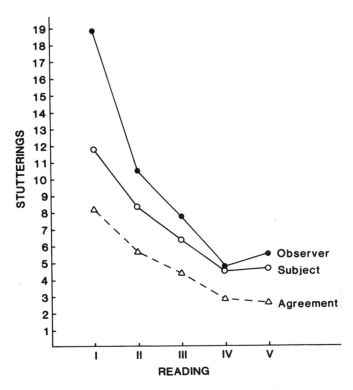

Figure 1. Mean number of stutterings counted by the observer, mean number of stutterings counted by the subject, and mean number of stutterings agreed upon by observer and subject for each of five successive readings.

minus 1-sec envelope. Comparable percentages of agreement for the second, third, fourth, and fifth readings are 67, 67, 62, and 55, respectively. On average, about two out of three times a subject identified a stuttering, the independent observer identified the same stuttering. There were, however, marked intersubject differences with regard both to total stuttering frequency counts and to subject-observer agreement for individual stutterings. As indicated in Figure 1, the observer counted about one third more stutterings than the subject for the first reading. By the fourth and fifth readings, however, the stutterer and observer were quite close in their counts of total stutterings on the reading. Interestingly, the subject-observer discrepancy in total stutterings for the first reading is due almost entirely to two subjects. Subject SS pushed his switch 22 times during the first reading, but the observer pushed his switch 39 times. In subsequent readings, these figures changed dramatically. In the second reading, for example, the switch pushes were 28 for the subject and 27 for the observer. Careful examination of SS's audio tape revealed two sources of the discrepancy during the first reading. Obviously, SS stuttered quite frequently during the first reading. On several occasions, SS held his breath for 3 or 4 sec before saying the word and immediately thereafter held his breath again on the very next word. Almost without exception, SS pushed his switch during the first breath holding but not during the second. The observer, on the other hand, consistently pushed his switch for both breath holdings. This, of course, resulted in a higher stuttering count by the observer. The second source of Subject SS-observer discrepancy in total stuttering counts is quite relevant to the Perkins definition. On nine occasions, SS held his breath for at least 4 sec prior to "exploding" a word or syllable but did not depress his hand switch. None of these episodes was involved in the back-to-back stutterings just described. Those stutterings for which SS did not depress his switch were very similar to those for which SS did depress his switch in terms of initial sound, duration of breath holding, and topography of struggle. Consistent with the Perkins explanation of stuttering, SS apparently experienced involuntary loss of control in one instance, but not in another, and this in spite of the fact that the externally observable behaviors in both instances were quite similar and somewhat abnormal.

Interestingly, by the second reading, SS emitted many fewer breath-holding stutterings and almost never stuttered on two successive words or syllables. As indicated earlier, SS and the observer's agreement improved dramatically (SS, 28; observer, 27).

The other subject who accounted for much of the first reading difference in total stuttering frequency counts between the stutterer and the observer was Subject TM. On the first reading, TM pushed his switch 22 times, but the observer pushed his switch 48 times when he subsequently listened to TM's tape recording. Later inspection of the tape revealed quite clearly the source of the discrepancy. Most of TM's stutterings were short repetitions with a few brief prolongations. Some of the repetitions were audibly forceful. During the first reading, this subject simply did not press his switch after many of the stutterings. It is the case, however, that TM sometimes pushed his switch and sometimes did not push his switch for behaviors that appeared essentially identical to the observer. This situation existed even for a number of repetitions that included obvious audible struggling. During the second reading, TM pushed his switch 22 times, and the observer pushed his switch 28 times. Careful inspection of the tape recording corroborated the marked reduction in both repetitions and prolongations during the second reading. At the end of the session, the experimenter asked TM if his stuttering frequency changed during the experiment. TM replied that his stuttering reduced "a lot" after the first reading. The lack of internal consistency in identifying stuttering demonstrated by SS and TM will be discussed later. The important point to be stressed here is that both individually and collectively, stutterers in the present study definitely demonstrated the adaptation effect both when they identified their own stuttering (loss of control) and when the observer identified moments of stuttering. With regard *solely* to the set of procedures that encompass the adaptation effect, whether stuttering is defined as specific speech disfluencies, as a perceptual instance of stuttering, or as an involuntary loss of speech control may be academic.

A second feature of the Perkins definition that may be influential in determining its ultimate usefulness relates to questions of reliability and validity. As Perkins indicates, defining stuttering in terms of the involuntary loss of speech control raises some especially bothersome questions about both validity and reliability. This situation is expressed quite succinctly in Perkins's statement that "the implication of the foregoing analysis is that a valid definition of stuttering precludes its being reliable" (Perkins, 1983, p. 247). To most researchers, this statement is a nonsequitur because the logic of scientific inquiry dictates that in order for a given explanation of behavior to be valid, the observations upon which that explanation is based must be accurate (reliable). The source of what Perkins calls this validity-reliability paradox resides in the involuntary nature of stuttering and in the notion that the involuntary loss of control is the only essential feature of every stuttering instance or "block." Presumably, whatever stimulation the stutterer uses to know for sure that an involuntary loss of control has been experienced is private and available only to that speaker. Additionally, this stimulation probably is highly transitory in the speech act. Because experiencing this stimulation is a private and transitory event, it is by definition impossible to assess the reliability of the speaker's report that an involuntary loss of control occurred.

The validity-reliability paradox makes it difficult to assess the utility of the Perkins definition of stuttering. It should be mentioned, however, that one potential source of the validity-reliability paradox rests with the manner in which Perkins uses the term validity. In the development and exposition of his proposed definition, Perkins appears to use validity to mean truth or reality. For example, Perkins states that "an *indisputable reality* [italics ours] for people who consider themselves to be stutterers is that they feel as if they lose control of their speech when they stutter" (Perkins, 1983, p. 247). This statement demonstrates quite clearly how Perkins's definition reflects the idea that the involuntary loss of control is what stuttering really is and that any conflicting definitions are invalid. In some senses, this reasoning is reminiscent of the Freudian logic that posits, "If you don't believe you're ill, you are."

To the degree that Perkins's definition rests rigidly on the assertion that stuttering really is the involuntary loss of speech control, then the definition probably will not prove too useful. To assert that the only valid definition of stuttering involves behaviors that by their very nature cannot be observed reliably simply precludes meaningful scientific inquiry. It is possible, however, that viewing the Perkins definition from a different perspective about validity might render the definition quite useful in terms of generating creative research. If validity is viewed not as truth or reality, but rather as explanations of observed events or behaviors or phenomena (that is, of facts), then validity describes a process more than it does absolute truth or reality. This notion of validity is outlined in some detail in the 1985 *Standards for Educational and Psychological Testing* published by the American Psychological Association (APA).

> The concept [validity] refers to the appropriateness, meaningfulness, and usefulness of the specific inferences made from test scores. Test validation is the process of accumulating evidence to support such inferences. A variety of inferences may be made from scores produced by a given test, and there are many ways of accumulating evidence to support any particular inference. Validity, however, is a unitary concept. Although evidence may be accumulated in many ways, validity always refers to the degree to which that evidence supports the inferences that are made from the scores. (1985, p. 9).

Consonant with the above cited APA standard, if the validity of the definition of stuttering is viewed as the process of gathering information supporting certain inferences about stuttering, then Perkins's definition constitutes a potentially fruitful area for creative and exciting research. If the inference proposes that stuttering involves the involuntary loss of speech control, then experiments can be designed to test many facets of this inference. Creative effort can be directed toward studies that attempt to operationalize and measure involuntary. Studies can be designed to explore if certain speech disfluencies are linguistic, or motor, or both. Studies can be generated to explore if the involuntary loss of control can be used to differentiate stuttered from nonstuttered repetitions and prolongations more accurately than observer perception or acoustic analysis.

Presumably, the more information that is obtained in support of the inference that stuttering is an involuntary loss of speech control, the more valid the inference will become. Similarly, other inferences about stuttering will become more valid as accumulated information appears to confirm these inferences. Within this framework, no inferences about, including definitions of, stuttering are valid or invalid. Inferences about stuttering and the definition of stuttering are more or less valid depending on the quantity and quality of information available at any given time that supports a particular inference.

Within this inference-process conception of validity, it is not necessary that the Perkins definition posit that either the speech disfluency or the perceptual explanation of stuttering is invalid. It is not necessary to insist that involuntary loss of speech control is the "indisputable reality" of stuttering. Instead, the Perkins involuntary loss of control notion should be viewed as a highly thoughtful, challenging, and creative inference about the nature of stuttering, and members of the professional discipline should set about the exciting task of testing the inference in the very best sense of the word. Rather than being discouraged about "barking up the wrong tree" in terms of the standard, consensus definition of stuttering, researchers and clinicians can now enjoy the challenge of sharpening their teeth on a new, juicy sapling.

REFERENCES

Goldiamond, I. (1965) Stuttering and fluency as manipulatable operant response classes. In L. Krasner & L. P. Ullmann (Eds.), *Research in behavior modification* (pp. 106–156). New York: Holt, Rinehart, & Winston.

Ingham, R. J., Adams, S., & Reynolds, G. (1978). The effects on stuttering of self-recording the frequency of stuttering or the word "the." *Journal of Speech and Hearing Research, 21,* 459–469.

James, J. E. (1981). Behavioral self-control of stuttering using time-out from speaking. *Journal of Applied Behavior Analysis, 14,* 25–37.

Johnson, W., Darley, F. L., & Spriestersbach, D. C. (1963). *Diagnostic methods in speech pathology.* New York: Harper & Row.

Martin, R. R., & Haroldson, S. K. (1982). Contingent self-stimulation for stuttering. *Journal of Speech and Hearing Disorders, 47,* 407–413.

Perkins, W. H. (1983). The problem of definition: Commentary on stuttering. *Journal of Speech and Hearing Disorders, 48,* 246–249.

Perkins, W. H. (1984). Stuttering as a categorical event: Barking up the wrong tree—A reply to Wingate. *Journal of Speech and Hearing Disorders, 49,* 431–433.

Standards for educational and psychological testing. (1985). Prepared by American Educational Research Association, American Psychological Association, and National Council on Measurement in Education. Washington, DC: American Psychological Association.

More Bite for a Bark: Epilogue to Martin and Haroldson's Letter

William H. Perkins

This is not so much a response to Richard Martin and Samuel Haroldson as it is an expression of gratitude that they have taken my bark and given it such scholarly bite. I am in complete agreement with almost every point they've made. I merely wish to nibble a bit more on the sapling on which they have already chewed.

They are correct in pointing out that unless the loss-of-control definition of stuttering makes a difference, then it will be merely an academic exercise. In this regard, they conclude that as far as the adaptation effect is concerned, no difference is found between using a listener definition or the stutterer's loss-of-control definition. In fact, I would carry their argument further and speculate that it probably makes no difference in the therapy of stuttering. Added to the evidence they cite is that of Costello and Hurst (1981) that different topographies of disfluency, including kernel and accessory features of stuttering, form a single response class. If the disfluencies that were behavioral manifestations of the feeling of loss of speech control had been included, as perhaps they were, they, too might have been in that response class. I would hypothesize, however, that the feeling of loss of control is separable from observable speech characteristics and would, therefore, be in a different response class. Presumably, this distinction was the basis of the late Joseph Sheehan's argument (cf. Sheehan & Sheehan, 1984) that establishing fluency is merely symptomatic treatment that results only in the suppression of stuttering. I make this presumption because, in our discussions of this issue, he agreed with my reply that fluency did more than suppress stuttering when it freed the speaker from the feeling of stuttering. Although stutterers seem able to identify their own moments of stuttering, some of which may not be observable by listeners, a more refined and reliable measure will have to be developed before my hypothesized difference between moments of stuttered speech can be distinguished from nonstuttered normal and abnormal fluency and disfluency.

Viewed from another angle, even if stuttering as loss of control is in a different response class from abnormal or normal disfluency, I would still argue that the choice of definition is immaterial to effective outcome, at least for fluency-skills therapy. My reason is that even though a listener-based disfluency definition may result in removal of some nonstuttered as well as stuttered disfluencies, no harm is done. Seen from a fluency-shaper's view, treatment resulting in greater-than-normal fluency is, if anything, a bonus associated with removing any disfluency that might possibly be considered to be stuttering.

To say that the loss-of-control definition may make no difference in therapy does not mean it has no clinical significance. I see it as having at least two important effects. One is that covert stuttering is as authentic a manifestation of the problem as is overt stuttering. An observation which helped lead me away from a listener-based-observable-disfluency definition was curiosity as to why many who complained most bitterly about stuttering were seldom or never heard to stutter. I have known clinicians who would not accept anyone for treatment of stuttering who did not manifest the disorder overtly because, by a listener definition, they did not stutter. Ironically, by offering fluency-skills therapy to these people who seem to need it least (after all, they are already fluent), it is our view that they are often the most satisfied with the outcome. Therapy seems to free them of the fear that they will stutter, which apparently is equivalent to freeing them of covert stuttering.

Another clinical effect of this new definition is in the advice to parents of young stutterers. The appropriate recommendation deriving from the semantogenic theory (which assumes that stuttering develops as children, misguidedly, learn to fear their normal disfluencies) has been to counsel acceptance and patience. By focusing on *what* children have to say and not on *how* they say it, the theory is that children will outgrow any hesitation to hestitate they may have acquired and will become normally disfluent speakers. True as this conception may be for up to 80 percent who appear to recover without formal assistance from what someone, often a parent, has judged to be early stuttering, the remaining 20 percent are at high risk of becoming chronic stutterers. Traditionally, this high-risk group has not been differentiated, and, even if it had been, the same advice to avoid direct early intervention would have applied.

Reprinted from *Journal of Speech and Hearing Disorders, 51*, no. 2, 190–191. Copyright © 1986 American Speech-Language-Hearing Association.

156

The loss-of-control definition adds theoretical support to the recommendation for early intervention being made by a growing number of clinicians. By this definition, it is not disfluency, normal or abnormal, that is frightening; it is the prospect of becoming helplessly stuck on a sound or syllable. Although I know of no formal research, I do know of many clinical reports that these at-risk children are keenly aware that they have a problem. Avoiding mention of it can make it seem even more frightening; it must be bad if no one will speak of it. Those who have intervened early not only have found no ill effects (e.g., Costello, 1983), they report instead that the younger the child when therapy begins, the greater the likelihood of full recovery.[1]

The problem of identifying the at-risk group is closely related to the validity-reliability paradox raised by Martin and Haroldson. Again I am in agreement, almost, with their analysis of my paradox: that if a valid moment of stuttering can only be known at the moment it is experienced, then by definition it cannot be repeated.

In truth, they dealt with me too gently for stating the paradox so strongly as to make it useless. I was too carried away by the realization that the only basis for validity provided by a listener definition is the high reliability obtained with measures of frequency of stuttering, such as in the adaptation procedures Martin and Haroldson used.

There is irony in using frequency count reliability as a basis for defining stuttering. What it says, in effect, is that listeners can reliably identify *stutterers*, but when asked to judge *stuttering*, they rarely exceed 50 percent agreement with themselves if independent listener judgments are maintained, let alone with each other (see Perkins, 1984, for details of this argument). Thus, listeners appear to have a very clear idea as to who is a stutterer, but only a fuzzy notion as to what stutterers do that is called stuttering. Nonetheless, it is the reliability of *stutterer* judgments (which can be inferred from frequency measures as well as measured directly) which have been taken as the basis for defining stuttering, rather than reliability of *stuttering* judgments, which have never come close to being acceptable.

I began to sort out this bit of definitional sleight of hand about the same time it began to dawn on me that what stutterers fear is loss of control of their speech. Seen from this perspective, I was so struck by our illogical use of frequency measure reliability as a basis for validating a listener definition of stuttering that I fell overboard on the other side by overstating a paradox in which a valid judgment of stuttering (as the transitory experience of loss of speech control) precludes a test of its reliability. Partly, too, I fell overboard because I did not see a clinically useful behavioral method of testing reliability of the new definition. I still do not, although I suspect one may eventually emerge as we get a clearer idea of what to look for. My guess is that we will find acoustic and physiological measures sooner than we find behavioral ones.

In any event, Martin and Haroldson are absolutely correct in taking me to task for using validity in a manner that excludes tests of reliability. As they point out, a definition based on the stutterer's subjective experience can only be validated by inferences that can be measured empirically. This is the point, however, at which I part company with them. They apparently would not use empirical results to *test* inferences but rather to *support* them. As they say, "Within this framework, no inferences about, including definitions of, stuttering are valid or invalid. Inferences about stuttering, and the definition of stuttering, are more or less valid depending on the quantity and quality of information available at any given time that support a particular inference."

I would submit that this use of evidence undercuts the power of the scientific method, and has become so traditional an approach in investigations of stuttering as to be the fundamental reason why our conception of the nature of this problem has hardly changed in half a century. Platt (1964), a biophysicist whose description of the method of strong inference has become a classic, maintains that this is the method used (as originally intended by Francis Bacon when the scientific method was formulated) by those fields that have advanced farthest fastest. The crux of the method is disproof, not proof. The purpose of the method is to devise crucial experiments by which hypotheses can be tested and excluded if they fail the test. In this view, an experiment that does not definitively exclude the weakest of two alternative hypotheses is not a crucial experiment.

I would argue, therefore, that validity of any sort, including definitions of stuttering, depends less on how much support has accumulated and far more on how strong the tests have been that it has survived. Just as in sports, the strength of a player or team cannot be determined by playing weak competition, similarly the strength of a definition (or hypothesis or theory) cannot be determined without vigorous attempts to disprove it. Although in science definitive disproof is possible, proof is not—as physicists discovered at the turn of the century when their conviction that Newton's theories answered all of the questions in physics was shattered by Einstein's theories. Nothing in science is ever proven.

I have philosophized at length to make clear why I disagree that mutually exclusive definitions of stuttering (or anything else) can be equally valid. The strength of the loss-of-control definition will not reside in how much support it accumulates but in how resistant it is to disproof. It may, and probably will, eventually be disproven. What can be said in its favor is that so far it has not been excluded. Not so with listener definitions that are intended to account for stuttering as the stutterer experiences it. The evidence of unacceptable reliability of judgments of stuttering would have wounded it decades ago if that evidence had been used for purposes of disproof. Although admittedly not definitive, it nonetheless stands in direct opposition to the adequacy of a listener definition. That its significance was virtually ignored is testimony to the long-prevailing conception that validity of an idea is determined by how much support it can muster. No idea was presented during this long period which unreliable judgments of stuttering would support. Had this evidence, which was at least partial disproof of a listener definition, been used to cast doubt on the adequacy of it, we might long ago have begun seeking a better definition, and explanation, of stuttering.

The different uses to which we would put evidence not lessen the importance of Martin and Haroldson's main point that unless empirically measurable inferences can be generated by my definition, then for practical purposes it will be useless. Much as I agree with the thrust of their point, I have one more quibble which has important ramifications. They object to my arguing that stuttering "really is" loss of speech control, which they take to be an argument for this being my statement of truth as well as of reality. I do intend it to be the latter, but not the former. "Truth" implies a level of absolute certainty far beyond any claim I would make, "Reality," however, is another matter. I take this term to refer to the real world, much of which cannot be known directly, such as what occurred at the instant of creation (the Big Bang) as well as what goes on when we think and perceive.

Saying that subjective experience can be measured only by inferences drawn from it (a statement with which I agree) does not mean that such experience is not real. Solipsistic philosophy, for example, holds that subjective experience is the only reality. For myself, and I assume for everyone else as well, how I experience the world determines how I respond to it. By the same token, I am hypothesizing that what is frightening to stutterers is the temporary feeling of loss of control of the flow of speech, and that their response to this feeling largely determines the topography of their stuttering.

If this hypothesis is correct, then it has particular significance for efforts to determine the physiology and acoustics of stuttering. By using a listener definition, what we have sought so far with these measures are correlates of disfluencies judged by listeners to be stuttering. But if the essence of stuttering is the stutterer's experience of momentary loss of speech control, then perhaps we should be looking for physiologic and acoustic correlates of different responses than we have sought to date. Not only would the correlates probably be different, but so would the credible conception of stuttering.

Inferences can be drawn from a listener definition that directly oppose those from the loss-of-control hypothesis. When they are pitted against each other as alternative hypotheses, empirical evidence will determine the victor, not so that both can continue to coexist, but so that efforts will be directed to testing the strongest. By vigorous testing will its flaws be determined. As its weaknesses are revealed, stronger alternatives will be developed that will raise our understanding to higher generations of hypotheses and theories.

NOTES

1. Measuring effectiveness of early intervention is confounded by the fact that about half of young children who are thought to stutter will stop within the first year after onset. Validity of the argument, therefore, requires evidence that likelihood of full recovery is improved by early intervention for those children at risk of becoming chronic stutterers. Such evidence, of course, will require valid and reliable measures of children at risk. Whether such measures are currently available is questionable.

REFERENCES

Costello, J. (1983). Current behavioral treatments for children. In D.E. Prins & R.J. Ingham (Eds.), *Treatment of stuttering in early childhood* (pp. 69–112). San Diego: College-Hill Press.

Costello, J., & Hurst, M. (1981). An analysis of the relationship among stuttering behaviors. *Journal of Speech and Hearing Research, 24,* 247–256.

Perkins, W. (1984). Stuttering as a categorical event: Barking up the wrong tree—Reply to Wingate. *Journal of Speech and Hearing Disorders, 49,* 431–434.

Platt, J. (1964). Strong inference. *Science, 146,* 347–353.

Sheehan, J.G., & Sheehan, V.M. (1984). Avoidance-reduction therapy: A response-suppression hypothesis. In W.H. Perkins (Ed.), *Current therapy of communication disorders. Stuttering disorders* (pp. 147–151). New York: Thieme-Stratton.

A Protocol for Differentiating the Incipient Stutterer

Rebekah H. Pindzola
Dorenda T. White

Speech-language pathologists are often asked to judge the fluency of preschool and school-age children's speech. The early identification of children who will require intervention for the development of fluent speech is important to both parents and professionals. Regardless of the directness or indirectness of the management program, it is important that the incipient, beginning stutterer be differentiated from the child experiencing only normal disfluencies. In clinical practice, many speech-language pathologists feel inadequate and ill-prepared to make important diagnostic decisions regarding fluency. However, the stuttering literature describes factors to consider in making these differential diagnoses (cf., Adams, 1977; Cooper, 1973; Van Riper, 1971, 1982) and clinicians can learn to organize, present, and interpret information regarding the child's fluency.

FORMAT OF THE PROTOCOL

The Protocol for Differentiating the Incipient Stutterer presented here (see Appendix) attempts to decrease the gap between theory and practice by synthesizing available information from the professional literature. The uniqueness of the Protocol lies in its format which has three advantages. First, it guides the speech-language pathologist in clinical observations of the client; second, the speech-language pathologist familiar with the Protocol knows exactly which behaviors to count or quantify. Areas in need of data collection are delineated; and third, the Protocol provides interpretive guidelines for normal behaviors and clinical signs. This third feature helps the clinician differentiate the child who experiences normal disfluencies from the incipient stutterer.

ADMINISTRATION OF THE PROTOCOL

To administer the Protocol one needs to obtain a sample of the child's natural speech. All auditory and visual behaviors,

sections I-II, should be observed during connected discourse. An audio or video tape-recording of the sample is valuable for reanalysis of the child's auditory behaviors; however, such data may be collected live-voice with the aid of mechanical counters or pencil tallies (Riley, 1980, 1972). To use the Protocol, the clinician interviews the child using open-ended questions, interesting discussion topics, and whatever other stimuli are necessary (e.g., sequencing pictures). The goal is to obtain a conversational, connected, and natural sample of speech with few responses that are single-item naming, or reciting. The length of the speech sample is not critical, but it is unlikely that adequate observational data can be collected from samples containing less than 3 min of talking time.

One may find it possible to discuss openly the child's feelings about speech, and what happens when his "voice gets stuck." The resulting information will be useful in completing section III of the Protocol.

The Protocol is arranged in four sections. Section 1 contains a record of auditory behavior, section 2 visual behavior, and section 3 covert psychological feelings and reported information. The fourth section allows the clinician to summarize the available evidence and clinical impressions and to arrive at a diagnostic decision.

AUDITORY BEHAVIORS

Eight categories of auditory behavior are assessed and marked on the Protocol (see Appendix). The literature supporting each category is reviewed below.

Type of Disfluency

The predominant type of disfluency influences listener judgments of normalcy (Perkins, 1971). Interjections (i.e., "uh," "er," "well") and hesitations typically are found in normal speakers, may serve various purposes and, by themselves, they do not accurately differentiate stutterers from nonstutterers (Ryan, 1974; Wingate, 1964a). Repetitions are disfluencies typical of both stutterers and nonstutterers, but the location of the repetition within the speech unit must be

Reprinted from *Language, Speech, and Hearing Services in Schools, 17,* no. 1, 2–15. Copyright © 1986, American Speech-Language-Hearing Association.

considered. For example, part-word repetitions were found by Yairi and Lewis (1984) to distinguish between stuttering and nonstuttering preschoolers. Finally, the presence of prolonged speech sounds (Yairi & Lewis, 1984) or speech attempts with coexisting physical signs of struggle (Ryan, 1974) strongly suggests fluency abnormalities. The type of disfluency should be marked on the appropriate grid on the Protocol.

Size of Speech Unit Affected

Perkins (1971) recognized that the size of the speech unit affected by the disfluency affects listener judgments of normalcy. Repetitions of whole phrases, for example, are more normal, and less severe, than repetitions of whole words. Similarly, whole-word repetitions are found among the disfluencies of both stutterers and nonstutterers, but part-word repetitions are more typical of stutterers (Yairi & Lewis, 1984; Ryan, 1974). Hesitations or pauses before phrases or before words may, likewise, be less innocuous than such gaps within words (i.e., preceding syllables or sounds). The rule of thumb suggested by Perkins (1971) is that the smaller the speech unit affected, the more abnormal the disfluency. The level at which disfluencies occur should be marked on the grid on the Protocol.

Frequency of Disfluencies

The frequency with which disfluency behaviors occur has long been recognized as important in the diagnosis of stuttering and in appraising its severity (cf., Bloodstein, 1981; Van Riper, 1971, 1982).

Metraux (1950) suggests that all kindergarten-aged children repeat. When the repetitions exceed 50 per 1,000 words spoken, a 5 percent disfluency rate, the disfluent speech may be a problem. Van Riper (1971, 1982) proposed that syllable repetitions on more than 2 words per 100 words are indicative of stuttering whereas syllable repetitions on less than 2 percent of words uttered may be considered to be within normal limits. The frequency of repetitions in the child's speech should be noted on the Protocol.

The presence of prolongations may indicate a fluency disorder. Van Riper's (1971, 1982) criterion of more than 1 prolongation per 100 words (1%) is used to differentiate stuttering from nonstuttering. The percentage of prolongations observed in the child's speech should be noted on the Protocol.

Overall rate of disfluency may also be used to differentiate the normal child from the incipient stutterer. Stutterers' total disfluencies average 10 or more per 100 words spoken (10%) (Adams, 1977), while normal childrens' disfluencies average no more than 5 or 6 per 100 words (5%). Adams does not discuss the interpretation of disfluency rates between 5 or 6 percent and 10 percent. Yairi and Lewis (1984) counted the mean number of disfluent syllables per 100 orthographic syllables in the speech of 2- and 3-year-old stutterers and nonstutterers. Stutterers were found to be three times more

disfluent than nonstutterers (means of 21.54 and 6.16 disfluencies per 100 syllables, respectively). The average number of syllables per English word is 2.5; therefore, one can extrapolate that the stuttering preschoolers were disfluent on an average of 9 percent of their words. The nonstuttering preschoolers were disfluent on only 2 to 3 percent of the words spoken spontaneously. This is consistent with the 10 percent figure suggested by Adams (1977).

The 2 to 3 percent disfluency rates of normal-speaking children in the Yairi and Lewis (1984) study is comparable to values reported by Van Riper (1971, 1982), for older speakers. The percentage of disfluencies observed in the child's speech should be noted on the Protocol.

Duration of Disfluencies

The duration of the disfluency may be expressed in two ways: (a) either as number of times for repetitions or (b) as length of time for prolongations. For example, in the sentence "My my my cat had kittens," the whole-word "my" is produced twice before being uttered meaningfully. Adams (1977), based on Egland's (1955) work, states that part-word repetitions of incipient stutterers consist of one to five reiterations (e.g., "b-ball" or "b-b-b-b-b-ball"). This is contrasted with the number of reiterations of nonstuttering children, which typically does not exceed three.

Van Riper's (1971, 1982) more stringent guidelines suggest that more than two syllable repetitions per word is abnormal, while less than two per word may be considered normal. Yairi and Lewis' (1984) data on part-word repetitions of 2- and 3-year-olds is in agreement with Van Riper's guidelines. Yairi and Lewis found the range of reiterations for stutterers to be 1 to 11 ($M = 1.72$) units but only 1 to 2 ($M = 1.12$) units for the nonstutterers. The typical number of reiterations detected in the sample should be marked on the Protocol.

Audible Effort

Audible signs of effort while speaking generally are not noted among normal speakers and are indicative of abnormality. A complete listing of these audible behaviors is not realistic but behaviors typically seen among stutterers are listed on the Protocol to be noted if present. (Adams, 1977; Bloodstein, 1981; Van Riper, 1971, 1982).

Rhythm/Tempo/Speed of Disfluencies

Van Riper (1971, 1982) provides clinical reports that normal disfluencies and perhaps very early stutterings are characterized by repetitions that preserve the normal rhythm and rate of speech. Not until the tempo of the reiterations speeds up or their rhythm becomes irregular and choppy is there substantial reason for concern. The clinician is asked to judge subjectively the child's rhythm, tempo, and the speed of disfluencies on the Protocol.

Intrusion of Schwa Vowel During Repetitions

Another feature that may distinguish the syllabic repetitions of stutterers from nonstutterers is the perceived presence of the schwa vowel. Van Riper (1971, 1982) provided anecdotal evidence that stuttering repetitions often have the neutral schwa vowel intruding on the intended vowel (e.g., "suh-suh-suh-soap" instead of "so-so-soap)". The repetitions of normal speakers presumably do not exhibit the inappropriate schwa vowel. The acoustic evidence to support this intrusion hypothesis seems lacking (cf., Allen, Peters, & Williams, 1975; Montgomery & Cooke, 1976), but some authorities support its perceptual reality as indicative of defects in coarticulatory transitions and of chronic stuttering (Adams, 1978; Cooper, 1973, 1976; Stromsta, 1965; Van Riper, 1971, 1982). Presence of schwa vowel instrusion may be indicated on the Protocol.

Audible Learned Behaviors

Behaviors such as those listed on the Protocol as audible learned behaviors are thought to develop as a means of minimizing stuttering and in 1963, Van Riper suggested a fivefold classification of such "concealment devices." Word substitutions or circumlocutions may be used to avoid feared words, postponement devices may consist of maneuvers (e.g., interjections) to delay attempts on a feared word, and starting tricks (e.g., "uh" prefixed to the feared word) may be used to assist in initiating feared words. These and other mannerisms may discriminate between stutterers and nonstutterers and, if detected, should be marked on the Protocol.

VISUAL EVIDENCE

Visual signs of effort suggest to the listener that the act of speaking is unduly difficult. Such signs may reflect the speaker's own opinion that speech is difficult and to be avoided if at all possible (Bloodstein, 1981). The excess tensing of muscles might also represent the speaker's attempts to "break an invisible hold" and force out the word. Whatever the motivation, such visual evidence is considered by listeners in judging speech normalcy. Furthermore, their presence indicates that (a) the child is aware of his speaking difficulties, (b) is trying to do something about the moments of difficulty, and (c) that the disfluency has developed into a more severe problem.

Facial Grimaces/Articulatory Posturing

The clinician should list on the Protocol all contortions and posturing observed in the facial region. Among the most frequently observed, according to Bloodstein (1981), are eye-blinks and wrinkling of the forehead. Also common are frowning, distortions of the mouth, especially tongue and lip movement, quivering of the nostrils, and mandibular tension.

Head Movements

Rhythmical head movements, conspicuous head jerks, and the more subtle head turnings to divert eye contact are observable in some stutterers and, if present, should be noted on the Protocol.

Body Involvement

Nonspecific movements such as fidgeting and shuffling and the more specific, rhythmical movements of swaying, swinging, and tapping may be readily observable and should be noted on the Protocol. Any part of the body may be involved, including the hands, arms, legs, feet, and torso. These movements are usually associated with a stuttering block, but may occur independently of a speech disruption.

HISTORICAL AND PSYCHOLOGICAL INDICATORS

The subjective evaluations made by a speaker while experiencing speech disfluencies and in reaction to them are diagnostically important. These covert reactions have been studied through the introspection of older stutterers, but may also be present to some degree in child stutterers. The child's perceptions of his problem should be explored whenever possible.

Additional information collected from parental reports, while useful, is often subject to errors of memory and interpretation. For this reason, historical accounts and parental opinions of how the child views the speech problem are considered subjective indicators on the Protocol.

Awareness and Concern

Bluemel's (1932) concept of the early or "primary stutterer" included the notion of the child's lack of awareness. Only when the speech difficulties became apparent and of concern to the youngster did the problem merit direct intervention; the client then was reclassified as a "secondary stutterer." Today it seems that early stutterers are more sophisticated than their predecessors. It is not uncommon for preschool children to be aware and concerned about their disfluent speech (Shine, 1980). Parents report examples of their child's being upset at peer teasing and even crying over not being able to talk. Clearly, this early concern is testimony to the reality of a disfluency problem. Sheehan and Martyn (1966) and Cooper (1976) suggest that those who have incorporated stuttering into their self-concept are likely to be chronic stutterers.

Glasner and Rosenthal (1957) found a relationship between parental concern and chronic stuttering in the child. While the level of awareness and presence of concern in both the child and the parents are not perfect indicators of true stuttering problems, they may be useful aids in differentiating chronic from benign disfluencies. Such information is best obtained from direct interviews of the parents and of the child in question, and should be summarized on the Protocol.

Length of Time Fluency Problem Has Existed

If stuttering develops from normal nonfluency, as proposed by Bloodstein (1981), then it is plausible that stuttering patterns become more ingrained with the passage of time. Furthermore, if normal children go through a period of normal disfluency, then this "period" should not be chronic nor progressive. Consequently, if the fluency problem has existed for some time, it would seem that it is not just a "phase" the child is going through, but a real problem which is likely to persist. Despite the superficial logic inherent in such a statement, it is not supported in the literature. Andrews and Harris (1964), in a longitudinal survey, found that nearly 80 percent of early disfluency cases recovered from their symptoms. Some children who eventually outgrew stuttering had symptoms for 1 or 2 years. Similarly, Wingate (1964b) found no relationship between recovery and duration of stuttering.

A related issue which may shed light on clinical interpretations is the child's age at the time of the initial evaluation. Jameson (1955) found that normal speech was achieved in 82 percent of children when advice was sought "early" by the parents. The prognosis for recovery was greatest when professional advice was provided before the child was 5 years old; this contrasts with only a 37 percent recovery rate for children evaluated after the age of 5. Panelli, McFarlane, and Shipley (1978) also compared the time of stuttering onset and the initial evaluation in recovered and nonrecovered stutterers. The subjects who recovered were evaluated within an average of 4 months post-onset. However the children who had not recovered were seen an average of 19 months after reported onset.

Clinically then, children exhibiting disfluencies for a longer period of time are (a) more likely to be stutterers rather than merely experiencing a period of normal disfluency; (b) more likely to have a chronic problem that resists spontaneous recovery; and (c) more apt to have a more severe fluency problem (e.g., greater frequency, conspicuous physical concomitants, covert reactions, etc.). Child disfluency cases receiving "early" evaluations and intervention strategies have better prognoses for normal fluency. For this reason a statement regarding the length of time the fluency problem has existed is requested on the Protocol.

Consistent versus Episodic Nature of Problem

Bloodstein's (1960, 1981) cross-sectional study of the developmental phases of stuttering suggests the importance of determining if the fluency problem is chronic. According to Bloodstein one of the best indicators that "stuttering is still in its most rudimentary form is that it appears for periods of weeks or months between long interludes of normal speech." Furthermore, he suggests that spontaneous recovery is probable during this episodic phase. Parental reports of chronic,

day-to-day disfluencies would, however, be a danger sign. Therefore the consistency of the problem should be noted on the Protocol.

Reaction to Stress

Bloodstein (1960, 1981), noted that children are most disfluent when they are excited or upset. Parents, too, are likely to report this about their child. Van Riper (1963) suggested that parents remove conditions of communicative pressure in the home environment to foster more fluent speech. Ryan (1974) used this knowledge in his diagnostic interview (Preschool, Form A). In his "Speed" task the child is asked to name as many things in the room as possible while the examiner counts to 10, or to tell the examiner what he did during the day and to do so in a hurry. Using a similar approach at some point in the diagnostic session, and recording on the Protocol the impact it had on the child's speech, is recommended. The stress reactions may make both stutterers and nonstutterers more disfluent, but the types of disfluency may be different. Normal disfluencies should predominate in the speech of normal children, while incipient stutterers will display more broken words, prolongations, part-word repetitions, and the like. In summary, what is important is not that the child increased his disfluency rate under stressful situations, but the form that these disfluencies took. Once again, the types of disfluency and size of the speech unit affected are seen as diagnostically important. Specific observations should be made on the Protocol regarding changes in frequency and type of disfluency during stressful situations.

Phoneme/Word/Situation Fears and Avoidances

As previously noted, sound and word fears develop into avoidance behaviors, such as the concealment devices discussed by Van Riper (1963). Tell-tale symptoms of fears and avoidances may be present in the child's overt speech; many times they are not easy to identify. Often the child or the parent will reveal, through probing interviews, evidence of emotional reactions to phonemes, words, and speaking situations. The presence of these reactions suggests a true stuttering problem and one that has progressed in its severity. Such fears or avoidance should be described on the Protocol.

Familial History

Evidence regarding the relationship between family history and stuttering is unclear. However, genetic research and clinical reports suggest that the disfluent child with a positive history of stuttering in the family is more likely to be an incipient stutterer than a child without such a background (cf., Bloodstein, 1981; Kidd, 1980; Van Riper, 1971, 1982). A familial history of disfluency should be noted on the Protocol.

Other Covert Factors

Space is provided for the clinician to record other features of the disfluency problem and the individual's reaction to it.

SUMMARY OF CLINICAL EVIDENCE AND IMPRESSIONS

The Protocol for Differentiating the Incipient Stutterer provides a systematic procedure for making specific observations regarding speech fluency. It categorizes eight types of auditory behaviors the clinician should identify. When the behavior is recorded on the Protocol, a grid allows the clinician to automatically determine whether it is normal, questionable, or likely to be indicative of stuttering. While failure in any particular category is not an indication of a fluency problem, a number of questionable symptoms suggests a possible disorder, or at least the need to monitor the child's fluency. The presence of several abnormal auditory behaviors would lead a clinician to a diagnosis of stuttering.

The eight auditory behaviors provide adequate information on which to make a diagnosis; the remaining sections on the Protocol (i.e., visual evidence and historical/psychological indicators) provide supportive information. Given our present understanding of incipient stuttering, it is not possible to weigh the importance of each of the eight auditory behaviors. Clinical common sense and face validity, however, suggest that the first five of the eight behaviors are the more indicative of incipient stuttering. It is conceivable, therefore, that a quick diagnostic impression can be formulated from an analysis of the child's overt speech on only these five dimensions. Continued research efforts and field testing are necessary to confirm such hypotheses.

For a thorough evaluation, the clinician should not stop with auditory behaviors, despite their primary role in the diagnostic, decision-making process. Visual evidences of speech effort such as the presence of facial grimaces, articulatory postures, head movements, or other body involvement can be systematically investigated and catalogued. These observations supplement auditory evidences of incipient stuttering.

Psychological indicators of disfluency can be accumulated through observation, direct interview, supplemental tests, etc. The Protocol is valuable in insuring that these indicators are not overlooked, but are routinely considered in an overall evaluation of the child's fluency.

CONCLUSION

The preceding report was an attempt to synthesize the literature with regard to the differential diagnosis of disfluent children. The Protocol organizes a body of knowledge in a clinically useful format to provide guidelines for intervention and service. It is to this end that the Protocol for Differentiating the Incipient Stutterer is presented.

REFERENCES

Adams, M. R. (1977). A clinical strategy for differentiating the normally nonfluent child and the incipient stutterer. *Journal of Fluency Disorders, 2,* 141–148.

Adams, M. R. (1978). Further analysis of stuttering as a phonetic transition defect. *Journal of Fluency Disorders, 3,* 265–272.

Allen, G. D., Peters, R. W., & Williams, C. L. (1975). *Spectrographic study of fluent and stuttered speech.* Paper presented at the Annual Convention of the American Speech and Hearing Association, Washington, DC.

Andrews, G., & Harris, M. (1964). *The syndrome of stuttering.* London: Heineman.

Bloodstein, O. (1960). The development of stuttering: Part II. Developmental phases. *Journal of Speech and Hearing Disorders, 25,* 366–376.

Bloodstein, O. (1981). *A handbook on stuttering.* Chicago: National Easter Seal Society.

Bluemel, C. S. (1932). Primary and secondary stammering. *Quarterly Journal of Speech, 18,* 187–200.

Cooper, E. B. (1973). The development of a stuttering chronicity prediction checklist for school age stutterers: A research inventory for clinicians. *Journal of Speech and Hearing Disorders, 38,* 215–223.

Cooper, E. B. (1976). *Personalized fluency control therapy.* Hingham, MA: Teaching Resources.

Egland, G. (1955). Repetitions and prolongations in the speech of stuttering and nonstuttering children. In W. Johnson (Ed.), *Stuttering in children and adults.* Minneapolis: University of Minnesota Press.

Glasner, P. J., & Rosenthal, D. (1957). Parental diagnosis of stuttering in young children. *Journal of Speech and Hearing Disorders, 22,* 288–295.

Jameson, A. M. (1955). Stammering in children—some factors in the prognosis. *Speech, 19,* 60–67.

Kidd, K. K. (1980). Genetic models of stuttering. *Journal of Fluency Disorders, 5,* 187–201.

Metraux, R. W. (1950). Speech profiles of the pre-school child 18 to 54 months. *Journal of Speech and Hearing Disorders, 15,* 37–53.

Montgomery, A. A., & Cooke, P. A. (1976). Perceptual and acoustic analysis of repetitions in stuttered speech. *Journal of Communication Disorders, 9,* 317–330.

Panelli, C. A., McFarlane, S. C., & Shipley, K. G. (1978). Implications of evaluating and intervening with incipient stutterers. *Journal of Fluency Disorders, 3,* 41–50.

Perkins, W. H. (1971). *Speech pathology an applied behavioral science.* Saint Louis: C. V. Mosby.

Riley, G. D. (1972). A stuttering severity instrument for children and adults. *Journal of Speech and Hearing Disorders, 37,* 314–320.

Riley, G. D. (1980). *Stuttering severity instrument for children and adults.* Tigaard, OR: C. C. Publications.

Ryan, B. P. (1974). *Programmed therapy for stuttering in children and adults.* Springfield, IL: Charles C. Thomas.

Sheehan, J. G., & Martyn, N. M. (1966). Spontaneous recovery from stuttering. *Journal of Speech and Hearing Research, 9,* 121–135.

Shine, R. E. (1980). Direct management of the beginning stutterer. *Seminars in Speech, Language, and Hearing, 1,* 339–350.

Stromsta, C. (1965). A spectrographic study of the dysfluencies labeled as stuttering by parents. *De Therapia Vocis et Loquelae*, *1*, 317–320.

Van Riper, C. (1963). *Speech correction: Principles and methods* (4th ed.). Englewood Cliffs, NJ: Prentice-Hall.

Van Riper, C. (1971). *The nature of stuttering*. Englewood Cliffs, NJ: Prentice-Hall.

Van Riper, C. (1982). *The nature of stuttering* (2nd ed.). Englewood Cliffs, NJ: Prentice-Hall.

Wingate, M. E. (1964a). A standard definition of stuttering. *Journal of Speech and Hearing Disorders, 29*, 484–489.

Wingate, M. E. (1964b). Recovery from stuttering. *Journal of Speech and Hearing Disorders, 29*, 312–321.

Yairi, E., & Lewis, B. (1984). Disfluencies at the onset of stuttering. *Journal of Speech and Hearing Research, 27*, 154–159.

APPENDIX

Protocol for Differentiating the Incipient Stutterer

Name _____   Date of birth _____

Address _____   Age _____ Sex _____

_____   Date of test _____

Clinician _____

I. AUDITORY BEHAVIORS

- **Type of Disfluency (mark the most typical)**

  Interjections   *Hesitations/Gaps-* *Repetitions-*   *Prolongations-* *Coexisting struggle*

PROBABLY NORMAL	QUESTIONABLE	PROBABLY ABNORMAL

- **Size of Speech Unit Affected (mark the typical level at which disfluencies occur)**

  Sentence/Phrase-   *Word-*   *Syllable/Sound*

PROBABLY NORMAL	QUESTIONABLE	PROBABLY ABNORMAL

- **Frequency of Disfluencies (compute from speech sample and mark values on continua)**

  - Frequency of Repetitions

    <------------------ *2%* ------------ *5%* ------------------>

PROBABLY NORMAL	QUESTIONABLE	PROBABLY ABNORMAL

  - Frequency of Prolongations

    <------------- *1%* ------------------------------->

PROBABLY NORMAL	PROBABLY ABNORMAL

  - Frequency of Disfluencies, in General

    <----------- *2%* --------- *5%* --------- *10%* ----------->

NORMAL	PROBABLY NORMAL	QUESTIONABLE	PROBABLY ABNORMAL

● **Duration of Disfluencies**

  • Typical Number of Reiterations of the Repetition =_____

Less than 2	*2 to 5*	*More than 5*
PROBABLY NORMAL	QUESTIONABLE	PROBABLY ABNORMAL

  • Average Duration of Prolongations =_____

Less than 1 Second	*One or More Seconds*
PROBABLY NORMAL	PROBABLY ABNORMAL

● **Audible Effort (mark those that apply)**

Lack of the Following:	*Presence of the Following:*
PROBABLY NORMAL	PROBABLY ABNORMAL

_____ hard glottal attacks
_____ disrupted airflow
_____ vocal tension
_____ pitch rise
_____ others:

● **Rhythm/Tempo/Speed of Disfluencies**

Slow/Normal; Evenly Paced	*Fast, Perhaps Irregular*
PROBABLY NORMAL	PROBABLY ABNORMAL

● **Intrusion of Schwa Vowel during Repetitions**

Schwa Not Heard	*Presence of Schwa*
PROBABLY NORMAL	PROBABLY ABNORMAL

● **Audible Learned Behaviors (mark those that apply)**

Lack of the Following:	*Presence of the Following:*
PROBABLY NORMAL	PROBABLY ABNORMAL

_____ word/phrase substitutions
_____ circumlocutions
_____ avoidance tactics (starters, postponers, and the like)

II. VISUAL EVIDENCE (list behaviors observed)

● **Facial Grimaces/Articulatory Posturing:**
● **Head Movements:**
● **Body Involvement:**

III. HISTORICAL/PSYCHOLOGICAL INDICATORS (comment on the following based on client and/or parent interviews, observations, and supplemental tests or questionaires, if any.)

- **Awareness and Concern (of child; of parents):**
- **Length of Time Fluency Problem Has Existed:**
- **Consistent versus Episodic Nature of Problem:**
- **Reaction to Stress:**
- **Phoneme/Word/Situation Fears and Avoidances:**
- **Familial History:**
- **Other Covert Factors:**

IV. SUMMARY OF CLINICAL EVIDENCE AND IMPRESSIONS

A Comparison of Stutterers' and Nonstutterers' Affective, Cognitive, and Behavioral Self-Reports

Jennifer Barber Watson

The relationship between stuttering and stutterers' communication attitudes has been of interest for a number of years. Investigators have examined: (a) stutterers' attitudes as prognostic indicators of successful therapy (Busta, Agnello, & Creaghead, 1980; Guitar, 1976, 1980); (b) the role of stutterers' communication attitudes in facilitating changes in speech behaviors (Cooper, 1973, 1976; Gregory, 1968, 1973, 1979; Perkins, 1979, 1981; Sheehan, 1968, 1970, 1979; Williams, 1968, 1979); and (c) the importance of attitude change in maintaining fluency (Ammons & Johnson, 1944; Andrews & Cutler, 1974; Boberg, 1981; Brutten, 1975, 1979; Erickson, 1969; Gregory, 1969; Guitar, 1979; Guitar & Bass, 1978; Ingham, 1979, 1981; Lanyon, 1967; Perkins, 1979, 1981; Shumak, 1955; Woolf, 1967; Young, 1981). Much of this research was attempted to obtain a better understanding of the relationship between stuttering and stutterers' communication attitudes and, thereby, improve treatment. Many such studies, however, used assessment procedures that were limited in one or more of the following ways: (a) minimal assessment of instruments' content, construct, and criterion validity; (b) limited attention to estimating reliability with adult stutterers; (c) response options (e.g., true/false, checklists) that dichotomize attitudinal domains; (d) little distinctions between reports of thoughts or feelings, and reports of behavior; (e) ambiguous or restricted items, such as items worded exclusively for one sex or for students; and (f) preliminary development and evaluation of the instrument (e.g., proposing "normative" guidelines based on a single administration of the instrument). Improved assessment procedures could increase our ability to describe adult stutterers' attitudes. It has been suggested that attitudinal domains are multidimensional (Gregory, 1979; Ostrom, 1969; Rosenberg & Hovland, 1960; Triandis, 1967, 1971), and an increased understanding of stutterers' attitudi-

nal domains and how these domains compare with those of nonstutterers may improve our understanding of stuttering as well as our clinical efforts in treating it. The purpose of this study was to compare the attitudes of stutterers and nonstutterers as measured by a newly developed procedure designed to examine adult stutterers.

PROCEDURES

Assessment Inventory

The development and evaluation of the Inventory of Communication Attitudes[1] was completed in two earlier investigations that examined the responses of 133 adult stutterers and 56 nonstutterers (Barber, 1981). The result of these investigations was an inventory based on a tripartite attitudinal model (Ostrom, 1969; Rosenberg & Hovland, 1960; Triandis, 1967, 1971). This model includes three classes of evaluative responses: (a) an affective component, associated with sympathetic nervous responses and verbal statements of affect; (b) a cognitive component, associated with perceptual responses and verbal statements of belief; and (c) a behavioral component, associated with overt actions and verbal statements concerning behavior. Although these components are not independent, responses within each category generally provide some unique information (Ostrom, 1969).

The Inventory of Communication Attitudes uses four response scales to measure these three classes of responses. These response scales, reported in Appendix A, include: Affective Scale 1, which obtains ratings of feelings of enjoyment/hate about speaking in designated situations; Behavioral Scale 2, which deals with ratings of one's speech skills in various situations; Cognitive-A Scale 3, which obtains ratings of one's perceptions of how most people feel about speaking in the situations; and Cognitive-B Scale 4, which requests ratings of one's perceptions of most people's speech skills in specific speaking contexts. Cognitive Scales 3 and 4 assess respondents' two belief systems of what is

Reprinted from *Journal of Speech and Hearing Research, 31*, no. 7, 377–385. Copyright © 1988, American Speech-Language-Hearing Association.

considered "usual" in affect and behavior. These scales are used to rate 39 speaking situations that comprise 13 situational subscales that represent different types of speaking contexts (see Appendix B). To determine if stutterers and nonstutterers encounter these situations with comparable frequency and to assess any relationship between reported frequency of meeting situations and communication attitudes, Frequency Scale 5 also was included (see Appendix A).

Subjects

Subjects were 76 stutterers and 81 nonstutterers who were monolingual English speakers. The stuttering group consisted of 57 men and 19 women who were clinically diagnosed stutterers. They ranged in age from 18 years to 71.17 years ($M = 32.81$; $SD = 10.56$), with educational status ranging from completion of the 10th grade to 6 years of graduate studies ($M = 15.50$; $SD = 2.54$). None had observable physical handicaps, clinically diagnosed psychological problems, hearing impairments, or speech and language problems other than stuttering as reported by a contact clinician. Fifty-three (69.7%) of the stutterers were receiving therapy at the time they completed the inventory. The total amount of reported speech therapy ranged from none to 25 years ($M = 3.56$; $SD = 4.42$; median = 2.00). Self ratings of stuttering severity ranged from 1 to 6 (on a 7-point scale with "1" indicating mild stuttering and "7" indicating severe stuttering), with a mean of 3.48 and a standard deviation of 1.27.

Nonstuttering subjects were 57 men and 24 women, ages ranging from 18 years to 73.83 years ($M = 35.03$; $SD = 15.02$). Educational status ranged from completion of the 12th grade to 9 years of graduate work ($M = 16.04$; $SD = 2.51$). None reported having current speech, language, or hearing problems.

Test Administration

Twenty-five institutions in 12 states and four Canadian provinces assisted in collection of stutterers' data. Clinicians at each institution were asked to distribute the inventory to subjects who met the criteria specified earlier. To identify nonstuttering respondents, students from two universities, one in the Southwest and the other in the Midwest, distributed packets to friends and family members who agreed to participate in a study involving communication attitudes and to complete the inventory in one day. Respondents mailed the completed inventory to the investigator. Two different randomized orders of the situational subscale items were distributed, and the order of response scale presentation was counterbalanced. The frequency scale always was administered last, because it was not considered part of the tripartite attitudinal model.

STATISTICAL ANALYSES AND RESULTS

Reliability Estimates

Estimates of the reliability of the internal consistency[2] of the inventory were computed from stutterers' responses to the situational subscales on Scales 1 through 4. The means and standard deviations for each situational subscale are reported in Table 1.

Standardized Cronbach's coefficient alphas were computed for the total inventory score, for the four response scales separately, and for each situational subscale in each response scale (see Table 2). In addition, item/situational subscale correlations revealed that no item had coefficients less than .50 in more than one scale. The coefficients indicate that the internal consistency of the inventory ranged from moderate to excellent.

TABLE 1. Means and standard deviations (in parentheses) of stutterers' responses to situational subscales for scales 1 through 4.

Situational subscale	Scale			
	1	2	3	4
1: Telephone Conversations	13.53 (4.82)	12.68 (4.83)	9.66 (3.80)	7.07 (3.82)
2: Argument/ Conflict With Friend	14.49 (4.13)	12.58 (4.44)	14.59 (4.36)	10.59 (4.88)
3: Argument/ Conflict With Stranger	13.96 (4.11)	12.27 (4.12)	13.09 (4.06)	9.68 (4.59)
4: One-to-One Conversation With Family	7.24 (4.01)	9.01 (3.91)	5.38 (2.69)	5.47 (3.44)
5: One-to-One Conversation With Authority	11.52 (3.83)	11.05 (3.79)	10.20 (3.48)	7.99 (3.57)
6: Informal Known Group Conversation	8.64 (4.53)	9.87 (4.16)	5.37 (2.51)	5.70 (3.13)
7: Informal Unknown Group Conversation	14.03 (4.71)	13.81 (4.37)	11.46 (3.99)	9.59 (4.43)
8: Formal Presentation	15.72 (5.16)	14.60 (4.73)	13.53 (3.99)	10.42 (4.33)
9: Questioning Friend/Family	10.36 (3.83)	9.57 (3.67)	9.75 (3.46)	7.38 (3.69)
10: Questioning Stranger	10.43 (3.86)	10.04 (4.22)	8.28 (3.32)	5.75 (2.68)
11: Questioning Authority	13.85 (4.24)	13.38 (4.00)	11.28 (3.61)	8.87 (3.86)
12: Time Constraint Situations	13.75 (4.26)	12.91 (4.23)	11.62 (3.92)	8.53 (4.34)
13: Unchangeable Content Situations	10.72 (4.54)	10.76 (4.77)	6.51 (3.42)	4.45 (2.50)

Note: Because there were three items in each subscale and item ratings could range from "1" to "7," subscale scores could range from 3.0 to 21.0.

TABLE 2. Cronbach's coefficient alpha for each situational subscale in scales 1 through 4, response scales 1 through 4, and total inventory.

Situational subscale	Scale			
	1	2	3	4
1	.889	.903	.855	.886
2	.887	.893	.870	.923
3	.833	.864	.849	.925
4	.848	.767	.734	.790
5	.774	.807	.791	.882
6	.871	.830	.810	.820
7	.880	.883	.848	.909
8	.930	.902	.833	.929
9	.750	.786	.671	.802
10	.808	.838	.770	.734
11	.822	.844	.797	.831
12	.865	.869	.832	.906
13	.833	.832	.918	.858
Response scales	.919	.941	.942	.964
Total inventory .968				

Assessment of Subscale and Scale Validity

The construct validity of the 13 situational subscales and the four response scales was studied by factor analyses. First, the dimensionality of each situational subscale was assessed. Each subscale should contain items that reflect the single dimension or construct defined by each speaking situation.

Principal axis factoring was performed on each situational subscale for each response scale separately. Results revealed that a single factor with an eigenvalue greater than or equal to 1.0 was extracted in each of the subscales. The percentage of variance accounted for by these single factors ranged from 60.3 percent to 87.9 percent. These findings indicate that each of the situational subscales represent a single construct.

To examine the dimensionality of the four response scales, a single factor analysis extracting four factors was completed.[3] This four-factor technique was used to document the presence of the four constructs that had been identified in earlier studies (Barber, 1981): an affective construct (Affective Scale 1), a behavioral construct (Behavioral Scale 2), and two cognitive constructs (Cognitive-A Scale 3 and Cognitive-B Scale 4). Principal axis factoring followed by varimax rotation was completed for all situational subscale scores on Scales 1 through 4. This analysis confirmed the presence of scale factors, which prior to rotation, accounted for 66.4 percent of the total variance. Correlations greater than or equal to $\pm.40$ of situational subscales by scale across the four factors are reported in Table 3. The correlations suggested that three of the four factors represent response scale constructs. Affective Scale 1 and Behavioral Scale 2, which involve reports of self-enjoyment and self-skill, respectively, both appeared on the first factor. Evidently, how well one speaks in a given situation is a good indicator of how one feels about speaking in that situation. Thus, these two scales represent a single self-assessment dimension.[4] Cognitive-A Scale 3 and Cognitive-B Scale 4 each loaded on a distinct factor. Factor 2

TABLE 3. Correlations of subscales by scale across four factors.

	Situational subscales												
	1	2	3	4	5	6	7	8	9	10	11	12	13
Factor 1													
Scale 1	.73	.52	.70		.75	.60	.66	.66	.54	.66	.87	.80	.64
2	.71	.66	.73		.86	.70	.72	.72	.62	.74	.87	.81	.62
3													
4													
Factor 2													
Scale 1													
2													
3						.40							
4	.84	.80	.81	.57	.76	.73	.78	.76	.81	.80	.81	.72	.64
Factor 3													
Scale 1													
2													
3	.80	.70	.66		.79		.64	.57	.68	.78	.86	.80	.58
4													
Factor 4													
Scale 1				.71		.44			.42				
2				.66		.49			.51				
3				.44									
4													

Note: Only those correlations greater than or equal to $\pm.40$ are reported.

correlations appear to reflect beliefs about others' feelings about speaking in the 13 types of situations covered by the inventory. Factor 3 represents a different belief dimension based on one's perceptions of how well others speak. Results suggest that the four response scales represent three constructs, one related to self-assessment and two related to beliefs about others. The fourth factor did not correlate with more than three situational subscales in any one scale, and, thus, did not seem to represent a scale construct.

A related issue is whether the inventory can distinguish stutterers and nonstutterers. Stutterers' and nonstutterers' responses to the four response scales and to the 13 situational subscales in each response scale were compared in a series of five multiple discriminant analyses. Response scale scores and situational subscale scores were calculated by summing all responses in each scale and in each subscale. Results are reported in Table 4. These findings indicate that the inventory can differentiate stutterers and nonstutterers on the basis of their responses to each of the response scales and to the situational subscales.

Stutterer and Nonstutterer Response Comparisons

Comparisons of the responses of stutterers and nonstutterers included examination of the four response scales, the 13 situational subscales, and the interrelationships among the four response scales plus the frequency scale. An examination was conducted to determine if the two groups encountered the various speaking situations with similar frequency. A discriminant analysis between stutterers and nonstutterers on the situational subscale scores on Frequency Scale 5 was significant [Wilks Lambda (13) = .741; χ^2 = 44.49; $p < .001$]. However, only three situational subscales had significant ($p < .001$) univariate F ratios and correlation coefficients between the discriminant functions and subscale scores greater than or equal to ±.30. Subscale 3, Argument or Conflict With a Stranger, Subscale 8, Formal Presentations, and Subscale 11, Questioning an Authority were encountered significantly less often by stutterers. These findings suggest that, with the exception of three types of

situations, there were no significant differences between stutterers and nonstutterers in terms of how often they encountered the various speaking situations.

Response Scale Comparisons. To compare responses across the four response scales, results of the significant discriminant analyses previously reported were examined further (see Table 4). Identification of correlation coefficients greater than or equal to ±.30 between the discriminant functions and response scale scores and significant ($p < .001$) F ratios revealed that stutterers and nonstutterers were best discriminated on the basis of their responses to the Affective and Behavioral Scales. Stutterers' scores were higher than nonstutterers' on both scales, indicating less enjoyment and poorer speech skills. Behavioral Scale 2 was statistically the more important contributor to this discrimination, suggesting that self-reports of speech skills were the primary differentiator. Respondents' scores were submitted to a Bayesian classification analysis (Klecka, 1975) that estimates group membership on the basis of responses on the four scales. Table 5 shows that 91.4 percent of the nonstutterers were classified on the basis of their response scale scores, compared with 77.6 percent of the stutterers. These findings suggest that reports of self-enjoyment of speaking, self-speech skills, and perceptions of others' enjoyment and speech skills may be somewhat more homogeneous among nonstutterers than among stutterers.

Situational Subscale Comparisons. As noted previously, stutterers and nonstutterers responded differently to situational subscales in all four response scales (see Table 4). In the Affective and Behavioral Scales, Situational Subscale 11, Questioning an Authority Figure to Obtain Information or to Elicit Action, best discriminated stutterers from nonstutterers (see Table 6). Four additional situational subscales also were identified as statistically important contributors to the discrimination of reports of self-enjoyment and self-speaking skills in these situations;

Subscale   1:   Telephone Conversations
Subscale   6:   Informal Known Group Conversations

TABLE 4. Summary of discriminant analyses performed on response scale scores and on situational subscale scores in scales 1 through 4.

Score	Function	Canonical Correlation	Wilks Lambda	Chi-Square	df	p
Scales 1–4	1	.72	.479	112.52	4	.001
Subscales: Scale 1	1	.73	.472	111.51	13	.001
Subscales: Scale 2	1	.80	.364	150.07	13	.001
Subscales: Scale 3	1	.51	.737	45.30	13	.001
Subscales: Scale 4	1	.55	.702	52.46	13	.001

TABLE 5. Classification results of response scales 1 through 4.

Actual group		Predicted group membership	
	n	Stutterers	Nonstutterers
Stutterers	76	59 (77.6%)	17 (22.4%)
Nonstutterers	81	7 (8.6%)	74 (91.4%)

Subscale 8: Formal Presentations
Subscale 13: Situations Involving Unchangeable Content

Stutterers reported significantly less enjoyment of speaking and significantly poorer speech skills than nonstutterers. The responses of stutterers to Behavioral Scale 2 indicated poorer speech skills in five additional situational subscales, including both one-to-one and group conversations with familiar and unfamiliar listeners.

In Table 7, stutterers' responses to Cognitive-A and Cognitive-B Scales can be seen to differ significantly from those of nonstutterers' on three situational subscales. Stutter-

ers rated others' enjoyment of speech significantly greater and others' speech skills significantly better. Stutterers also rated others' speech skills significantly better than did nonstutterers in five additional situational subscales including telephone conversations and conversations with strangers or authority figures.

Response Scale Interrelationship Comparisons. Two factor analyses extracting four factors were performed separately on stutterers' and nonstutterers' situational subscale scores on each of the five response scales. Correlations greater than or equal to ±.40 of situational subscales across the four factors for stutterers and nonstutterers are reported in Tables 8 and 9, respectively. As indicated by Factor 1 for stutterers and by Factor 2 for nonstutterers, both groups' self-reports of enjoyment of speaking and speech skills in the various situations were related. However, for stutterers, additional correlations with subscales on Frequency Scale 5 indicated that frequency of encountering situations was related both to enjoyment of speech and to reported speech skills. Frequency was not related to nonstutterers' perceptions of speaking proficiency or to enjoyment of speech. Nonstutterers' cognitive reports on Cognitive-A Scale 3 and Cognitive-B Scale 4 also were related (see Factor 1), which

TABLE 6. Correlations between discriminant function and subscale scores and univariate *F* ratios on subscales in Affective Scale 1 and Behavioral Scale 2.

Situational subscale	Affective Scale 1 correlation		Behavioral Scale 2 correlation	
	F	p	F	p
1: Telephone Conversations	.449 34.91	.001	.537 78.19	.001
4: One-to-One Conversation With Family			.404 44.14	.001
5: One-to-One Conversation With Authority			.439 52.25	.001
6: Informal Known Group Conversation	.401 27.95	.001	.406 44.70	.001
7: Informal Unknown Group Conversation			.396 42.37	.001
8: Formal Presentation	.523 47.47	.001	.605 99.22	.001
10: Questioning Stranger			.491 65.24	.001
11: Questioning Authority	.625 67.70	.001	.717 139.10	.001
12: Time Constraint Situations			.541 79.15	.001
13: Unchangeable Content Situations	.538 50.14	.001	.699 132.30	.001

Note: Only subscales with correlation coefficients greater than or equal to ±.30 and Univariate *F* ratios with *p* less than or equal to .01 are reported.

TABLE 7. Correlations between discriminant function and subscale scores and univariate *F* ratios for subscales in Cognitive-A Scale 3 and Cognitive-B Scale 4.

Situational subscale	Cognitive-A Scale 3 correlation		Cognitive-B Scale 4 correlation	
	F	p	F	p
1: Telephone Conversations			.367 8.82	.004
2: Argument/ Conflict With Friend	.393 8.53	.004	.536 18.86	.001
3: Argument/ Conflict With Stranger			.366 8.80	.004
5: One-to-One Conversation With Authority			.556 20.26	.001
7: Informal Unknown Group Conversation	.511 14.44	.001	.498 16.25	.001
9: Questioning Friend/Family Member	.370 7.57	.007	.417 11.43	.001
10: Questioning Stranger			.441 12.77	.001
12: Time Constraint Situations			.376 9.29	.003

Note: Only subscales with correlation coefficients greater than or equal to ±.30 and Univariate *F* with *p* less than or equal to .01 are reported.

TABLE 8. Correlations of subscales by scale across four factors for stutterers.

	Situational subscales												
	1	2	3	4	5	6	7	8	9	10	11	12	13
Factor 1													
Scale 1	.76	.47	.67		.74	.57	.64	.63	.50	.68	.84	.79	.65
2	.73	.61	.69		.86	.67	.70	.68	.58	.76	.84	.82	.63
3													
4													
5	.49		.45		.41	.51	.45	.51		.50	.47		.49
Factor 2													
Scale 1									.41				
2													
3						.41	.40						
4	.85	.83	.84	.57	.75	.75	.75	.77	.84	.79	.81	.73	.65
5													
Factor 3													
Scale 1													
2										.43			
3	.81	.62	.57	.45	.78		.60	.56	.66	.82	.85	.77	.64
4													
5													
Factor 4													
Scale 1													
2		.42		.49					.46				
3				.46		.42			.42				
4													
5		.53				.54			.55				

Note: Only those correlations greater than or equal to ±.40 are reported.

TABLE 9. Correlations of subscales by scale across four factors for nonstutterers.

	Situational subscales												
	1	2	3	4	5	6	7	8	9	10	11	12	13
Factor 1													
Scale 1		.43											
2													
3	.67	.54	.60		.67		.58	.65	.62	.68	.64	.65	.52
4	.74	.77	.78	.41	.77		.74	.71	.79	.63	.79	.76	.47
5													
Factor 2													
Scale 1	.73			.49	.62		.59	.55	.63	.67	.81	.73	.47
2	.69		.52	.58	.60	.45	.52	.41	.48	.55	.64	.55	.40
3													
4													
5													
Factor 3													
Scale 1													
2													
3													
4													
5		.69			.48		.48			.54	.58	.58	
Factor 4													
Scale 1													
2				.41		.59				.56			.55
3						.63							
4				.53		.59							
5				.41		.49							

Note: Only those correlations greater than or equal to ±.40 are reported.

suggests that nonstutterers' believe that most people's enjoyment of speech and most people's speech skills are related, just as one's own feelings and behavior reports are related. In contrast, stutterers' beliefs about others' enjoyment of speech and speech skills were unrelated (Factors 2 and 3).

DISCUSSION

This investigation examined the communication attitudes of adult stutterers through the use of the Inventory of Communication Attitudes. Findings raise issues regarding stutterers' avoidances, attitude multidimensionality in the perceptions of speaking situations, differences in stutterers' and nonstutterers' belief systems, and stuttering group homogeneity.

Only 3 of the 13 situational subscales were encountered significantly less by stutterers. Two of these three infrequently met situations were also rated more negatively by stutterers, which suggests that these contexts may be avoided because of negative feelings and anticipated poor speech skills. The premise that frequency is related to stutterers' self-ratings of affect and behavior was further supported by the correlational analyses summarized in Table 8. These findings are consistent with clinical observations that speech anxieties or fears lead to avoidances. Like nonstutterers, stutterers may need to learn to disassociate their feelings and perceptions from their tendency to enter various speaking contexts thereby reducing avoidance of feared situations.

Stutterers' ratings of the various speaking situations suggest that their attitudes are multidimensional. All of the situational subscales differentiated stutterers and nonstutterers in one or more of the attitude scales. Moreover, no situational subscale differentiated the two groups of respondents on all four response probes. However, two situations, telephone conversations and unknown group conversations, differentiated stutterers and nonstutterers on three of the four response scales. In addition to these specific situational differences, five of the eight discriminating situations in Cognitive-B Scale 4 also were discriminating situations in Behavioral Scale 2. These findings suggest that stutterers' perceptions of others' speech skills are inversely related to their own speech skills in these situations. Thus, as stutterers rate their own speech skills negatively, they tend to rate most people's speech skills positively.

Nonstutterers' reports of others' enjoyment of speech were related to perceptions of others' speech skills. Similarly, their ratings of self-enjoyment of speaking and of their own speech skills also were related. Stutterers did not believe that most people's enjoyment is related to how they speak in the situations. Stutterers may need to understand that, just as with themselves, nonstutterers' feelings are related to reported speech skills. Through this increased understanding, stutterers may be more realistic about others' attitudes and, in turn, adopt more realistic self-expectations.

Comparisons of stutterers' and nonstutterers' responses also suggested that nonstutterers' response scale scores were more homogeneous than were those of stutterers (see Table 5). This variability in the stuttering group may be expected and could be accounted for in subsequent empirical investigations by identifying subgroups of stutterers within this clinical population. Patterns of responding characteristic of subgroups of stutterers may be based on variables such as current speech behavior, pretreatment severity, therapy status, and perceived therapy effectiveness. In the current study, stutterers of varying therapy status and severity were included. Additional empirical work examining the possible relationships among such variables as those mentioned and reported communication attitudes are needed.

Bandura (1969) and others have suggested that changes in attitude will affect behavior and that behavioral response patterns become more stable over time when accompanied by cognitive supports. The importance of attitude change in the long term maintenance of fluency has been recognized by many clinical researchers (Boberg, 1981). For the stutterer, the gap between sounding normal and feeling normal may be a matter of attitude (Perkins, 1979). To "bridge the gap," specific attitudes may need to be identified, reinforced, or modified. Findings of this study suggest that attitudes are multidimensional and that clinicians may expect both similarities and differences in stutterers' and nonstutterers' attitudes. If one goal in therapy is to "normalize" attitudes, then those communication attitudes common to stutterers and nonstutterers may warrant reinforcement. Attitudinal domains that differentiate these two groups may be targeted for change. Attudinal similarities should not be disregarded, because changes in one domain may affect other domains. As research examining the relationship between attitude change and maintenance of the therapy gains continues, further assessment of these self-reports will be valuable. More comprehensive descriptions of stutterers' and nonstutterers' communication attitudes should result in increased understanding of these covert aspects of stuttering and may lead to increased long-term effectiveness of stuttering therapy.

ACKNOWLEDGMENTS

Preparation of this article was supported in part by Texas Christian University Research Fund Grant 523727 to Jennifer Barber Watson.

The author would like to express her appreciation to the numerous individuals and institutions who so kindly cooperated in data collection. Without their assistance and interest, this research would not have been possible. In addition, she gratefully acknowledges the help of Bennett Fletcher, Hugo Gregory, and Doris Kistler in the preparation of this manuscript.

NOTES

1. For detailed descriptions of all statistical analyses and results obtained in the development and evaluation of this Inventory, contact the investigator.

2. According to Borhnstedt (1970), measures of stability and measures of equivalence are basic types of reliability measurements. Stability measures examine the consistency of repeatability of responses across time, e.g., test-retest methods. Equivalence measures focus on determining the equivalence of each item as an indicator of an underlying construct. In the initial development of the attitude scale, the emphasis should be primarily on item equivalence and not item repeatability (Borhnstedt). It should be noted, however, that adequate test-retest reliability is essential for clinical use of such scales.

3. In addition to the reported analysis, other analyses were completed extracting all factors with eigenvalues greater than or equal to 1.0 and the factor loadings were examined. Even though up to nine factors had eigenvalues that met this criterion, factor loadings were similar to those obtained with the four-factor technique. These additional factors, therefore, did not appear to represent anything of either theoretical or practical value.

4. Earlier analyses (Barber, 1981) had suggested that some unique information was obtained by Affective Scale 1. However, the present analysis revealed that this affective scale did not account for enough unique variance to be present in the four extracted factors. The relationship between Affective Scale 1 and Behavioral Scale 2 may be due in part to obtaining ratings of feelings about *speaking* in situations, rather than feelings about the situations themselves.

Four factors were extracted in this analysis that reflect the three constructs identified in previous analyses (self-assessment of feelings and behaviors and two belief systems) plus a frequency dimension.

REFERENCES

Ammons, R., & Johnson, W. (1944). Studies in the psychology of stuttering: XVII. The construction and application of a test of attitude toward stuttering. *Journal of Speech and Hearing Disorders, 9,* 39–49.

Andrews, G., & Cutler, J. (1974). Stuttering therapy: The relation between changes in symptom level and attitudes. *Journal of Speech and Hearing Disorders, 39,* 312–319.

Bandura, A. (1969). *Principles of behavior modification.* New York: Holt, Rinehart, & Winston.

Barber, J. (1981). *The development and evaluation of an instrument assessing stutterers' communication attitudes.* Unpublished doctoral dissertation, Northwestern University, Evanston, IL.

Boberg, E. (1981). *Maintenance of fluency.* New York: Elsevier.

Borhnstedt, G. (1970). Reliability and validity assessment in attitude measurement. In G. Summers (Ed.), *Attitude measurements* (pp. 80–99). Chicago: Rand McNally.

Brutten, G. (1975). Stuttering: Topography, assessment, and behavior-change strategies. In J. Eisenson (Ed.), *Stuttering: A second symposium* (pp. 199–262). New York: Harper & Row.

Brutten, G. (1979). *Behavioral assessment and the strategy of therapy.* Unpublished manuscript, Southern Illinois University.

Busta, K., Agnello, J., & Creaghead, N. (1980). Stutterers' scaled attitudes and their prognostic significance in therapy. *Journal of Fluency Disorders, 5,* 373–381.

Cooper, E. (1973). The development of a stuttering chronicity prediction checklist: A preliminary report. *Journal of Speech and Hearing Disorders, 38,* 215–223.

Cooper, E. (1976). *Personalized fluency control therapy: An integrated behavior and relationship therapy for stutterers.* Austin, TX: Learning Concepts, Inc.

Erickson, R. (1969). Assessing communication attitudes among stutterers. *Journal of Speech and Hearing Research, 12,* 711–724.

Gregory, H. (1968). *Learning theory and stuttering therapy.* Evanston, IL: Northwestern University Press.

Gregory, H. (1969). *An assessment of the results of stuttering therapy.* (Final Report, Research & Demonstration Project 1725-S.) Washington, DC: U.S. Department of Health, Education, & Welfare, Social & Rehabilitation Service.

Gregory, H. (1973). *Stuttering: Differential evaluation therapy.* Indianapolis: The Bobbs-Merrill Company.

Gregory, H. (1979). *Controversies about stuttering therapy.* Baltimore: University Park Press.

Guitar, B. (1976). Pretreatment factors associated with the outcome of stuttering therapy. *Journal of Speech and Hearing Research, 19,* 590–600.

Guitar, B. (1979). A response to Ingham's critique. *Journal of Speech and Hearing Disorders, 44,* 400–403.

Guitar, B. (1980, November). *Prediction of stuttering treatment long-term outcome.* Presented at the annual meeting of the American Speech-Language-Hearing Association, Detroit, MI.

Guitar, B., & Bass, C. (1978). Stuttering therapy: The relationship between attitude change and long-term outcome. *Journal of Speech and Hearing Disorders, 43,* 392–400.

Ingham, R. (1979). Comment on "Stuttering therapy: The relation between attitude change and long-term outcome." *Journal of Speech and Hearing Disorders, 44,* 397–400.

Ingham, R. (1981). Evaluation and maintenance in stuttering treatment: A search for ecstasy with nothing but agony. In E. Boberg (Ed.), *Maintenance of fluency* (pp. 179–218). New York: Elsevier.

Klecka, W. (1975). Discriminant analysis. In N. Nie, C. Hull, J. Jenkins, K. Steinbrenner, & D. Bent (Eds.), *Statistical package for the social sciences* (pp. 434–467). New York: McGraw-Hill.

Lanyon, R. (1967). The measurement of stuttering severity. *Journal of Speech and Hearing Research, 10,* 836–843.

Ostrom, T. (1969). The relationship between the affective, behavioral, and cognitive components of attitudes. *Journal of Experimental Social Psychology, 5,* 12–30.

Perkins, W. (1979). From psychoanalysis to discoordination. In H. Gregory (Ed.), *Controversies about stuttering therapy* (pp. 97–127). Baltimore: University Park Press.

Perkins, W. (1981). Measurement and maintenance of fluency. In E. Boberg (Ed.), *Maintenance of fluency* (pp. 147–178). New York: Elsevier.

Rosenberg, M., & Hovland, C. (1960). Cognitive, affective, and behavioral components of attitude. In M. Rosenberg, C. Hovland, W. McGuire, K. Abelson, & J. Brehm (Eds.), *Attitude organization and change* (pp. 1–14). New Haven, CT: Yale University Press.

Sheehan, J. (1968). Stuttering as a self-role conflict. In H. Gregory (Ed.), *Learning theory and stuttering therapy* (pp. 72–83). Evanston, IL: Northwestern University Press.

Sheehan, J. (1970). *Stuttering: Research and therapy.* New York: Harper & Row.

Sheehan, J. (1979). Current issues on stuttering and recovery. In H.

Gregory (Ed.), *Controversies about stuttering therapy* (pp. 175–207). Baltimore: University Park Press.

Shumak, I. (1955). A speech situation rating sheet for stutterers. In W. Johnson (Ed.), *Stuttering in children and adults* (pp. 341–347). Minneapolis: University of Minnesota Press.

Triandis, H. (1967). Toward an analysis of the components of interpersonal attitudes. In C. Sherif & M. Sherif (Eds.), *Attitude, ego-involvement and change* (pp. 227–270). New York: John Wiley.

Triandis, H. (1971). *Attitude and attitude change.* New York: John Wiley.

Williams, D. (1968). Stuttering therapy: An overview. In H. Gregory (Ed.), *Learning theory and stuttering therapy* (pp. 52–66). Evanston, IL: Northwestern University Press.

Williams, D. (1979). A perspective on approaches to stuttering therapy. In H. Gregory (Ed.), *Controversies about stuttering therapy* (pp. 241–268). Baltimore: University Park Press.

Woolf, G. (1967). The assessment of stuttering as a struggle, avoidance, and expectancy. *British Journal of Disordered Communication, 2,* 158–171.

Young, M. (1981). A reanalysis of "Stuttering therapy: The relation between attitude change and long-term outcome." *Journal of Speech and Hearing Disorders, 46,* 221–222.

APPENDIX A

Response Scales of the Inventory of Communication Attitudes

Affective Scale 1
1—I definitely enjoy speaking in this situation.
2—
3—
4—
5—
6—
7—I hate speaking in this situation.

Behavioral Scale 2
1—My speech skills are excellent in this situation.
2—
3—
4—
5—
6—
7—My speech skills are poor in this situation.

Cognitive-A Scale 3
1—Most speakers definitely enjoy speaking in this situation.
2—
3—
4—
5—
6—
7—Most speakers hate speaking in this situation.

Cognitive-B Scale 4
1—Most speakers' speech skills are excellent in this situation.
2—
3—
4—
5—
6—
7—Most speakers' speech skills are poor in this situation.

Frequency Response Scale

Frequency Scale 5
1—I meet this situation 2 or 3 times a day, or more, on the average.
2—
3—
4—
5—
6—
7—I never meet this situation.

APPENDIX B

Thirteen Situational Subscales and Associated Items of the Inventory of Communication Attitudes

Subscale 1: Telephone Conversations
  Item 01 Telephoning to ask a price, train fare, etc.
  Item 02 Telephoning to make an appointment with a stranger.
  Item 03 Talking with a salesperson on the telephone.
Subscale 2: Argument/Conflict With a Friend
  Item 04 Refusing a friend a favor
  Item 05 Confronting a friend who has failed to fulfill an agreement.
  Item 06 Criticizing a friend for a mistake he has made.
Subscale 3: Argument/Conflict With a Stranger
  Item 07 Arguing with a salesperson about an overcharge.
  Item 08 Arguing with a serviceman to provide additional service or to lower the cost of service.
  Item 09 Complaining to a waiter/waitress about poor service.
Subscale 4: One-to-One Conversation With a Family Member
  Item 10 Talking with my father.
  Item 11 Talking with my mother.
  Item 12 Talking with a family member while riding in a car.
Subscale 5: One-to-One Conversation With an Authority Figure
  Item 13 Telling my doctor what is ailing me.
  Item 14 Talking with a lawyer.
  Item 15 Talking with a store manager.

Subscale 6: Group Conversation With Known Group (Informal)

Item 16 Telling a funny story to a group of 2 to 8 friends.

Item 17 Talking with a group of 2 to 8 friends at a party.

Item 18 Carrying on a conversation with 2 to 8 friends during a card, golf, or other game.

Subscale 7: Group Conversations With Unknown Group (Informal)

Item 19 Talking with 2 to 8 strangers during dinner.

Item 20 Taking part in a discussion group of 2 to 8 strangers.

Item 21 Starting off a discussion in a group of 2 to 8 strangers.

Subscale 8: Formal Presentations

Item 22 Making a short speech (1 or 2 minutes) at work or in a class.

Item 23 Making a 5- to 10-minute speech at work or in a class.

Item 24 Acting as a spokesperson or representative of a group in a meeting at work or in a class.

Subscale 9: Questioning a Friend or Family Member to Obtain Information or to Elicit Action

Item 25 Asking a friend for a ride.

Item 26 Asking a family member for money (a small loan).

Item 27 Asking a family member for advice.

Subscale 10: Questioning a Stranger to Obtain Information or to Elicit Action

Item 28 Asking a stranger for the time of a movie or other event.

Item 29 Asking for stamps at the post office.

Item 30 Asking a waiter/waitress for help.

Subscale 11: Questioning an Authority Figure to Obtain Information or to Elicit Action

Item 31 Asking a policeman for directions or information.

Item 32 Asking a question of a boss at work or an instructor in class.

Item 33 Asking a question of an authority at a forum or a meeting.

Subscale 12: Situations Involving Time Constraints

Item 34 Asking a secretary to see her employer when I am late for an appointment.

Item 35 Asking for flight or bus information when I am late for that plane or bus.

Item 36 Talking to a store clerk when a number of other customers are waiting for help.

Subscale 13: Situations Involving Memorized Content or Unchangeable Content

Item 37 Telling someone my address.

Item 38 Telling someone my telephone number.

Item 39 Telling someone my name.

CHAPTER 4 ADDITIONAL READINGS

Adams, M.R. (1982). Fluency, non-fluency, and stuttering in children. *Journal of Fluency Disorders, 7,* 171–185.

Andrews, G., & Harvey, R. (1981). Regression to the mean in pretreatment measures of stuttering. *Journal of Speech and Hearing Disorders, 46,* 204–207.

Conture, E.G. (1982). Youngsters who stutter: Diagnosis, parent counseling, and referral. *Journal of Developmental and Behavioral Pediatrics, 3,* 163–169.

Cooper, E.B. (1987). The chronic perseverative stuttering syndrome: Incurable stuttering. *Journal of Fluency Disorders, 12,* 381–388.

Costello, J.M., & Hurst, M. (1981). An analysis of the relationship among stuttering behaviors. *Journal of Speech and Hearing Research, 24,* 247–256.

Craig, A.R., Franklin, J.A., & Andrews, G. (1984). A scale to measure locus of control of behaviour. *British Journal of Medical Psychology, 57,* 173–180.

Cullinan, W.L. (1988). Consistency measures revisited. *Journal of Fluency Disorders, 13,* 1–9.

Curlee, R.F. (1981). Observer agreement on disfluency and stuttering. *Journal of Speech and Hearing Research, 24,* 595–600.

Fields, T.A. (1980). An individualistic approach to the evaluation and remediation of stuttering. *Journal of Fluency Disorders, 5,* 115–136.

Gottwald, S.R., Goldbach, P., & Isack, A.H. (1985). Stuttering: Prevention and detection. *Young Children, 41,* 9–14.

Greiner, J.R., Fitzgerald, H.E., Cooke, P.A., & Djurdjic, S.D. (1985). Assessment of sensitivity to interpersonal stress in stutterers and nonstutterers. *Journal of Communication Disorders, 18,* 215–225.

Hall, D.E., Lynn, J.M., Altieri, J., & Segers, V.D. (1987). Inter-intrajudge reliability of the stuttering severity instrument. *Journal of Fluency Disorders, 12,* 167–173.

Kully, D., & Boberg, E. (1988). An investigation of interclinic agreement in the identification of fluent and stuttered syllables. *Journal of Fluency Disorders, 13,* 309–318.

Ladoucer, R., & Saint-Laurent, L. (1986). Stuttering: A multidimensional treatment and evaluation package. *Journal of Fluency Disorders, 11,* 93–103.

Madison, L.S., Budd, K.S., & Itzkowitz, J.S. (1986). Changes in stuttering in relation to children's locus of control. *Journal of Genetic Psychology, 147,* 233–240.

McDonough, A.N., & Quesal, R.W. (1988). Locus of control orientation of stutterers and nonstutterers. *Journal of Fluency Disorders, 13,* 97–106.

Mowrer, D.E., Fairbanks, C., & Cantor, A.B. (1980). How school-aged students define stuttering and stammering. *Journal of Fluency Disorders, 5,* 331–344.

Myers, F.L., & Wall, M.J. (1981). Issues to consider in the differential diagnosis of normal childhood nonfluencies and stuttering. *Journal of Fluency Disorders, 6,* 189–196.

Ornstein, A.F., & Manning, W.H. (1985). Self-efficacy scaling by adult stutterers. *Journal of Communication Disorders, 18,* 313–320.

Perkins, W.H. (1984). Stuttering as a categorical event: Barking up the wrong tree: Reply to Wingate. *Journal of Speech and Hearing Disorders, 49,* 431–434.

Ratner, N.B., & Benitez, M. (1985). Linguistic analysis of a bilingual stutterer. *Journal of Fluency Disorders, 10,* 211–219.

Riley, G.D., & Riley, J. (1979). A component model for diagnosing and treating children who stutter. *Journal of Fluency Disorders, 4,* 279–294.

Schiavetti, N., Sacco, P.R., Metz, D.E., & Sitler, R.W. (1983). Direct magnitude estimation and interval scaling of stuttering severity. *Journal of Speech and Hearing Research, 26,* 568–573.

Seymour, C.M., Ruggiero, A., & McEneaney, J. (1983). The identification of stuttering: Can you look and tell? *Journal of Fluency Disorders, 8,* 215–220.

Ulliana, L., & Ingham, R.J. (1984). Behavioral and nonbehavioral variables in the measurement of stutterers' communication attitudes. *Journal of Speech and Hearing Disorders, 24,* 288–291.

Watson, J.B., Gregory, H.H., & Kistler, D.J. (1987). Development and evaluation of an inventory to assess adult stutterers' communication attitudes. *Journal of Fluency Disorders, 12,* 429–450.

Wells, G.B. (1983). A feature analysis of stuttered phonemes. *Journal of Fluency Disorders, 8,* 119–124.

Wingate, M.E. (1981). Knowing what to look for: Comments on stuttering identification—standard definition and moment of stuttering. *Journal of Speech and Hearing Research, 24,* 622–624.

Wingate, M.E. (1984). Definition is the problem. *Journal of Speech and Hearing Disorders, 49,* 429–431.

Wingate, M.E. (1984). Fluency, disfluency, dysfluency, and stuttering. *Journal of Fluency Disorders, 9,* 163–168.

Wingate, M.E. (1986). Adaptation, consistency and beyond. I: Limitations and contradictions. *Journal of Fluency Disorders, 11,* 1–36.

Wingate, M.E. (1986). Adaptation, consistency, and beyond. II: An integral account. *Journal of Fluency Disorders, 11,* 37–53.

Wingate, M.E. (1987). Fluency and disfluency: Illusion and identification. *Journal of Fluency Disorders, 12,* 79–101.

CHAPTER FIVE

Treatment of Stuttering

An outgrowth of a comprehensive evaluation of the stuttering behavior will be the development of a treatment program that fits the needs of the client. The clinician is faced with the responsibility of developing an appropriate treatment program for each stutterer in his or her caseload. Regimented, highly structured treatment programs that are used for all stutterers will not produce effective results. Clinicians need to plan carefully the goals and objectives of therapy for each client based on findings from the assessment process. Only then will the steps and procedures in the program be grounded in a well-defined rationale for each phase of the program.

Over the past several decades a vast number of approaches have been developed for the treatment of stuttering. Advocates of each method have proclaimed that their method is "successful" in treating stuttering, but no one has suggested that any one approach is effective with all stutterers. For the reader who wants a complete historical review of the management of stuttering, the chapters on treatment in the books by Wingate (1976) and Bloodstein (1987) are must readings. (See references at end of this introduction.)

In this chapter, the first article, by Guitar and Peters, provides us with a general overview of the basic stuttering treatment philosophies. Although there are many treatment approaches to choose from, the method chosen usually depends on the treatment philosophy that a speech-language pathologist adopts. In 1979, Gregory proposed that the majority of the approaches for the treatment of stuttering could be summarized into three major philosophies. The titles for these treatment methods included: (1) "speak more fluently"; (2) "stutter more fluently"; and (3) a combination of "speak and stutter more fluently."

The "speak more fluently" philosophy, oftentimes referred to as "fluency shaping therapy," is based on the notion that a stutterer should be taught to achieve immediate, controlled, fluent speech in one- to two-word utterances. These fluent responses are then positively reinforced by the clinician. By gradually increasing both the length and the linguistic and motoric complexity of an utterance, a clinician can help a stutterer achieve improved fluency in conversation. Manipulation of the length of the utterance is combined with various instructional techniques such as airflow management, gentle onsets of phonation, speech rate reduction, and continuous phonation patterns through the aid of a delayed auditory feedback (DAF) unit. Any one or a combination of these techniques is used to facilitate the establishment of fluency. Once perceptually fluent or stutter-free speech is established, it is then shaped to approximate normal-sounding speech.

It is important to add that this basic approach does not provide any information to the stutterer about any features of stuttering. Rather, information about the components and mechanics of fluent speech becomes the major focus of discussion in this type of therapy.

Moreover, this approach does not attend to stutterers' negative emotional reactions or feelings about stuttering or about being a stutterer. Advocates of this method believe that the emotional aspects of the problem will improve once fluency replaces stuttering on a consistent basis. Programs such as Webster's Precision Fluency Shaping Program (1974), the "Stutter-Free Speech" program developed by Shames and Florance (1980), and Goebel's (1986) Computer-Aided Fluency Establishment Trainer" (CAFET) are examples of this treatment approach.

By contrast, the "stutter more fluently" approach (also called "stuttering modification therapy") is usually referred to as the traditional method for treating stuttering. This approach was advocated by Joseph Sheehan and Charles Van Riper, two prominent scholars and clinicians in the area of stuttering. Years ago, Sheehan and Van Riper developed separate programs based on the rationale that stuttering results from avoidance and struggle behavior associated with the stuttering and/or feared words or situations. Therefore, in this approach stutterers are encouraged to reduce their anxiety and fear of stuttering in order to manage the fluency failures that occur in conversation. This is accomplished by having stutterers identify, analyze, explore, and familiarize themselves with the stuttering behavior before any specific attention is directed toward modifying the client's disfluent behavior.

Initially, this approach is designed to help stutterers acquire an objective attitude toward their fluency problem. Once a stutterer's feelings and attitudes about the stuttering have improved through a desensitization process such as voluntary stuttering and pseudostuttering, the next step is to modify the stuttering behavior. During this phase of the program, a stutterer learns to stutter with less effort, tension, and struggle through the use of new speech preparatory sets, pull-outs and cancellations of stuttering blocks, and smooth articulatory contacts to reduce the amount of force used to produce the syllabic units. Thus, the major goals of this approach are to have stutterers develop an improved attitude about their stuttering and be able to speak with less stuttering as well as be able to control and modify the stutterings as they arise in spontaneous speech. Proponents of this approach feel strongly that this is an effective way to reduce a stutterer's avoidance of speaking and sensitivity to the stuttering behavior.

To help us understand the differences and similarities as well as the advantages and disadvantages of the speak-more-fluently and stutter-more-fluently treatment methods, the first article in this chapter, by Guitar and Peters, provides a review of each method in some detail. Given the nature of each treatment philosophy, it can be seen that there would be some stutterers who would not fit the philosophy of either approach. Moreover, the trend in the last few years is that most clinicians would prefer to choose a treatment philosophy that combines the best features of each approach. For example, a clinician may believe that most stutterers need some training in analyzing and modifying their stuttering behavior through pull-outs, cancellations, negative practice, and voluntary stuttering so as to reduce avoidance behaviors. Following that, stutterers could then be taught a variety of fluency-enhancing skills such as easy onsets of phonation and rate control in order to produce improved fluency rather than modified stuttering. It is thought that a combined approach of adjustments in perception and attitudes about stuttering along with improved fluency skills will create longer-lasting effects than either the speak-or-stutter-more fluently approaches employed separately. A detailed discussion of a model of therapy that incorporates a combined approach to treatment is provided by Williams (1979) and in the Speech Foundation of America publication by Guitar and Peters.

Even though the treatment methods described above would accomodate adults, adolescents, and young children who stutter, any treatment of stuttering should be tailored to meet the needs of the individual client. For some, a fluency-shaping program would be sufficient.

Nevertheless, there has been a strong trend in the last decade toward the use of a fluency-shaping approach or a combination of speak-and-stutter-more-fluently methods with young children who stutter. Increased attention in the last few years has also focused on the language skills of young stutterers (Adams, 1988).

Some treatment programs have been developed specifically for children and those procedures have been provided by Ryan (1974), Gregory and Hill (1984), Nelson (no date), and Shine (1980). In keeping with the relationship between language abilities and stuttering, a common element among these treatment programs is the manipulation of the child's length and complexity of an utterance in order to enhance the number of fluent responses, as discussed in the excerpted portion of Adam's (1980) article. However, as Bernstein-Ratner and Sih (1987) point out, changes in utterance length and complexity do not influence a young child's fluency in similar ways. The syntactic complexity of an utterance appears to have a much greater effect on stuttering than does the length of the message.

Thus, the basic approach with young preschool stutterers usually involves the positive reinforcement of fluency through the control of the utterance. Most young stutterers tend to develop only minimal awareness or avoidance behaviors about their speech. Therefore, direct therapeutic attention to a young child's negative attitudes about stuttering may not be warranted. When appropriate, clinicians can supplement the basic reinforcement for fluency program with instruction in rate reduction and easy onset of phonation techniques (Costello, 1983).

In the article by Runyan and Runyan in this chapter, the authors present an innovative approach to the treatment of young stutterers. They describe the development and implementation of a fluency training program that incorporates the use of seven "fluency rules." These rules are clearly defined, easy to follow, easy for young children to comprehend, and based on sound rationale. Clinicians who treat elementary school-aged stutterers will find a number of helpful clinical tips in this article.

In addition to the direct management of a child's fluency problem, most clinicians would agree that parent counseling is an important part of any stuttering therapy program for young children. Typically, parent counseling involves discussions of how to improve interpersonal communication and reduce communicative pressures in the home environment (Cooper, 1979; Gregory, 1984). Starkweather (no date) recommends that parents use a slow, easy style of talking when conversing with their disfluent child. In this way, parents can understand how less rapid and linguistically complex forms of communication facilitate increased fluency for the child as well as improved parent-child interactions.

In contrast to the young, preschool disfluent child, stutterers in the upper-elementary, junior-high, and high-school grade levels could be considered much like adult stutterers in terms of the consistency of their stuttering pattern. However, there are many unique characteristics associated with this age group that makes the therapy slightly different from stutterers who are older or younger. Some of the factors that are unique to these age groups include the extent to which the social environment influences the disorder, the degree of parental reaction to the fluency problem, the number of maladaptive attitudes associated with the stuttering, and the child's willingness to actively use the methods taught to them in a treatment program. Recently, a publication by Fraser and Perkins (1987) discusses the unique aspects of being a teenage stutterer. Their publication contains valuable information about stuttering and shows the teenage stutterer how to cope with the problem. This is must reading for any clinician treating stutterers in this age group.

Another important aspect of the treatment of teenagers is the clinician's attitude toward stuttering and his or her confidence in treating this disorder. Daly's article in this chapter addresses this important issue in stuttering treatment. A clinician's attitude about stuttering and preconceived notions about stutterers can directly influence the outcome of the therapy. Thus, in order to work effectively with stutterers, it is beneficial for the clinician to have good listening skills and adopt a positive attitude toward helping stutterers achieve improvements in their stuttering.

Much of what was said above about teenagers who stutter is applicable to adults who stutter. Adults, however, have longer histories of avoidance behaviors, negative attitudes, and perceptions of the problem than do those in their teens. Because of this, some adult stutterers may be difficult to treat or the process of changing the stuttering pattern might involve an extensive period of therapy. Some stutterers make only minimal improvements in their stuttering despite several years of treatment. Nevertheless, there are adult stutterers who are extremely motivated to improve their fluency for personal reasons. These clients usually respond well to treatment and experience dramatic improvements in their fluency in a variety of speaking situations. Daly suggests that improved fluency involves a combination of learning the mechanical aspects of properly coordinating breathing, voicing, and articulatory activities as well as developing an improved mental image of being a fluent speaker. Cognitive activities such as positive self-talk, guided relaxation, and positive mental imagery are helpful in bringing about an effective outcome of sustained fluency.

Although a stutterer might be able to sustain fluency or develop the capability of controlling stuttering through a variety of methods, the main goal of any treatment program is to help the client maintain the newly learned speech behaviors outside of the clinical environment. Thus, both the transfer and the maintenance of improved speaking behaviors become paramount issues in stuttering therapy. Many clinicians assume that in-clinic speech improvements will naturally maintain themselves and generalize to situations out of the clinical environment. However, experts in the field of stuttering now agree that transfer of maintenance activities must become an integral portion of any treatment program (Gregory, 1986).

Generally, extensive training in self-monitoring and self-evaluation is important to transfer and maintenance so that a stutterer can bring about the necessary changes in the speech behavior without a clinician being present. Role-playing a variety of speaking situations in therapy is another helpful transfer method that is used prior to the client performing a speaking task outside of therapy. Regardless of which therapy techniques are used, it is clear that in order for the maintenance of fluency to occur, there must be some planned activities for transfer of the new speech behaviors outside of the immediate clinical environment. Clinicians should also bear in mind that parents, teachers, spouses, and friends become important adjuncts to the transfer and maintenance process.

One other important aspect of stuttering therapy that cannot be ignored is the quality of a stutterer's speech following treatment. Onslow and Ingham (1987) review various approaches that have been used in the evaluation of speech quality following the management of stuttering. The issue of how "natural" or normal-sounding a stutterer's speech is during and after treatment is an important one since many fluency-enhancing techniques used in therapy might contribute to "fluent" but abnormal-sounding speech. The use of speech naturalness ratings of stutterers' speech may allow a clinician to determine which acoustic or physiological factors need attention in therapy before the client is dismissed from the treatment program.

As we have seen, it is important for clinicians to provide not only direct attention to the transfer and maintenance of fluency but also a means by which the quality of a stutterer's speech behavior can be measured following therapy. These are factors that all clinicians should bear in mind when treating adult and children who stutter. Moreover, these issues are germane to any treatment approach.

However, despite the fact that we know that there are many ways of addressing these issues in a stuttering therapy program, we are interested also in knowing which stuttering therapy programs report long-term effectiveness in creating changes in stutterers' speaking behavior. Although determining the long-term effectiveness of stuttering therapies has been a difficult problem in the past, Andrews, Guitar, and Howie found that a mathematical technique called *meta-analysis* could simplify the problem. Thus, in their article in this chapter, they show us how they used data from previously published studies dealing with the treatment of stuttering in order to reach some conclusions about the long-term effectiveness of treatment and which treatments were most effective. From the meta-analysis technique, Andrews and colleagues found that the treatments that focused on prolonged speech and gentle onset of phonation produced the best short- and long-term gains than did either attitude or airflow procedures. Nevertheless, the authors point out that for an individual client, there is not one treatment that is necessarily or predictably "best." What is best will depend on a number of factors, including the characteristics of the stutterer seeking treatment and the skills of the clinician.

The article by Andrews and co-workers is informative too for its coverage and summary of many of the published approaches to the treatment of stuttering in the 1960s and 1970s. Many of these treatment programs are still in use today and continue to be beneficial in treating the disorder. As new programs and techniques for the treatment of stuttering emerge, it will be necessary to conduct a systematic evaluation of the effectiveness of these new methods.

Finally, given the recent trends in the treatment of stuttering, it is possible to try to predict some of the directions that will be taking place in the near future. Adams (1988) predicts that there will be continued attention paid to the study of stutterers' speech naturalness following therapy. Other important management issues are discussed by Cooper in the last article of this chapter. Cooper predicts that the future treatment of stuttering will involve (1) a client becoming a more active participant in establishing therapy goals; (2) an increase in the number of early intervention programs for young stutterers; (3) a decrease in the number of short-term intensive treatment programs; and (4) a greater visibility and number of support groups for stutterers. In short, the treatment of stuttering will become more focused, responsive to the client's needs, and more effective than we have seen in the past.

The future for stuttering therapy looks bright, given our increased understanding of stuttering in the past few years and our ability to objectively measure improvement in stutterer's fluency skills before and after therapy. Moreover, through the early identification and verification of childhood stuttering, it is hoped that clinicians will be increasingly effective in their efforts. Realistically, we will never be able to successfully treat every client's stuttering. Therefore, our goal in treatment should be to provide stutterers with the most effective form of fluency control or modified stuttering that they can achieve without excessive effort.

REFERENCES

Adams, M.R. (1988). Five-year retrospective on stuttering theory, research, and therapy: 1982–1987. *Journal of Fluency Disorders, 13,* 399–406.

Bernstein-Ratner & Sih, C.C. (1987). Effects of gradual increases in sentence length and complexity of children's dysfluency. *Journal of Speech and Hearing Disorders, 52,* 278–287.

Bloodstein, O. (1987). *A handbook on stuttering.* Chicago: Easter Seal Society.

Cooper, E. (1979). *Intervention procedures for the young stutterer.* In H. Gregory (Ed.), *Controversies about stuttering therapy.* Baltimore: University Park Press.

Costello, J.M. (1983). *Current behavioral treatments for children.* In D. Prins & R. Ingham (Eds.), *Treatment of stuttering in early childhood.* San Diego: College-Hill Press.

Fraser, J., & Perkins, W.H. (1987). *Do you stutter? A guide for teens.* Speech Foundation of America, Publication No. 21.

Goebel, M. (1986). *A computer-aided fluency establishment trainer.* Falls Church, VA: Annandale Fluency Clinic.

Gregory, H.H. (1979). *Controversies about stuttering therapy.* Baltimore: University Park Press.

Gregory, H.H. (1984). *Prevention of stuttering: Management of early states.* In R. Curlee & W. Perkins (Eds.), *Nature and treatment of stuttering.* San Diego: College-Hill Press.

Gregory, H.H. (1986). Stuttering: A contemporary perspective. *Folia Phoniatrica, 38,* 89–120.

Gregory, H.H., & Hill, D. (1984). Stuttering therapy for children. In. W. Perkins (Ed.), *Stuttering disorders.* New York: Thieme-Stratton.

Nelson, L. (no date). *Language formulation related to disfluency and stuttering.* In *Stuttering therapy: Prevention and intervention with children.* Speech Foundation of America, Publication 20.

Onslow, M., & Ingham, R. (1987). Speech quality measurement and the management of stuttering. *Journal of Speech and Hearing Disorders, 52,* 2–17.

Ryan, B. (1974). *Programmed therapy for stuttering in children and adults.* Springfield, IL: Charles C. Thomas.

Shames, G.H., & Florance, C.L. (1980). *Stutter-free speech: A goal for therapy.* Columbus, OH: Charles E. Merrill.

Shine, R. (1980). *Direct management of the beginning stutterer*. In W. Perkins (Ed.), *Strategies in stuttering therapy*. New York: Thieme-Stratton.

Starkweather, C.W. (no date). *Talking with the parents of young stutterers*. In *Counseling stutterers*. Speech Foundation of America, Publication 18.

Webster, R.L. (1974). *Behavioral analsysis of stuttering: Treatment and theory*. In M. Calhoun (Ed.), *Innovative treatment methods in psychotherapy*. New York: John Wiley.

Williams, D.E. (1979). A perspective on approaches to stuttering therapy. In H. Gregory (Ed.), *Controversies about stuttering therapy*. Baltimore: University Park Press.

Wingate, M.E. (1976). *Stuttering theory and treatment*. New York: Irvington Publishers.

Comparison of Stuttering Modification and Fluency Shaping Therapies

Barry Guitar
Theodore Peters

DEFINITIONS

Stuttering Modification Therapy

In this book stuttering modification therapy refers to an approach to stuttering based on the theory that most of the stutterer's problems in speaking are the result of avoiding or struggling with disfluencies (repetitions and/or prolongations), avoiding feared words, and/or avoiding feared situations. The process of therapy includes reducing avoidance behaviors, speech related fears, and negative attitudes toward speech. It also includes helping the stutterer learn to modify the form of his stuttering.[1] This can be done in a variety of ways. For example, the stutterer can reduce his struggle behavior and smooth out the form of his stuttering. He can also reduce the tension and rapidity of his stuttering to stutter in a more relaxed and deliberate manner. The reader is referred to Luper and Mulder (1964), Sheehan (1970), Van Riper (1973), Williams (1971), and previous Speech Foundation of America publications (1974, 1978) for discussions of stuttering modification approaches to treatment.

Fluency Shaping Therapy

Fluency shaping therapy is based on operant conditioning and programming principles (e.g., successive approximations of antecedent stimulus events, use of reinforcement of appropriate responses, and so on). In a fluency shaping therapy program some form of fluency is first established in a controlled stimulus situation. This fluency is reinforced and gradually modified to approximate normal conversational speech in the clinical setting. This speech is then generalized to the person's daily speaking environment. For a description of several representative fluency shaping therapy programs

the reader is referred to Perkins (1973), Ryan (1974), Webster (1974), and *Conditioning in Stuttering Therapy (1970).*

BASIC SIMILARITIES AND DIFFERENCES

Stuttering modification therapy and fluency shaping therapy can be compared in many ways. We feel, however, that the following six comparisons are the most important with regard to the treatment of stuttering. Four of these comparisons pertain to the goals of therapy, and two are concerned with clinical procedures. The four goal comparisons relate to: (1) feelings and attitudes, (2) speech behaviors, (3) fluency maintaining strategies, and (4) general communication skills. The two clinical procedure comparisons deal with: (1) structure of therapy and (2) data collection. First, we will compare the two therapy approaches with regard to their goals.

Feelings and Attitudes

Stuttering modification therapy places a great deal of emphasis upon reducing the fear of stuttering. Much of the therapy is concerned with reducing the fear of stuttering and eliminating the avoidance behavior associated with this fear. Stuttering modification therapy adherents are also interested in developing positive attitudes toward speaking. They encourage the stutterer to develop an approach attitude toward speaking situations, rather than an avoidance attitude. Stutterers are encouraged to seek out speaking situations that they formerly avoided. Finally, many stuttering modification therapy clinicians are concerned with improving the stutterer's overall adjustment. They attempt to improve the stutterer's social and vocational skills within the limits of their clinical abilities.

Fluency shaping therapy clinicians do not directly attempt to reduce the stutterer's fear and avoidance of words and speaking situations. This is not one of their stated goals.

---

1. We will use the masculine pronoun when referring to stuttering clients and female pronouns for speech-language pathologists.

Reprinted from *Stuttering: An Integration of Contemporary Therapies,* Speech Foundation of America, Publication No. 16.

We feel, however, that often their programming leads to a reduction in fear. Further, fluency shaping therapy clinicians usually do not make direct attempts to improve the stutterer's attitudes. Again, however, we feel that often the stutterer develops a positive attitude toward speaking as a by-product of this therapy. Through generalization of the stutterer's fluency to previously feared speaking situations, the fears and avoidances associated with these situations are often reduced. Finally, fluency shaping therapy clinicians usually do not make direct attempts to improve the stutterer's social or vocational adjustment, though this may happen as a by-product of therapy.

Speech Behaviors

Before we outline the speech behavior goals of each approach, we first need to define some terms we will be using. These terms are *spontaneous fluency, controlled fluency*, and *acceptable stuttering*.

By *spontaneous fluency* we mean a normal level of speech flow that contains neither tension nor struggle behaviors, nor does it contain more than an occasional number of repetitions and prolongations. This fluency is not maintained by paying attention to speech or by changing speaking rate; rather, the person just talks and pays attention to his ideas. It is the fluency of the normal speaker.

Controlled fluency is similar to spontaneous fluency except that the speaker must attend to his manner of speaking to maintain relatively normal sounding fluency. He may do this by monitoring the auditory and/or proprioceptive feedback of his speech. He may monitor his speech rate, or he may use preparatory sets and pull-outs to maintain his fluency. Whether he uses these or other techniques, the speaker exhibits normal sounding speech by paying attention to how he is talking.

Finally, *acceptable stuttering* refers to a level of speech flow where the speaker exhibits noticeable but not severe disfluency and feels comfortable speaking despite his disfluency. As with controlled fluency, the stutterer may be attending to his manner of speaking to maintain this acceptable level of stuttering.

Now, with these definitions in mind we can discuss the speech behavior goals held by each of the two approaches. We believe that the stuttering modification therapy advocates see their ultimate goal for the stutterer to be spontaneous fluency. If this is unobtainable, then for some stuttering modification clinicians controlled fluency would be the next goal. For these clinicians, if a stutterer is unable to obtain this controlled fluency, then acceptable stuttering would become the goal. Other stuttering modification clinicians, however, do not advocate controlled fluency; rather, they advocate acceptable stuttering when spontaneous fluency cannot be achieved.

We believe that the adherents of fluency shaping therapy also have as their ultimate goal the attainment of spontaneous fluency. If this is not possible, then controlled fluency would become their goal. Acceptable stuttering, however, would not be a goal for many fluency shaping therapy adherents. This would be regarded as a program failure.

Both stuttering modification and fluency shaping approaches attempt to achieve spontaneous fluency or controlled fluency, helping the stutterer become more fluent by teaching him to talk, at least temporarily, in a modified, controlled, or purposeful fashion. The methods used to achieve spontaneous or controlled fluency, however, differ somewhat for the two approaches. Stuttering modification therapy reduces fears and avoidances as one means of enhancing fluency. In addition, the stutterer is taught that he can talk more fluently if he uses certain techniques to modify his stuttering. Fluency shaping therapy, on the other hand, usually focuses on speech behavior alone, not fears and avoidances. This approach is characterized by establishing stutter-free speech in a controlled speaking situation. It is the manner of speaking rather than the moment of stuttering that is modified.

We have observed that these two approaches may produce speech patterns that often sound similar. As clients in each therapy become more spontaneously fluent, they pass through a stage of controlled fluency in which words are spoken with a prolonged, gradual onset. The pull-outs and preparatory sets of stuttering modification therapy may be indistinguishable from the gentle onsets or slow prolonged patterns of some fluency shaping therapies.

Fluency Maintaining Strategies

Stuttering modification and fluency shaping approaches employ different techniques to help the stutterer maintain his fluency. Stuttering modification clinicians urge their clients not to avoid words or situations. They stress the importance of nonavoiding. Along with nonavoiding, they stress the importance of keeping speech fears at a minimum level. Stuttering modification clinicians also teach their clients strategies or techniques to cope with feared words. They teach the stutterer how to approach feared words or how to ease out of words on which they have already begun to stutter.

Many stuttering modification clinicians also try to foster maintenance of fluency by enhancing the stutterer's social and emotional adjustment. These clinicians will counsel the stutterer in particular problem areas and may refer him to another professional if problems are serious. The stutterer's morale and self-esteem are seen as important considerations for fluency maintenance.

Fluency shaping clinicians, on the other hand, do not generally deal with the stutterer's fears, attitudes, or general adjustment. Rather, they stress maintenance of fluency by such techniques as slowing speech rate, monitoring speech carefully, or paying particular attention to the easy onset of speech. In fluency shaping programs the client is also expected to be as fluent as he possibly can in a given stimulus situation.

If the above techniques break down, the stutterer is expected to use programming principles in addition to the above techniques to reinstate his fluency. For example, if a stutterer generalizes his fluency to his employment setting, but then relapses, he is expected to practice fluency in easier speaking situations, gradually proceeding through successively more difficult situations until he has re-established fluency at work. In other words, in fluency shaping therapy, maintenance procedures consist essentially of having the stutterer recycle himself through the same steps that he went through in his original therapy.

The fluency shaping clinician may also want to explore environmental contingencies for stuttering. Some stutterers may be living or working in environments which have rewarded their stuttering in the past and which continue to do so after treatment. One example is the spouse who does most of the speaking for the stutterer he or she is married to. In such cases, environmental contingencies for stuttering and fluency must be rearranged, through mutual planning, to reinforce fluency rather than stuttering.

General Communication Skills

Before we discuss the goals of each approach with regard to communication skills, it might be best to discuss what we have in mind in this area. We mean a variety of things. First of all, many who stutter also have other speech and language disorders. In some cases children are referred for stuttering and upon evaluation are found to have delayed speech and/or language development in addition to their stuttering. In other cases, a child referred for an articulation or language disorder may be come markedly disfluent while in therapy. Most experienced speech-language pathologists have encountered children like these. A second consideration under the heading of general communication skills is the enhancement of speech flow. Some clinicians recommend that stutterers in therapy need work on such aspects of speech as phrasing, pausing, intonation patterns or organization of their verbal output in addition to fluency. Finally, and less obvious, however, are communication problems that remain or are sometimes created after the stutterer becomes more fluent as a result of therapy. We have seen stutterers who have become quite fluent following therapy, but who still lack conversational skills. A typical example would be the young man who is no longer afraid to talk to a young woman, but who doesn't know what to say when he meets one. Another problem we have seen is the stutterer who, fluent for the first time in his life, begins to monopolize conversations. This is like a child with a new toy who will not give anyone else a chance to play with it. In some cases these now fluent stutterers carry this behavior to such an extreme that they begin to irritate their listeners. These stutterers need a short course in conversational skills. These are the types of considerations we have in mind when we talk about communication skills in this section.

We believe that neither the stuttering modification nor the fluency shaping approach has addressed itself to these areas of communication skills. Stuttering modification therapy has given only minimal consideration to one of these areas: enhancement of speech flow after stuttering behavior is reduced. A number of stuttering modification clinicians suggest that the stutterer should work on a smooth flow of verbal output after moments of stuttering have been reduced or eliminated. Interpersonal communication is not addressed. We are unable to find in the stuttering modification literature much discussion dealing with treatment considerations for children who have articulation and language problems accompanied by disfluency or stuttering.

Some fluency shaping clinicians also suggest that organization and flow of verbal output may be an important consideration for treatment. As far as we can tell, advocates of fluency shaping have not written about other aspects of general communication skills.

It is our belief that communication problems in a general sense should receive more consideration by clinicians working in either framework with stutterers of all ages.

Structure of Therapy

Stuttering modification therapy is usually conducted within a teaching/counseling situation. The stutterer and the clinician typically interact in a loosely structured manner. Fluency shaping therapy, on the other hand, is usually performed in a highly structured situation. Specific instructions and materials are prescribed. Specific responses are called for from the stutterer with specific reactions to these responses required from the clinician. In summary, the two approaches differ substantially with regard to the use of programming principles.

Data Collection

Traditionally, stuttering modification clinicians do not put a great deal of emphasis upon the collecting and reporting of objective data (e.g., the frequency of stuttering before and after therapy). Stuttering modification clinicians tend to regard as more valid their and the client's descriptions and impressions of the client's stuttering. Fluency shaping clinicians, on the other hand, with their roots in behavior modification, put a great deal of emphasis upon the collection and reporting of objective and reliable data.

Summarizing this section, stuttering modification and fluency shaping therapies are similar in some important ways and different in others. With regard to therapy goals, stuttering modification therapy emphasizes the reduction of speech fears and avoidance behaviors, as well as modifying the stuttering behavior. Fluency shaping therapy focuses on establishing and generalizing stutter-free speech. Although fluency shaping clinicians do not directly attempt to modify the stutterer's fears and attitudes, we suspect that their programs often accomplish this.

These approaches appear to use quite different procedures to develop and maintain fluency. In spite of this, we feel that the posttreatment speech of successful clients of these two therapies is often similar. Stuttering modification clinicians tend to use a less structured approach to therapy and to consider as more valid global descriptions of the client's stuttering problem. Fluency shaping clinicians prefer the structure of programmed therapy and tend to collect more objective and reliable data. See Table 1 for an overview of the similarities and differences of these two approaches

PROS AND CONS OF EACH APPROACH

The pros and cons of each approach will be considered with regard to the stutterer, to the clinician, and to the college or university training program. These considerations are important because they can and do affect daily decisions of stutterers and their clinicians. The advantages and disadvantages of each approach to the client will be discussed first.

Stuttering modification therapy is more attractive to some stutterers because it does not require the stutterer to speak in an abnormal pattern during part of his therapy. On the other hand, some fluency shaping therapy programs do require the stutterer to use slow prolonged speech for part of their therapy program; and some stutterers find this manner of speaking rather unpleasant. Thus, stuttering modification therapy would be preferred for this reason by some stutterers. Stuttering modification therapy, however, does have a real disadvantage on another level. In most stuttering modification therapy the stutterer needs to confront his speech fears. He needs to perform fear-producing tasks. He needs to eliminate his avoidance behaviors and get his stuttering out in the open. Some stutterers find this extremely unpleasant and resist therapy at this point. This resistance can be overcome with the help of an unusually supportive clinician. Unfortu-

nately, however, this skill comes only with considerable experience. In fluency shaping therapy, however, stutterers usually are not required to confront their fears as directly as they are in stuttering modification therapy. This is because of its highly structured nature and its gradual sequencing of speech tasks. In these programs the stutterer usually confronts his fear in small doses. Thus, many stutterers prefer a fluency shaping therapy approach to confronting fears rather than the stuttering modification approach.

Both approaches also have some pros and cons for the clinician. Stuttering modification therapy tends to be less structured and more spontaneous than fluency shaping therapy. Because of this the clinician may find it more enjoyable. Fluency shaping therapy, because of its highly structured nature can be boring at times. The data collection often used in fluency shaping programs can also be time consuming and laborious. The less structured nature of stuttering modification therapy, however, can be a disadvantage to the clinician, especially the beginning clinician. It involves difficult clinical decisions. Procedures are not laid out in as organized a fashion. Fluency shaping therapy, on the other hand, because of its highly structured nature requires less insight and less clinical sensitivity. Specific procedures are prescribed as to what to do and when to do it. Also, especially with commercially available programs, there is less planning time needed by the clinician. These two approaches also differ on one other dimension that is important for the clinician. As noted earlier, stuttering modification therapy traditionally has not emphasized the collection of data relative to the stutterer's progress. This may be because the measurement of attitudes and the assessment of the quality of changes in stuttering are difficult. Fluency shaping, however, has placed a great deal of emphasis upon the collection of data. With today's emphasis upon accountability, data keeping has become

TABLE 1. Similarities and differences of stuttering modification and fluency shaping therapies.

Stuttering modification therapy	Fluency shaping therapy
A. Therapy goals	**A. Therapy goals**
1. Considerable attention given to reduction of speech fears and avoidance behaviors.	1. Little attention given to reduction of speech fears and avoidance behaviors.
2. Development of spontaneous fluency, controlled fluency, or acceptable stuttering. Client taught to be more fluent by various techniques to modify his stuttering.	2. Development of spontaneous or controlled fluency. Client taught stutter-free speech in clinical and outside situations.
3. Maintenance of fluency by maintaining reduction of fears and avoidance behaviors. Use of various techniques to modify stuttering.	3. Maintenance of fluency by modifying the manner of speaking, and if necessary the reinstatement of fluency by recycling through original program. Management of contingencies for stuttering and fluencies.
4. Minimal attention given to general communication skills.	4. Minimal attention given to general communication skills.
B. Clinical procedures	**B. Clinical procedures**
1. Structure is characterized by a teaching/counseling interaction.	1. Structure is characterized by conditioning and programming principles.
2. Data collection in terms of global impression of client's stuttering problem.	2. Data colletion in terms of objective data regarding client's speech.

TABLE 2. Pros and cons of stuttering modification and fluency shaping therapies with regard to: (A) client, (B) clinician, and (C) training program.

Stuttering Modification Therapy		Fluency Shaping Therapy	
A. Client		**A. Client**	
PRO	CON	PRO	CON
1. Does not require speaking in abnormal pattern.	1. Needs to confront and perform fear producing tasks.	1. Less need to confront and perform fear producing tasks.	1. May require speaking in abnormal pattern for a period of time.
B. Clinician		**B. Clinician**	
PRO	CON	PRO	CON
1. Therapy tends to be more spontaneous and enjoyable.	1. Therapy is nonstructured, more difficult decisions need to be made.	1. More structured programs available. Thus, less planning needed.	1. Therapy can be boring.
	2. Less data kept for measuring progress for IEP, etc.	2. More data kept for measuring progress for IEP, etc.	2. More charting of data needed.
C. Training program		**C. Training program**	
PRO	CON	PRO	CON
	1. More difficult to teach to clinicians.	1. Easier to teach to clinicians. There are fewer individual differences, clearer defined decisions based on observed behavior.	

more and more important for the clinician who must write an Individual Education Program (IEP) for each child.

Finally, these programs have different implications for college and university training programs. It is more difficult to train a student thoroughly in the stuttering modification approach. The student needs to be trained to respond differentially to many more individual differences in their clients. They must learn to provide emotional support at appropriate times. Although training students in the fluency shaping approach is not without problems, the skills to be taught are more clearly defined and less ambiguous. Table 2 summarizes the pros and cons to the client, the clinician, and the training program of each of these two approaches.

REFERENCES

Conditioning in Stuttering Therapy. (1970). Memphis: Speech Foundation of America.

If Your Child Stutters: A Guide for Parents. (1978). Memphis: Speech Foundation of America.

Luper, H. L., & Mulder, R. L. (1964). *Stuttering: Therapy for Children.* Englewood Cliffs, NJ: Prentice-Hall.

Perkins, W. (1973). Replacement of stuttering with normal speech. II. Clinical procedures. *Journal of Speech and Hearing Disorders, 38,* 295–303.

Ryan, B. (1974). *Programmed Therapy for Stuttering in Children and Adults.* Springfield, IL: Charles C Thomas.

Sheehan, J.G. (ed.) (1970). *Stuttering: Research and Therapy.* New York: Harper & Row.

Therapy for Stutterers. (1974). Memphis: Speech Foundation of America.

Van Riper, C. (1973). *The Treatment of Stuttering.* Englewood Cliffs, NJ: Prentice-Hall.

Webster, R.L. (1974). A behavioral analysis of stuttering: Treatment and theory. In K. Calhoun et al. (eds.), *Innovative Treatment Methods in Psychopathology.* New York: John Wiley and Sons.

Williams, D.E. (1971). Stuttering therapy for children. In L.E. Travis (ed.), *Handbook of Speech Pathology.* New York: Appleton-Century-Crofts.

A Fluency Rules Therapy Program for Young Children in the Public Schools

Charles M. Runyan
Sara Elizabeth Runyan

The effectiveness of using a stuttering treatment program designed specifically for children in a public school environment has not been extensively investigated. A notable feature often associated with providing therapy in public schools is the large number of children for whom each clinician provides service. Runyan and Bennett (1982) found that in Virginia the average caseload for a public school speech-language clinician was 60 children. They also found that a large caseload and the factors associated with its size (i.e., travel between schools, IEP meetings, parent conferencing, etc.) significantly contributed to the amount of services scheduled for each child. In fact, a typical child in this study was enrolled in therapy on the average of only two 30-min therapy sessions per week. Based on these findings, a stuttering treatment program to be considered for public school use would have to be effective given the therapeutic time limitations inherent in this job setting. Therefore, the purpose of this study was to develop and then test a stuttering treatment program designed specifically for preschool and early grade school children in a public school environment.

METHOD

The Fluency Rules Program (FRP) was devised 5 years ago with the intent to teach early grade school stuttering children to speak fluently. The FRP rules were developed to instruct these children, in language they could comprehend, about the physiologic concepts associated with fluent speech production.

The following is a description of the fluency rules that comprise the current FRP along with some comments and suggestions regarding their use.

Reprinted from *Language, Speech, and Hearing Services in Schools, 17,* no. 4, 276–284. Copyright © 1986, American Speech-Language-Hearing Association.

Rule 1—Speak Slowly

The child is instructed in a slow rate of speech production (Purcell & Runyan, 1980). This is intended to allow additional time for the child to remember the fluency rules as well as provide time to develop self-monitoring skills necessary for the acquisition of the physiological skills required for fluent speech. The use of symbolic therapy materials such as turtles and snails in conjunction with a desk level metronome can be helpful in establishing the child's comprehension of slow rate. In fact, in a follow-up study an ear-level metronome was used successfully on one fifth-grade male. This child, as well as those using the desk metronome, were instructed not to talk with each beat of the metronome. Instead, they were told to let the beat of the metronome remind them to talk slowly as well as to remind them of any other designated fluency rule. Of course, once fluency is well-established the child's conversational speech will be returned to an age appropriate rate.

Rule 2—Use Speech Breathing

Explain to the child the difference between regular and speech breathing. For speech breathing our explanation includes breathe in quickly, then slowly let the air out, speak on "out" breaths, begin speaking shortly after the "out" breath starts, and keep the air moving (i.e., do not hold your breath!). Having the child trace the outline of a breathing cycle as described above on a blackboard or a piece of paper has been useful in establishing this rule.

Rule 3—Touch the "Speech Helpers" Together Lightly

Illustrate that the speech helpers (i.e., lips, tongue, and teeth) are parts of the mouth and are used to make speech sounds. The use of cartoon characters of each speech helper has increased the child's awareness of these structures. Explain that it is necessary to touch the speech helpers together very lightly and if pressed together too hard airflow will stop. The concept of light contact has been effectively presented by contrasting this manner of speech production with a demonstration of trying to say a word with the lips pressed tightly together. Another treatment procedure used effectively to illustrate this concept involved squeezing the child's arm as he speaks. That is, as the child speaks fluently the clinician holds the stutterer's arm lightly, then when a stuttering block occurs that involves excessive oral tension, the clinician squeezes the arm gently but firmly. The amount of pressure applied to the arm should be subjectively proportional to the amount of tension exhibited.

Rule 4—Use Only the Speech Helpers to Talk

This rule explains to the child that fluent speech is produced by moving the speech helpers and it is not necessary or helpful to move other muscles or body parts when speaking. The intent of Rule 4 was to eliminate any secondary behaviors that may have developed. It has been our experience that the use of a mirror during therapy has been successful in eliminating secondary behaviors. Usually the children were unaware of these extraneous movements and once these behaviors were pointed out they were quickly eliminated. On occasion we have targeted a particular persistent behavior and had the child produce this motor response in an attempt to initiate speech. The purpose of this therapy technique was to illustrate to the child that he can perform a great number of motoric responses (e.g., head turns) but that speech is not begun until the speech helpers are moved and airflow begins.

Rule 5—Keep Your Speech Helpers Moving

Explain to the child that fluent talkers do not "hold on to" or prolong sounds when they speak; that fluent speech is made up of "short" sounds that are connected together to form words and sentences.

One effective clinical approach used to teach the concepts of long and short words employed the use of a long and short piece of rough material (e.g., Velcro), (Minor, 1983). These different lengths of rough material were used in therapy by instructing the child to rub his finger across the surface of each in order to feel the difference between long and short. Then, when the child produces a long sound (i.e., prolongation) he is required to rub his finger across the long piece of material as he repeats the prolonged word. This procedure is repeated several times with the intent to make the child aware of his length of production. Next, the child is asked to rub his finger across the short pieces of material as he produces the target word more quickly. Hopefully, this therapy procedure will improve the child's ability to understand and then self-monitor the feeling of using the more appropriate "short" word method of speech production.

Rule 6—Keep "Mr. Voice Box" Running Smoothly

By the use of a cartoon character or other illustrations, show the child that "Mr. Voice Box" is in the neck and when it is running you can feel the voice box vibrate. Of course, this can be demonstrated by having the child hum while holding his neck. We also explain to the child that it is the "out breaths" (see Rule 2) that makes "Mr. Voice Box" run and it is very important that when the voice box starts running it is done very smoothly with an easy or gentle onset of vocal-fold vibration. If a further demonstration of voice onset is needed we have the child contrast the physiological feelings associated with two distinctly different modes of initiating phonation. First, the child should feel the tension of abrupt phonation by phonating while pulling up on or pushing against a heavy object. Next, the child monitors easy onset by starting the phonatory process with a breathy voice and then increases vocal fold vibrations until the appropriate pitch and intensity has been reached. The practice of easy onset of voice often creates a prolonged method of speech production. Therefore, the final stage of this rule is to shorten the duration of the onset to an appropriate length for conversational speech.

Rule 7—Say a Word Only Once

Inform the young stutterer that to speak fluently and be understandable a talker does not have to repeat words. The most effective treatment procedure used for Rule 7 involved two railroad trains. The first train contained different cars and represents fluent speech. The second train had a number of similar cars in a row and represented speech that contained repetitions. The concept learned from this example demonstrates that the train can run smoothly with only one of each type train car. The duplicates (repetitions) are unnecessary.

To implement these fluency rules the FRP was structured in the following manner. First, as part of the diagnostic sessions, a determination is made regarding which fluency rules have been broken. Next, the appropriate fluency rules are explained to the child. Often this explanation includes teaching the child language concepts necessary for full comprehension of the various fluency rules (e.g., say a word only *once* and *slowly*). In order for the child to apply the new fluency rules, a self-monitoring program is used. This self-monitoring program is based on interdiscrimination and intradiscrimination and consists of three steps. First, the stutterer is asked to determine when the clinician, who through imitation, is breaking the designated fluency rules. Once the child is successful at identifying the clinician's disfluencies (interdiscrimination) he is asked to listen to tape-recorded samples of his speech to detect any occurrence of broken fluency rules. Finally, the stutterer is asked to determine when instances of broken fluency rules or stuttering occur during conversational speech. When the stutterer successfully completes the self-monitoring phase the intensive practice portion of the program is commenced. During this phase, the child converses with the clinician and is instructed to compare and contrast the physiologic feelings of fluency and stuttering. When the child breaks a fluency rule he practices the fluent version a designated number of times to again distinguish the feeling of fluency from that associated with stuttering.

Occasionally, a child has difficulty with a particular rule. To assist the child apply the difficult rule and then transfer its application to conversational speech it has been helpful to alter the position of the words associated with the target rule within the sentence framework. That is, the child either through reading or reciting after the clinician produces the target word fluently; first at the end of a sentence, then in the middle position and finally to the more difficult initial position (e.g., I see the *bear*; The large *bear* is fuzzy; *Bears* are large animals). As in the other phases of therapy, the child is instructed to physiologically feel and report how the target word is produced fluently using the fluency rules.

The final phase of the FRP involves the carry-over or the transfer of the fluency rules to the home and classroom. Obviously to accomplish this transfer it is paramount the child remembers the fluency rules in these new speaking environments. The most effective procedure used to facilitate this carry-over has been to place a discriminative stimulus in each environment. In the school the speech-language pathologist, the classroom teacher, subject teacher, and the student meet to select a small unobtrusive item to be placed in each room as a reminder of the fluency rule (i.e., stickers on notebooks or refrigerator magnets on the edge of chalk boards). Only the teacher and the student need be aware of the item. Then, if the child should forget to use a fluency rule the teacher can subtly provide a reminder by glancing in the direction of the stimulus item. At home, basically the same procedure is recommended. By placing the stimulus items in conversation areas (e.g., the family room, kitchen, bedroom, and dining room) and having family members use these stimuli with the stutterer when needed has been helpful. The subtle nature of the use of these stimuli has a secondary benefit in that it negates or reduces the need for direct confrontations when fluency rules are not used. This procedure can reduce the chance of family conflicts arising from the possible need for constant reminding of the fluency rules sometimes associated with the early stages of transfer. Ideally the transfer segment of therapy will result in the fluency rules being generalized to areas away from the therapy room and ultimately lead to fluent speech in these environments. The following is an outline of the Fluency Rules Program.

1. Determine fluency rules broken.
2. Teach language concepts necessary for complete understanding of instructions.
3. Self monitoring phase to determine when to apply the fluency rule.
4. Practice fluent speech production using the fluency rules.
   (a) Physiologically contrast the stuttered with the fluent speech productions.
   (b) For difficult to learn rules use the altered word position in sentence program.
5. Carry over to the home and classroom.

The therapeutic procedure outlined and explained above was used with nine young stutterers contained in the caseload of the public school clinician who had been trained by the authors in the use of the FRP. These nine stutterers were treated in two groups. The first group of five stutterers ranging in age from 4:6 to 6:5 was followed for 2 years. In the first year, these children were evaluated and then enrolled in the FRP. During the second year therapeutic instruction was not provided but the children were monitored for any sign of relapse by the speech-language pathologist, the classroom teacher, and the family. At the conclusion of this second year, each child's speech was again recorded and analyzed. A second group of four less severe stutterers ranging in age from 3:8 to 7:1 was enrolled in the FRP at the beginning of the second year of the investigation. That is, when the first group of stutterers was entering the monitoring year this second group was just beginning the active therapy portion of the program. At the beginning of each school year, the children were evaluated by the public school clinician and the first author and only those instances of stuttering agreed upon by both professionals were included in the subsequent evaluation. These agreed upon instances of stuttering were used to determine both pre and posttreatment frequency of words stuttered and to complete the three components of the Stuttering Severity Instrument: frequency, duration, and physical concomitants (Riley, 1972). Also evaluated was the child's speaking rate at the time of the diagnostic and at the end of each school year.

RESULTS

Table 1 provides a summary of the frequency of stuttering and speaking rate for both groups of stutterers over the 2-year period of the investigation. Statistical analysis using a t test for correlated data (Downie & Heath, 1970) indicated that a significant reduction in the frequency of stuttering [$t = 4.8$, $p = .01$, $df = 8$] was noted at the end of the first year of the therapeutic program. Examination of the speaking rates of the children demonstrates that the improvement in fluency did not occur because of a reduced speaking rate. Only one child did not increase his speaking rate as the first year concluded while a second child, who was in the group followed for 2 years, exhibited a slight reduction in rate at the end of the second year. It should be noted that this child, as was true for all the children, was speaking at an age appropriate rate at the conclusion of this investigation (Purcell & Runyan, 1980).

TABLE 1. Listed are the two groups of stutterers with their age, sex, frequency of words stuttered during a 5-min sample, and their speaking rates which were calculated in words per minute.

Subjects sex		Age	Speaking rate			Number stuttered words in a 5-min speech sample		
			Pretreatment	End of 1 yr	End of 2 yrs	Pretreatment	End of 1 yr	End of 2 yrs
1	M	4–8	92	135	138	46	2	1.67[1]
2	F	4–6	74	100	120	74	1.67[1]	1.67[1]
3	M	5–4	98	130	133	54	1.67[1]	1.67[1]
4	F	6–5	63	104	114	66	2	2
5	F	6–1	52	140	132	65	2	3
6	M	7–1	140	145	—	14	5	—
7	M	7–0	120	130	—	10	2	—
8	M	6–3	130	130	—	20	2	—
9	F	3–8	125	138	—	25	1.67	—

[1] These frequency scores were obtained for 3 min and extrapolated to 5 min for statistical analysis.

Table 2 contains the results of the Stuttering Severity Instrument (Riley, 1972) and the therapy schedule used with each child during the period of the investigation. Evaluation of the three subsections of the Stuttering Severity Instrument data demonstrates that improvement occurred on all three measures. These combined results seem to be consistent with the desired effect for an acceptable treatment program.

DISCUSSION

The outcome of this study indicated that the FRP was an effective therapy program when used in a public school environment to reduce stuttering in young children. The children's speaking rates and the frequency of words stuttered demonstrated that the newly acquired fluency did not occur because of a reduction in verbal output. The results of the Stuttering Severity Instrument (SSI) indicated that not only was there a reduction in the frequency of stuttered words, but that the severity of those remaining blocks was minimal. That is, both the duration of the blocks and the struggle behavior (i.e., physical concomitants) were eliminated or reduced. Further inspection of the data illustrates that this improvement in fluent speech production occurred during the first year of therapy and was maintained during the follow-up period. It should also be noted that even though each child demonstrated an improvement in the amount of fluent speech production, all the children's speech contained slight residual effects of the stuttering disorder. These residual effects were in the form of two or three iterations of a syllable and were noted in the duration section of the SSI. These iterations did not occur frequently enough nor were

TABLE 2. Total score and subtest scores for each subject on the Stuttering Severity Instrument (Riley, 1972) calculated during the diagnostic evaluation, 1 year, and 2 years after the diagnostic evaluation. Also included is the therapy schedule used for the entire school year following the diagnostic.

Subject	Total SSI[2]			Subtests of Stuttering Severity Instrument									Number and length of therapy session scheduled per week
				Frequency			Duration			Physical concomitants			
	Pretreatment	1	2	Pretreatment	1	2	Pretreatment	1	2	Pretreatment	1	2	
1	17	1	1	14	0	0	3	1	1	0	0	0	3–30 min sessions
2	27	2	2	16	0	0	4	2	2	7	0	0	2–30 min sessions
3	20	2	1	14	0	0	4	2	1	2	0	0	2–30 min sessions
4	21	3	2	16	0	0	4	2	2	1	1	0	2–30 min sessions
5	28	3	3	16	0	0	4	3	3	8	0	0	3–30 min sessions
6	11	1	—	6	0	—	2	1	—	3	0	—	3–20 min sessions
7	7	1	—	4	0	—	3	1	—	0	0	—	2–20 min sessions
8	16	4	—	6	0	—	4	2	—	6	2	—	3–20 min sessions
9	14	4	—	8	0	—	2	2	—	4	2	—	3–20 min sessions

Note: The Stuttering Severity Instrument is a 45-point scale that consists of three sections: frequency (instances of stuttering), duration (length of the three longest blocks), and physical concomitants (overt or noticeable secondary behaviors). The range of severity points assigned to each section of the scale depending upon the stutterers severity are as follows: frequency 0–18, duration 0–7, and physical concomitants 0–20.

they accompanied by any secondary behaviors to be scored in these respective columns. These remnants of stuttering are a lingering concern and should be followed to determine what impact they will have on the child's fluency at some later date.

An unexpected factor that was not considered during the design of this treatment program appeared to have played an important role in its success and versatility. This unexpected factor was the children's thorough understanding of the concept of "rules." Recall, that an integral component of the FRP was to develop treatment strategies in a language framework that a child could easily comprehend. It was apparent that all the children in this study knew, without supplementary instruction, the concept of not breaking or the importance of obeying rules. This familiarity with what constitutes a rule made the implementation of the program considerably more effective and efficient.

Of course efficiency and adaptability were important factors in the design of FRP because the treatment schedule used was a typical public school therapy format. Thus as Table 2 illustrates the children in both groups were seen in therapy two or three times a week with each session lasting 20 to 30 min. Therefore, the use of FRP in a public school environment seems to be effective in reducing the occurrence of disfluencies, duration of the blocks, and struggle behavior while maintaining an appropriate speaking rate even considering the time constraints of the therapeutic setting. And,

more importantly the beneficial effects of the program have been maintained over a reasonable period of time. It is also noteworthy that, although no formal assessment was made, the parents of all the children reported a significant improvement in fluent speech production at home. To date, this program has been used with only a small number of children and the therapeutic benefits documented for a relatively short period of time. Therefore, the FRP's ultimate effectiveness and versatility can only be demonstrated when a larger and more diverse group of stuttering children are treated over a longer time period.

REFERENCES

Downie, N.M., & Heath, R.W. (1970). *Basic statistical methods*. New York: Harper & Row.

Minor, B. (1983). Personal communications.

Purcell, R., & Runyan, C.M. (1980). A normative study on the speaking rates of children. *Journal of the Speech and Hearing Association of Virginia, 21*, 6–14.

Riley, G.D. (1972). A stuttering severity instrument for children and adults. *Journal of Speech and Hearing Disorders, 37*, 314–322.

Runyan, C.M., & Bennett, C.W. (1982). Results of a survey of public school speech-language pathologists in Virginia. *Journal of the Speech and Hearing Association of Virginia, 23*, 91–95.

The Young Stutterer: Diagnosis, Treatment, and Assessment of Progress

Martin R. Adams

For many years, speech-language pathologists have taken a passive approach to the treatment of young, preschool, or early, primary-grade stutterers. The traditional point of view had been that many of the stutterers in this age group would recover from their stuttering without any intervention from a formal stuttering-therapy program. Speech-language pathologists began to discover, however, that many young stutterers would not recover on their own and would later become chronic stutterers. Thus, in the early 1970s, clinicians began to take a more active role in the direct management of stuttering for children in the initial stages of the disorder. The focus of treatment for this age group has typically involved restructuring the child's speaking environment, systematically reducing the stutterer's speaking rate, and manipulating the length and complexity of the child's utterances to facilitate a fluent response.

In the excerpted portion of this article, Adams provides a detailed account of the structure of therapy for young stutterers who exhibit a lack of control and regulation of the breathstream for fluency. In another case, Adams provides an example of treatment for a young stutterer who does not exhibit any observable difficulty in initiating or sustaining vocalization.

CONSTRUCTION OF THERAPY: RATIONALE AND PROCEDURES

Since 1971, considerable time and effort has been expended in carefully studying the vocal tract behaviors associated with stuttering in adults (Hutchinson, 1973; Ford & Luper, 1975; Freeman & Ushijima, 1975; Lewis, 1975; Conture et al., 1977). This research has been viewed as showing that part-word repetitions and sound prolongations, the universally demonstrable features of stuttering (Wingate, 1964) are the most obvious peripheral manifestations of the stutterers'

underlying difficulty of the stutterers' underlying difficulty in starting and sustaining voicing or air flow for speech, and especially in coordinating voicing and articulation (Adams, 1974). The idea here is that articulatory postures and gestures are repeated and prolonged as the stutterer strives unsuccessfully to commence and sustain phonation. This interpretation that articulation becomes halting and repetitive when voicing cannot be started quickly or maintained follows logically from certain basics of speech production. In that regard, we all know that the voice is the acoustic "raw material" that gets shaped by the articulators into intelligible speech sounds and syllables. Simply put, speech is a series of articulatory movements made audible by the presence of phonation or at least air flow. When voicing cannot be initiated or sustained, there is no point in articulating because these movements will not be heard. That, in turn, markedly reduces the speaker's chances of communicating what he wants to say to the listener. Thus, the stutterer starts, stops, and repeats movements of the lips, mandible, and tongue as he strives to coordinate articulatory activity with a voice source that does not always start promptly or cannot be maintained.

There is an imposing array of evidence that supports this line of thinking (Adams & Reis, 1971, 1974; Adams & Hayden, 1976; Perkins et al., 1974, 1979) especially as it applies to adults. The very limited experimentation involving young stutterers (Stromsta, 1965; Agnello et al., 1974; Cross & Luper, 1979) indicates that the foregoing interpretation may apply to them as well. Indeed, it was this research with children, coupled with my repeated clinical observations, that led me to include "difficulty in starting and sustaining voicing or air flow for speech" as one of the five differential diagnostic criteria offered in Table 1.

I believe that when a young stutterer exhibits problems in commencing and sustaining voicing or air flow for speech he is, in effect, evincing deficiencies in the control and regulation of the breathstream. Consequently, this child needs a treatment that is directed toward helping him acquire breathstream management skills. A therapy regimen of this type has been developed and used with good effect by Perkins (1973a, 1973b, Perkins et al., 1974). This rehabilitative program includes techniques for normalizing fluency,

From Adams M, The Young Stutterer: Diagnosis, Treatment, and Assessment of Progress, in *Seminars in Speech, Language, and Hearing, 1*, no. 4. New York, 1980 Thieme Medical Publishers, Inc. Reprinted by permission.

TABLE 1. Criteria and guidelines for making a differential diagnosis between the normally nonfluent child and the incipient stutterers.*

Criterion	Guidelines for interpretation	
	Normally nonfluent	Incipient stutterer
Total frequency of disfluency, regardless of type, per 100 words spoken	Nine or fewer disfluencies per every 100 words spoken	At least 10 disfluencies per every 100 words spoken
Majority type(s) of disfluencies	Whole-word, phrase repetitions, interjections and revisions predominate	Part-word repetitions, audible-silent prolongations and broken words predominate
Number of unit repetitions per part-word repetition	No more than two unit repetitions per part-word repetition (e.g., "b-b-ball," but "b-b-b-ball")	At least three unit repetitions per part repetition (i.e., b-b-b-ball)
Perception of the schwa instead of the vowel normally heard in the word being marked by a part-word repetition	The schwa is not perceived; thus the normally nonfluent child's part-word repetitions will sound like "bee-bee-beet," but not "buh-buh-buh-beet")	The schwa will be perceived. Therefore, the incipient stutterer's part-word repetitions will sound like "buh-buh-buh-beet"
Difficulty in starting and/or sustaining voicing or air flow for speech, often heard in association with part-word repetitions, prolongations, and broken words	Little if any such difficulty evident; as a consequence, the normally nonfluent child's disfluencies are brief and effortless, and there is usually continuous voicing or air flow between units in a repetition (e.g., "beebeebeet" or "amamam," but not "buh--buh--buh--beet" or "am--am--am")	Frequent difficulty in starting and/or sustaining voicing or air flow for speech—most often heard in association with part-word repetitions, prolongations, and broken words; as a result, these disfluencies are of longer duration, more effortful, and may occur at transitions from voiceless to voiced speech sounds (e.g., "s-s-s-s-sun" or "ssssun")

*(After Adams, M.; *Journal of Fluency Disorders*, 2, 141–148, 1977.)

rate, breathstream management skills, and prosody. My preference has been to expose each child patient to the portion of the breathstream management regimen that seems best suited to eliminate his abnormal speech behavior. For example, if the youngster's stuttering is associated exclusively with difficulty in starting voicing, then only procedures for teaching the easy onset of phonation are prescribed for his therapy. If the child's sole problem is in sustaining voicing, treatment will emphasize techniques specifically chosen to remedy that deficit only. In still other cases, if a stutterer has trouble both in starting and maintaining voicing, methods designed to alleviate these abnormalities are thoughtfully selected and applied in combination.

There can be little doubt that *normal* breathstream management depends upon a speaker's execution of several complex motor behaviors, and on his ability to coordinate them. The young stutterer in a breathstream management program is working to acquire some or all of the same behaviors and coordinations. These goals are easier to attain if the clinician simplifies the motor timing and linguistic aspects of the child's responses in treatment. The simplification of motor timing is achieved by having the patient make each of his responses at a slower rate. More needs to be said about this matter because it is not enough to merely tell the child to "slow down" or "make each response slowly." Healey (1977) found that when told nothing more than to "slow down," the majority of the young stutterers he sampled

complied by both pausing for longer periods between words, and by prolonging the durations of the phonetic constituents in their utterances, the vowels in particular. For example, a child using this two-part or combined rate reduction strategy might say "Ill . . . aaaamm . . . aaa . . . mmaaaann."

Although this combined strategy of pausing and prolonging does indeed reduce speaking rate, it may not be the approach that will provide the greatest benefit to the child clinically. In his breathstream management procedures, Perkins advocates rate reduction by exclusive use of the prolongation tactic. To help induce a patient into this form of slow speech, Perkins routinely employs a delayed auditory feedback (DAF) apparatus, at least with adults. I strongly support Perkins' preference for the prolongation strategy but have encountered major difficulties in getting most young stutterers to tolerate the DAF device. Some have become frightened and tearful. Others have frequently and repeatedly interrupted their responses to laugh as soon as they heard the delayed speech signal. Taking these experiences into account, I have abandoned the DAF equipment. Instead, the child is given specific instructions and a behavioral model to follow, so that he will adopt the prolonged speech pattern and thus produce his clinical responses at a slower rate. As stable and reliable breathstream management skills are attained, appropriate directions and modeling are combined with operant reinforcement procedures to shape the speech rate back to within normal limits.

The rationale for using rate reduction to simplify response and to hasten the acquisition of complex breathstream management behaviors and coordinations is a straightforward one. In that regard, the stutterer learning breathstream management skills and coordinations is likened to any other individual who is attempting to develop proficiency at some complex, refined, highly integrated motor activity (for example, tennis; golf). Early in the learning process, the "pupil" will find it easier to effect and coordinate the component parts of the act if allowed to organize his behavior and execute it in "slow motion." If readers have ever taken golf or tennis lessons, they will doubtless recall that during their first several sessions, swings, strokes, and serves were always undertaken at reduced rates. Then, as the constituent parts of these acts were perfected and properly coordinated, the rate of movement was gradually increased.

If rate reduction serves to uncomplicate motor timing, how can linguistic aspects of the child's responding also be simplified? The answer that I have developed to this inquiry involves weaving the basic principles of Ryan's "Gradual Increase in Length and Complexity of Utterance" (GILCU) program (Ryan, 1974) into the framework of breathstream management. That is, the length and linguistic complexity of patients' responses in therapy will be carefully controlled by the judicious use of appropriate eliciting stimuli. For example, reading materials, starting with single common words organized in list fashion, will be presented first. Then, progressively longer and more elaborate phrases and sentences will be introduced systematically for reading by patients. At each length complexity level, children are instructed to use the aforementioned slow, prolonged speech pattern as they work on the breathstream management skills they are striving to master.

The justification for simplifying patients' responses by monitoring the length-complexity of their utterances derives from two sources: There have been (1) repeated clinical observations and (2) reports by stutterers that they are more likely to be fluent when effecting short, simple utterances. By requiring these sorts of responses early in treatment, we can more nearly maximize patients' chances of competently executing the intricate behaviors that are at the heart of breathstream management, and enjoying high levels of fluency in the process.

To summarize, here is the approach prescribed for the young stutterer whose disorder is characterized by trouble in starting or sustaining phonation: Breathstream management including rate reduction by the prolongation method, is used in combination with the principles and procedures that make up Ryan's GILCU program. The specific breathstream management techniques employed are the ones that seem to deal directly with the patient's particular deficits in regulating and controlling the breathstream.

All that said, attention must now be devoted to the rationale and procedures used with young stutterers who present a somewhat different diagnostic picture. Reference is made here to those children whose stuttering exists in the *absence* of problems in commencing and maintaining vocalization. In light of this last qualifying characteristic, I have begun to suspect that the immediate determinants and the actual stuttering of such children are quite different from those of patients who do exhibit problems in starting and sustaining voicing. The stuttering of the youngsters with voicing difficulties is, in large part, a motor problem involving deficiencies, excesses, and incoordinations of diverse behaviors at various levels in the vocal tract. In contrast, the children who lack these motor determinants may have stuttering problems that derive exclusively from slowness and uncertainty in the operation of various aspects of the language encoding process (for example, word retrieval). In light of that possibility, there is only equivocal evidence pointing to the existence of language deficits in large numbers of children who stutter. Some studies are supportive of the presence of language impairments (Weuffen, 1961; Telser, 1971; Murray & Reed, 1977), whereas others are not (Peters, 1968; Taylor et al., 1970; Boysen & Cullinan, 1971). One simple way of interpreting these results is to conclude that language deficiencies are not widespread among young stutterers, but also to acknowledge that there may be at least one subgroup in the population of stuttering children who are in possession of such problems. If this is indeed true, then we must entertain the hypothesis that the stuttering of the members of this subgroup may derive from their language dysfunctions and *not* from difficulty in commencing and maintaining phonation.

Interestingly, treatment for both the motor- and language-impaired groups of stutterers is much the same, *though for different reasons.* As already noted, patients who are experiencing difficulty in starting and sustaining voicing are offered a combination of breathstream management, rate reduction by the prolongation method, and Ryan's GILCU program. The last two components of this tripartite regimen are employed because they are presumed to simplify the motor aspects of speech production. Similarly it is my bias to take children whose stuttering may be tied to slowness in the management of central language functions, and expose them also to treatment involving rate reduction by means of the prolongation strategy and the GILCU procedures. This two-part program is constructed so as to give the child more time to manage the central integrative aspects of communication. Note, however, that breathstream management techniques are omitted since these youngsters present no behavioral evidence that they are in need of them. Obviously, it would be uneconomical to introduce into treatment methods that seem unnecessary, or that do not fit the patient's problem.

REFERENCES

Adams, M. (1974). A physiologic and aerodynamic interpretation of fluent and stuttered speech. *Journal of Fluency Disorders, 1,* 35–47.

Adams, M., & Hayden, P. (1976). The ability of stutterers and nonstutterers to initiate and terminate phonation during the production of an isolated vowel. *Journal of Speech and Hearing Research, 19,* 290–296.

Adams, M., & Reis, R. (1971). The influence of the onset of phonation on the frequency of stuttering. *Journal of Speech and Hearing Research, 14,* 639–644.

Adams, M., & Reis, R. (1974). The influence of the onset of phonation on the frequency of stuttering: A replication and re-evaluation. *Journal of Speech and Hearing Research, 17,* 752–754.

Agnello, J., Wingate, M., & Wendell, M. (1974). Voice onset and voice termination times of children and adult stutterers. Paper presented at the annual Convention of the Acoustical Society of America, St. Louis, Missouri.

Boysen, A., & Cullinan, W. (1971). Object-naming latency in stuttering and nonstuttering children. *Journal of Speech and Hearing Research, 14,* 728–738.

Conture, E., McCall, G., & Brewer, D. (1977). Laryngeal behavior during stuttering. *Journal of Speech and Hearing Research, 20,* 661–668.

Cross, D., & Luper, H. (1979). Voice reaction time of stuttering and nonstuttering children and adults. *Journal of Fluency Disorders, 4,* 59–78.

Ford, S., & Luper, H. (1975). Aerodynamic, phonatory and labial EMG timing relationships during fluent and stuttered speech. Paper presented at the annual Convention of the American Speech-Language and Hearing Association, Washington, D.C.

Freeman, F., & Ushijima, T. (1975). Laryngeal activity accompanying the moment of stuttering: A preliminary report of EMG investigations. *Journal of Fluency Disorders, 1,* 36–47.

Healey, C. (1977). Temporal relationships and strategies used by normal and stuttering children and adults in the self-regulation of speaking rate. Ph.D. diss., Purdue University.

Hutchinson, J. (1973). The effect of oral sensory deprivation on stuttering behavior. Ph.D. diss., Purdue University.

Lewis, J. (1975). An aerodynamic study of "artificial" fluency in stutterers. Ph.D. diss., Purdue University.

Murray, H., & Reed, C. (1977). Language abilities of preschool stuttering children. *Journal of Fluency Disorders, 2,* 171–176.

Perkins, W. (1973a). Replacement of stuttering with normal speech: I. Rationale. *Journal of Speech and Hearing Disorders, 38,* 283–294.

Perkins, W. (1973b). Replacement of stuttering with normal speech: II. Clinical procedures. *Journal of Speech and Hearing Disorders, 38,* 295–303.

Perkins, W., Rudas, J., Johnson, L., Michael, W., & Curlee, R. (1974). Replacement of stuttering with normal speech: III. Clinical effectiveness. *Journal of Speech and Hearing Disorders, 39,* 416–428.

Perkins, W., Bell, J., Johnson, L., & Stocks, J. (1979). Phone rate and effective planning time hypothesis of stuttering. *Journal of Speech and Hearing Research, 22,* 747–755.

Peters, T. (1968). Oral language skills of children who stutter. *Speech Monographs* (abstract), *35,* 325.

Ryan, B. (1974). *Programmed Therapy for Stuttering in Children and Adults.* Springfield, IL: Charles C Thomas.

Stromsta, C. (1965). A spectrographic study of disfluencies labelled as stuttering by parents. *Therapia Vocis et Loquelae, 1,* 317–320.

Taylor, W., Lore, J., & Waldman, I. (1970). Latencies of semantic aphasics, stutterers and normal controls to close items requiring unique and non-unique oral responses. *Proceedings of the Annual Convention of the American Psychological Association, 78,* 75–76.

Telser, E. (1971). An assessment of word finding skills in stuttering and nonstuttering children. *Dissertation Abstract International, 32*(6-B), 3693–3694.

Weuffen, M. (1961). Untersuchung der wortfindung bei normalsprechenden und stotterden kindern und jugendlichen im alter von 8 bis 16 jahren. *Folia Phoniatrica, 13,* 255–268.

Wingate, M. (1964). Standard definition of stuttering. *Journal of Speech and Hearing Disorders, 29,* 484–488.

A Practitioner's View of Stuttering

David A. Daly

As a speech-language pathologist with a thriving private practice specializing in stuttering, I have changed my theoretical and clinical perspectives about the treatment of stuttering considerably over the last few years. Rather than adhering to a specific program, I now use a combination of motor-training, positive mental imagery, and self-instruction techniques with most clients who are chronic stutterers. I agree with Van Riper's (1971) statement that "clinicians must deal with more than the speech of stutterers" (p. 213).

In addition to the significant role of client motivation in the therapy process, three variables stand out as crucial for successful treatment of stuttering: (1) the attitudes and expectations of the clinician; (2) the value of committing to a plan and schedule; and (3) supplementing speech treatment procedures with cognitive and self-instructional strategies.

THE CLINICIAN'S ATTITUDES AND EXPECTATIONS

The clinician's attitudes toward stuttering and people who stutter have as much to do with the successful treatment of this disorder as the methods selected for therapy. Clinical experience has convinced me that the clinician must believe in the client, just as the client must believe in the clinician.

The words we choose, and the way we say them, in answering even our clients' simplest questions have clinical implications. For example, our response to "Can my stuttering be cured?" is never a simple "No." Instead, we explain that no pill or therapy exists which will guarantee a cure. I, however, quickly add that our current treatment programs are helping those who are chronic stutterers to communicate more efficiently and effectively. I point out that some people who stutter do indeed become fluent; others achieve higher levels of fluency control although they may still stutter periodically. Some clients continue to speak in a predominantly disfluent manner, but we strive to help them speak as effectively as possible. That is our goal—to help each client develop the best fluency possible.

Some colleagues have asked whether we are promoting false hopes in our clients who stutter. I think not. An insightful book on terminally ill cancer patients suggests that "a positive attitude toward treatment was a better predictor of response to treatment than was the severity of the disease" (Simonton & Simonton, 1978, p. 82). This view has been advocated by other clinicians. Mowrer (1960), for example, maintained that hope is absolutely necessary if any learning is to be accomplished. Since we cannot predict which clients will make significant improvements in their fluency and which will not, I avoid making specific predictions about future gains. Instead, I am positive and enthusiastic with every client who stutters. I would rather err in the direction of optimism than pessimism.

I stuttered until my mid-20s. I was turned down for jobs because of my speech. Stuttering clients whom I was treating as part of my graduate school training complained to the clinic director that my stuttering was worse than theirs. They requested (and got) a more fluent clinician.

Fortunately, I received help from a sensitive and sincere faculty member who did not prejudge my potential for fluency. That clinician's attitude was a turning point in my quest for fluency. Thus I have a personal investment in urging clinicians to be positive, patient, and persistent with their stuttering clients.

At least one reviewer of the psychological literature dealing with the client's attitudes toward and expectations of therapy maintains that the effectiveness of therapy is closely linked to those expectations (Lazarus, 1971). Lazarus contends that the client enters therapy with preconceived ideas about the treatment and if the procedures do not make sense to the client, therapeutic impasse is likely to result.

Could a similar phenomenon occur in speech-language pathology treatment for the person who stutters? Might our clients detect any insecurities or uncertainties in the clinician's attitudes or feelings about the treatment advocated? Clinical experience repeatedly demonstrates that intelligent persons will expend effort and energy in treatment only when they expect substantial results. When the clinician concentrates on negative behaviors or problems rather than positive objectives, clients are apt to get discouraged. Such incongruity between the clinician's expectations and the client's expectations may account for the high dropout rate among our stuttering clients. Roughly one-third of stuttering clients withdraw from treatment prior to completion (Martin, 1981). We have expended tremendous effort studying clients who stutter. Perhaps it is time we study ourselves.

Reprinted from *ASHA, 30,* no. 1, April 1988, 34–35. Copyright © 1988, American Speech-Language-Hearing Association.

COMMITTING TO A THERAPY PLAN AND A SCHEDULE

The clinician should select one of the data-based treatment programs described in our literature and adhere to it. I recommend sticking to a treatment plan for a minimum of 16 sessions (Daly, 1984). Successful treatment of chronic stuttering takes time.

We favor the fluency-enhancing programs which teach components or targets of fluent speech behavior. For some clients, however, even the most basic task may need to be simplified. For example, not everyone automatically shifts to a deliberate, slower, more-fluent manner of speaking when talking on a delayed feedback machine. Some clients need repeated modeling or practice in producing the "drone-like" speech. Many people who stutter try to use the highly phonated, drone-type speech without decreasing the number of words in their sentences. Droning expends so much air that some clients can not complete their sentences without straining or taking a second breath. This recurrent faulty pattern is remedied by using structured therapy materials requiring shorter segments of speech.

All clients (even people in their 40s and 50s) initially practice lists of word-pairs. The first few lists contain no plosive phonemes (e.g., "man-fan" or "know-show"). Controlling the length of utterance allows close monitoring of breathing patterns, smooth onset of speech, and continuous phonation (droning). Enthusiastic feedback is given for correct productions. I insist on a 95 percent success rate on two-word productions before three-word lists are introduced. Again, specially designed lists are utilized (e.g., "foam-home-roam"; "you-flew-through"). The objective is to provide hundreds, perhaps thousands, of opportunities for the client to perfectly execute correct breathing, voicing, and speech onset patterns. When a criterion of 95 percent is reached, conversation is introduced. Here again the length of utterance is controlled. Initially, no sentence from either the client or the clinician exceeds four words. Performance of 95 percent or greater enables the client to move to structured reading material with sentences of five or six words.

Repeated failures have taught me that treatment once a week is unrealistic for most people who are chronic stutterers. I advocate treatment at least twice a week. I feel so strongly about the schedule that I will no longer see chronic stuttering clients once a week. We must load the probabilities for success in our favor. More frequent treatment in the beginning also serves to motivate our clients.

The quality of practice is as important as the quantity. Fluency skills must be executed precisely, and the correct performances must be accurately reinforced. Clients should not be sent out on assignments before they had had enough therapy to deliver the desired performance (Sheehan, 1980). Role-playing and periodically seeing two clients together facilitates transfer of newly acquired speech skills.

SUPPLEMENTING SPEECH TREATMENT: COGNITIVE AND SELF-INSTRUCTIONAL STRATEGIES

Too many of our clients get fluent in their mouths but not in their heads. Despite success, they feel threatened and helpless when trying their new skills alone. I have found mental rehearsal, guided relaxation, and positive mental imagery activities extremely valuable. Before clients can change, they must first see themselves in a new role (Maltz, 1960). Imagining the achievement of a goal actually facilitates achieving it in reality (Lazarus, 1984). Combining relaxation and mental imagery techniques has been effective in confronting and altering cancer patients' feelings of hopelessness and helplessness (Simonton & Simonton, 1978). Teaching positive self-talk behaviors leads to greater treatment efficacy, more generalization, and longer persistence of treatment effects (Meichenbaum & Cameron, 1974).

I have tried each of these strategies with people who are chronic stutterers. All have been successful with some clients, but not every technique works with every client. I advocate a combination of techniques. In my view, the value of helping clients picture themselves as fluent in future speaking situations cannot be overestimated. Before clients go out on speaking assignments, we instruct them to practice imagery activities at home. I have designed rating sheets for them to record the clarity of their images. With repeated practice most clients report picturing themselves more clearly. I then instruct them to continue imagery assignments by focusing on the sound of their fluent voice. Our goal is to change the image from visual to auditory. Finally, I ask them to sense how the new fluency "feels." The goal is to accentuate the speaker's awareness to more than one sensory modality. Interested readers are referred to Lazarus's (1981) discussion of multimodal therapy.

SUMMARY

In private practice (perhaps more than in other clinical settings), the proof is in the pudding. If your procedures do not produce the expected outcome, you are not in practice very long. My experience suggests that clients who stutter are helped to communicate more effectively and more fluently by combining speech treatment strategies with cognitive and self-instructional procedures.

REFERENCES

Daly, D.A. (1984). Treatment of the young chronic stutterer: Managing stuttering. In R.F. Curlee & W.H. Perkins (Eds.), *Nature and treatment of stuttering: New directions*. San Diego: College-Hill Press.

Lazarus, A.A. (1971). *Behavior therapy and beyond*. New York: McGraw-Hill.

Lazarus, A.A. (1981). *The practice of multi-modal therapy*. New York: McGraw-Hill.

Lazarus, A.A. (1984). *In the mind's eye*. New York: Guildford Press.

Maltz, M. (1960). *Pscho-Cybernetics*. Englewood Cliffs, NJ: Prentice-Hall.

Martin, R.R. (1981). Introduction and perspective: Review of published research. In E. Boberg (Ed.), *Maintenance of fluency*. New York: Elsevier.

Meichenbaum, D., & Cameron, R. (1974). The clinical potential of modifying what clients say to themselves. *Psychotherapy: Theory, Research, and Practice, 11,* 103–117.

Mowrer, O.H. (1960). *Learning theory and behavior*. New York: John Wiley.

Sheehan, J.G. (1980). Problems in the evaluation of progress and outcome. *Seminars in Speech, Language, and Hearing, 1,* 389–401.

Simonton, O.C., & Simonton, S.M. (1978). *Getting well again*. New York: Bantam Books.

Van Riper, C. (1971). *The nature of stuttering*. Englewood Cliffs, NJ: Prentice-Hall.

Meta-Analysis of the Effects of Stuttering Treatment

Gavin Andrews
Barry Guitar
Pauline Howie

There have been a large number of articles and books published in the last 20 years that suggest how stuttering might be treated. About one in five have also provided information about effectiveness of the proposed treatment. Despite availability of relevant information, speech pathologists often lack specific knowledge and training in how to treat stutterers (Thompson, 1977) and are often afraid that their attempts will do more harm than good (Wingate, 1971). Indeed there seems to be a prevailing idea, certainly reflected in media accounts of the condition, that stuttering is a mysterious and ill understood complaint that does not respond to treatment. In both the United States and in England stutterers are organizing, not for treatment, but to provide mutual support in bearing their affliction.

The idea that stuttering is ill understood and difficult to treat seems at variance with the literature. A considerable amount is known about the condition. We know about the onset, the clinical picture, and the likely outcome. We know how other people feel about stutterers and how stutterers feel about themselves. We know to a considerable degree the similarities between stutterers and nonstutterers, and we have reliable information about specific ways in which they differ. In the genetic and auditory-motor processing fields we may have good clues to the cause of stuttering. By using information about late development of speech, frequency of articulation problems, and family history of stuttering, we can probably identify many who are likely to stutter before they even begin to do so (Andrews & Harris, 1964).

In the past, determining the relative effectiveness of the different stuttering therapies has been difficult. It is, however, possible to compare the results of different treatments using a new mathematical technique: meta-analysis. With this technique it is possible to answer questions about the benefits likely to accrue from a therapy and to make comparisons among therapies, while taking into account the influences of such complex factors as stability of outcome, clinician and client acceptability, and cost-effectiveness. Answering such questions is the purpose of this paper.

The need to aggregate evidence from previous studies is a traditional problem in the accumulation of scientific knowledge. The existence of many individual studies in the literature makes such a step highly desirable, but procedures for reviewing the literature have not been developed in a methodologically rigorous way (Yin, Bingham, & Heald, 1976). Two of the issues that confound reviews of other clinical conditions do not exist in stuttering. First, stuttering can be reliably diagnosed and measured so that valid treatment research designs are possible. Second, the size of treatment effects usually reported make it likely that most treatment studies are reported and hence do not languish in Rosenthal's (1979) mythical file drawer.

In the field of psychotherapy, Smith and Glass (1977) employed a technique of synthesizing results (Glass, 1976) to compare effects of different types of psychotherapy and behavior therapy across a wide spectrum of psychological disorders. A strength of their technique, meta-analysis, is that it allows integration of diverse research through statistical analysis of the results of individual studies. The dependent variable is the magnitude of treatment effect or effect size (ES), and it is calculated from the difference between treated and control group mean scores, standardized by the variability of the control group scores. Smith and Glass (1977) chose only studies in which the treated group were compared with a control group, and were thus able to control for regression to the mean in scores of subjects seeking treatment, that is, the improvement that often occurs because persons with chronic problems seek therapy during severe phases of their disorder.

The literature on the treatment of stuttering is not sufficiently large to allow only randomized treatment/control studies to be used. Some workers have established a control group (Boudreau & Jeffrey, 1973; Öst, Götestam, & Melin, 1976; Peins, McGough, & Lee, 1972) and some have simply demonstrated a stable baseline before treatment (Webster, 1979; Ingham, Andrews, & Winkler, 1972; Gregory, 1972),

Reprinted from *Journal of Speech and Hearing Disorders, 45*, no. 3, 287–307. Copyright © 1980 American Speech-Language-Hearing Association.

but most appear to have presumed that spontaneous improvement is unlikely.

The data in the six studies cited do show a slight improvement in untreated subjects but in no group was it statistically significant. An improvement trend of similar size, but now significant because of the larger numbers, was evident in data on 132 stutterers waiting for treatment at the Prince Henry Hospital. For each pair of measures taken on two pretreatment assessment occasions separated by some months, an effect size statistic was calculated. The mean effect size for the 15 observations on adult stutterers (nine from the cited studies and six from the Prince Henry data) was 0.22 (SE = 0.04). Based on these data, neither regression to the mean nor spontaneous improvement appears to be a confounding problem of serious proportion in evaluating the treatment of adult stutterers. In treatment outcome studies where spontaneous improvement is a serious problem, untreated control groups, random allocation of patients to groups, and blind assessment are vital features of research design. Where spontaneous improvement is not a problem, as in the present situation, a pre/post design is valid as long as there is no blatant selection of subjects likely to do especially well and as long as reliable and valid measures are used. The results of such research should be as meaningful as those obtained from randomized treatment/control designs.

In respect to meta-analysis, the pre/post design offers a further advantage—the size of the improvement will be standardized by the variability of the subjects' own pretreatment scores rather than those of an unrelated group of subjects. Thus, in the present study, the measure of the effect of treatment (effect size) will be calculated as the difference between the mean pretreatment score on a measure and the mean posttreatment score on the same measure, divided by the standard deviation of the pretreatment scores:

$$\frac{\text{pretreatment} - \text{posttreatment mean}}{\text{standard deviation of pretreatment scores}}$$

Thus a study with an effect size of 1 indicates that the average posttreatment score is one standard deviation better than was the average score before treatment. Assuming that the frequency distribution of the symptom scores of untreated subjects is normal, the average stutterer in posttreatment would then score better than 84 percent of stutterers before treatment, a percentile gain of 34. This effect size statistic allows different treatments to be compared and different outcome measures to be related. The technique is exact when the distribution of scores is normal and all studies use the same measures. Violation of these assumptions do not invalidate the technique, and in fact nonparametric calculations of effect size produce answers similar to those produced by the more widely applicable Glass parametric technique. The present paper is an attempt to use the Glass methodology to answer three questions: (1) How effective is stuttering treatment? (2) What are the attributes of treatments reporting

the best results? and (3) What are the implications for treatment?

METHOD

The method followed that outlined by Glass (1976), Smith and Glass (1977), and Smith, Glass, and Miller (1980). In brief, the literature was searched for reports of stuttering treatment. An effect size was calculated for each outcome measure reported and the features of each study were coded for authors' characteristics, client characteristics, principal treatment, ancillary treatment, format of treatment, and characteristics of outcome measurement (Appendix). These features were used as the independent variables in the meta-analysis, while effect sizes became the dependent variables.

Selection of Studies for Analysis

Four journals were searched (*Journal of Speech and Hearing Disorders; Journal of Speech and Hearing Research; Journal of Communication Disorders; Journal of Fluency Disorders*) and documents mentioned in four reviews of stuttering therapy perused (Ingham & Andrews, 1973; Van Riper, 1973; Bloodstein, 1975; Ingham & Lewis, 1978). In addition, other recent books, periodicals, and proceedings of conferences held before August 1979 and likely to contain accounts of stuttering therapy were searched. Dissertations and some unpublished material were also included. The results should be representative of published reports of stuttering treatments.

To be included, a report had to give an account of treatment applied to three or more stutterers who had been measured before and after treatment. If the experimenter referred to his procedure as a treatment, the document was analyzed; no a priori decisions of what constitutes treatment were made. Studies in which a procedure was used to manipulate the frequency of stuttering were not included if the focus of the study was not clinical treatment; for example, Guitar (1975) was excluded because treatment was only considered in the case of the one subject who had prolonged follow-up. Studies were included only if it was possible to calculate effect sizes, that is, if the before and after treatment data included either means and standard deviations or information from which these could be calculated (*t* test, analysis of variance, or raw data). Additional data were obtained from a number of authors.

Some 100 publications were located but effect sizes were calculable in only 29. Many of these publications gave data on more than one group of clients; these were kept distinct if the client or treatment characteristics differed. Thus, 42 studies of treatment, comprising 756 stutterers, were used from which 116 effect sizes were computed. Table 1 lists each study analyzed, the principal treatment used, and the number of effect sizes generated from that study. The list

TABLE 1. List of studies analyzed, arranged alphabetically by principal treatment and chronologically by year of publication. In some studies additional data was obtained from the author or from other documentary sources.

Study no.	Author(s)	Year	No. of stutterers	Principal treatment	No. of effect sizes calculated
1.	Azrin and Nunn	1974	14	Airflow	1
2.	Weiner	1978	12	Airflow	1
3.	Azrin, Nunn, and Frantz	1979	21	Airflow	3
4.	Cypreanson	1948	3	Attitude therapy	1
5.	Martin and Haroldson	1969	10	Attitude therapy	3
6.	Gregory	1972	16	Attitude therapy	5
7.	Peins, McGough, and Lee	1972	12	Attitude therapy	1
8.	Burgraff	1974	9	Attitude therapy	1
9.	Lanyon	1978	4	Biofeedback	4
10.	Boudreau and Jeffrey	1973	8	Desensitization	2
11.	Burgraff	1974	9	Desensitization	1
12.	Azrin, Nunn, and Frantz	1979	17	Desensitization	2
13.	Webster, R. L.	1974	20	Gentle onset	1
14.	Daly and Darnton	1976	9	Gentle onset	4
15.	Schwartz and Webster, L. M.	1977	29	Gentle onset	2
16.	Webster, R. L.	1979	100	Gentle onset	2
17.	Andrews and Ingham	1972b	23	Prolonged speech	6
18.	Perkins	1974	25	Prolonged speech	2
19.	Perkins	1974	15	Prolonged speech	2
20.	Ryan	1974	8	Prolonged speech	2
21.	Ryan	1974	8	Prolonged speech	2
22.	Ryan	1974	7	Prolonged speech	2
23.	Guitar	1976	20	Prolonged speech	2
24.	Boberg and Sawyer	1977	13	Prolonged speech	9
25.	Frayne, Coates, and Marriner	1977	10	Prolonged speech	2
26.	Helps and Dalton	1979	44	Prolonged speech	7
27.	Howie, Tanner, and Andrews	1980	36	Prolonged speech	6
28.	Howie, Tanner, and Andrews	1980	43	Prolonged speech	5
29.	Martin and Haroldson	1969	10	Reinforcement	3
30.	Andrews and Harris	1964	5	Rhythm	3
31.	Andrews and Harris	1964	10	Rhythm	4
32.	Andrews and Harris	1964	20	Rhythm	4
33.	Brady	1971	23	Rhythm	1
34.	Ingham, Andrews, and Winkler	1972	20	Rhythm	2
35.	Ingham, Andrews, and Winkler	1972	10	Rhythm	2
36.	Andrews and Ingham	1972a	27	Rhythm	2
37.	Öst, Götestam, and Melin	1976	15	Rhythm	2
38.	Helps and Dalton	1979	21	Rhythm	7
39.	Culatta and Rubin	1973	6	Self-contol	1
40.	Kondas	1967	17	Shadowing	1
41.	Öst, Götestam, and Melin	1976	15	Shadowing	2
42.	Peins, McGough, and Lee	1972	12	Slow speaking	1

is organized alphabetically by principal treatment, and within each treatment type by date of publication.

Calculating the Effect Size

Effect size was calculated on any outcome variable the researcher measured before and after treatment. In most cases a study yielded several effect sizes, since improvement was often measured at more than one time and on more than one type of outcome measure. A limit of nine effect sizes per study was instituted, but only one study exceeded this limit. The mean number of effect sizes per study was 2.76 (SD 4.1).

Coding the Features of the Study

Each study was scored as to the presence of the features listed in the Appendix. The features used to describe the authors' characteristics and the characteristics of each group of clients are self-explanatory.

Defining the classes of treatment was less difficult than appeared initially. There were 22 treatment components used in the 42 studies. Each study could be characterized as having a principal treatment, and most used several ancillary treatments as well. Five publications compared different principal treatments. They were analyzed as separate studies, and the important comparative information that they contained will be further discussed.

Describing the nature and circumstances of the outcome measure was important since changes in these measures would be the basis for calculation of effect size. The type of outcome measure used was classified on a 9-point ordinal scale that broadly moved from reliable and unbiased measures of behavior such as stuttering frequency, to measures of speech rate, judgments of severity of stuttering, self reports of stuttering severity, questionnaires of attitude and speech related behavior, and finally, to the experimenter's opinions of the degree of improvement and other subjective measures. Duplicate measures of the same type taken at the same time and measures of reading were discarded.

The reliability of each measure was classified on a 3-point scale, based either on data or on the coders' judgment of the probable reliability of the particular measure used.

Obviously, studies that assess stutterers 6–12 months after treatment are preferred, but outcome measures taken at the end of treatment were included, the duration between treatment and the time of the outcome measure being recorded as zero. *Treatment to assessment interval* became another of the variables to be related to effect size. Many treatments included after-care or maintenance activities to maximize the retention of improvement, which poses a difficult question: When does treatment stop? Even in programs with no planned maintenance component, subjects experiencing relapse often seek further help. For the purpose of this analysis, treatment was deemed to end when that part of treatment designed to produce maximum fluency ended. Procedures intended to help the subject maintain this improvement were regarded as posttreatment. The presence of maintenance activities was entered as a further variable to be related to effects of treatment.

Another variable that may influence a treatment's effect size is the number of subjects lost during the study. It should be presumed that drop-outs are usually failures; thus the percent of clients lost was a variable of interest.

The internal validity of the research design was not a selection criterion but rather became another independent variable to be related to the reported effects of treatment. The five factors rated as important in a pre/post research design were (1) no bias in subject selection, (2) client drop-out of less than 15 percent, (3) clear description of treatment, (4) reliable objective measures, and (5) an outcome measure taken 6 months or more after treatment. Studies were scored one point for the presence of each factor, and the total score was entered as the internal validity of the research design.

The publications were coded in the following way: GA and BG rated each study independently, then met to reconcile the differences. PH used a written description of the coding form to rate a randomly selected 10 percent of the studies. Agreement between PH and the joint ratings of the other two authors exceeded 80 percent across all categories; mean agreement was 89 percent. Analyses of the data followed the model of Smith and Glass (1977) and included descriptive statistics for the body of data as a whole, descriptive statistics for the comparison of therapy types and outcome types, and a regression analysis in which the independent variables were used as predictors of the treatment effect size.

RESULTS

Characteristics of the Studies

The authors of the 42 studies were speech pathologists (52%), psychologists (33%), or physicians (14%). Eighty percent held a doctorate at the time of the report, and one-third of the cases were conducted in private practice settings. The 756 subjects were usually (86%) regular clinic clients; 80 percent were male and the median age range was 20–29 years, with the median IQ slightly above average. The average severity before therapy was 16 percent of syllables stuttered. The possibility of spontaneous remission accounting for the improvement was judged to be remote in 90 percent of the subjects.

In the 42 studies, the most frequently used principal treatments were prolonged speech (29%), rhythm (21%), and attitude therapy (12%). In the remaining studies, the principal treatment was gentle onset (10%), airflow (7%), densensitization (7%), and the other techniques listed in Table 1 (14%). Assertive training, behavioral rehearsal, daily practice, drugs, easy stuttering, masking, negative practice, relaxation, self report, social support, and psychotherapy were not reported as principal treatments, although many were used as ancillary treatments. Seventy-six percent of the studies incorporated transfer activities, and 46 percent, maintenance activities. The average treatment duration, including any transfer, was 80 hours and was completed in 8 weeks, though the standard deviations for both these variables were large.

Seventy-eight percent of the effect sizes were based on changes in speech measures and 22 percent on changes in attitude measures. The average treatment to assessment interval was 6 months (range 0–25 months). Forty-nine percent of the measures evidenced reliabilities in excess of 0.9, with 46 percent between 0.6 and 0.9. Three-quarters of the authors had been able to follow up more than 85 percent of their clients. A large proportion of the studies were therefore well designed, used reliable and appropriate measures, employed an adequate follow-up interval, and had a low rate of client loss.

Is Stuttering Treatment Effective?

The mean of the 116 effect sizes was 1.3, indicating a 1.3 standard deviation improvement of stutterers after treatment when compared with their scores before treatment. Thus, if pretreatment scores were normally distributed, the average treated stutterer was now more normal-speaking than 90 percent of his/her untreated fellows, a gain of 40 percentiles. This finding is depicted in Figure 1. The two curves represent the hypothetical distributions of pre- and posttreatment measures in the population from which the 756 stutterers were drawn. As in the Glass (1976) report, the curves are drawn as two normal distributions, although no conclusion about the distributions of scores is intended. For ease of representation, the assumption of normality has much justification and allows comparison with the Smith and Glass (1977) report.

The standard deviation of effect sizes was 0.8, skewness + 0.9, median 1.2, and range −0.13–3.72. Only four effect sizes were negative, whereas if stuttering treatment were ineffective and design/measurement flaws immaterial, one would have expected 58, or half the effect size measurements, to be negative. Clearly stuttering treatment is effective.

The size of the average treatment effect is of some interest, but of more interest is the time course of the improvement. In Figure 2 the mean effect size over time is displayed, with effect sizes classified in blocks of 3 months since treatment. The bars joined by broken lines represent the standard errors of the means. The number of data points vary as the treatment to assessment intervals lengthen, and this is

reflected in the fluctuating size of the standard errors. The length of treatment is represented as 2 months, with an effect size of 0.22 at the beginning of treatment. These two data points are based on the calculated average length of treatment, and the earlier noted average effect size of 0.22 ± 0.04 observed in stutterers while waiting for treatment represents the average extent of spontaneous improvement.

The graph shows that improvement after treatment reaches a maximum effect size of 1.67 within the first 6 months, and this is followed by some suggestion of relapse thereafter. On the basis of a linear regression analysis of mean effect sizes on months since treatment, the estimated decay of mean effect sizes is 0.35 of a standard deviation per year.

Which Treatments Report the Best Results?

The average effect sizes for the six most common principal treatment types are presented in Table 2. The 47 effect size measures for prolonged speech average 1.65, the nine for gentle onset, 1.53. Taken together they represent data from 410 subjects in 16 studies. Judging by the standard errors (SE), their results are significantly better than those obtained with stutterers treated by any other technique except for rhythm.

The other treatments, rhythm apart, have a mean effect size of 0.77, and all but desensitization produce effects greater than that due to any improvement likely to be observed in untreated adult stutterers over time. In Table 2 the judged internal validity of the research designs associated with each treatment is shown together with the average treatment to assessment time. These data suggest that the

Figure 1. Meta-analysis model representing the effect of treatment. The left-hand curve represents the assumed normal-frequency distribution of pretreatment stuttering measures in the population of stutterers from which the 756 subjects in the meta-analysis were drawn. The curve 1.3 standard deviation units to the right of the first curve represents the assumed normal posttreatment distribution of stuttering scores of that same population. The model therefore reflects the meta-analysis finding that following treatment the average stutterer will have shifted 1.3 standard deviation units away from his/her pretreatment score in the direction of fluency, and will therefore, under the assumption of the model, be more fluent than were 90% of the stutterers in the population represented before treatment.

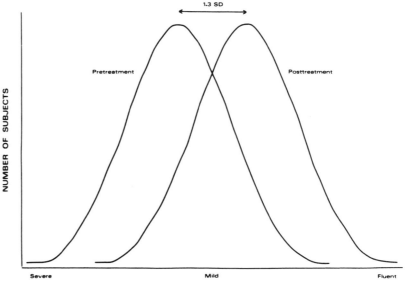

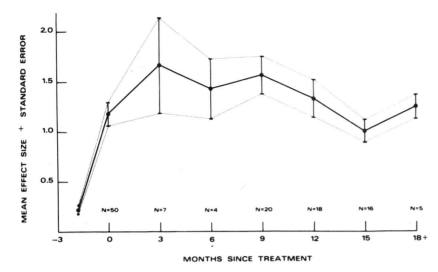

Figure 2. Mean effect sizes for all treatments combined, for treatment to assessment intervals from zero (immediately after treatment) to 18 months, classified in blocks of 3 months. The pretreatment level of 0.22 allows for regression to the mean in stuttering severity while clients wait for treatment. The average duration of treatment was 2 months. These two points are taken as the starting points of the graph. The bars joined by broken lines represent the standard errors of the means, and the N values indicate the number of effect sizes used to calculate each mean.

apparent superiority of prolonged speech and gentle onset treatments cannot be attributed to poor research design or inadequate duration of follow-up.

To what extent do prolonged speech and gentle onset treatments differ? The average codings of various components of treatment used in the two techniques are indicated in Table 3. Clearly both treatments have much in common; each uses something of the other's principal technique, and both share a number of other ancillary treatments. Until comparative studies of rate of onset of vocalization, syllable duration, pause time, and utterance length are measured and shown to be different in the two techniques, the possibility exists that they may both be ways of training the subjects to attain a common speech skill that seems conducive to fluent speech.

Decisions about effectiveness of a treatment should not depend solely on the average effect size. Effects of an initially strong treatment may be transient, whilst effects of an initially less powerful treatment may be more beneficial in the longer term. Effect sizes of the separate treatments at differing points after end of treatment are displayed in Figure 3. The scale and conventions are as in Figure 2.

Prolonged speech and gentle onset techniques appear the strongest treatments both in the short and long term. These effects of treatment diminish over time at a rate of one-third of a standard deviation per 12 months. Rhythm exerts a strong effect on fluency, but after 12 months fades rapidly. Both attitude and airflow appear to have weaker effects although their rates of relapse are slower than with rhythm. None of the less frequently used treatments were demonstrably superior to the five major treatments.

Which Features Predict Effect Size?

In the Appendix, the possible predictors of effect size are organized into six sections: author characteristics, client characteristics, principal treatments, ancillary treatments, format of treatment, and characteristics of outcome measures. The first two categories may be of value prognostically, but knowledge of them does not help a clinician with

TABLE 2. The effect sizes, validity of research design, and mean treatment to assessment interval for the main types of treatment.

Treatment	No. of stutterers	Effect Size					Validity of research design 1 = low 5 = high		Treatment to assessment interval (Months)	
		N	Mean	SE	Min	Max	Mean	SE	Mean	SE
Prolonged	252	47	1.65	0.12	0.60	3.72	4.4	0.10	7.6	1.0
Gentle onset	158	9	1.53	0.20	0.95	2.40	3.3	0.24	6.2	2.8
Rhythm	151	27	1.27	0.14	0.10	3.22	4.9	0.04	7.0	1.0
Airflow	47	5	0.92	0.11	0.74	1.36	3.0	0.00	4.2	3.0
Attitude	50	11	0.85	0.27	−0.13	2.70	4.1	0.37	3.3	1.4
Desensitization	34	5	0.54	0.22	0.01	1.07	4.0	0.45	5.0	3.8
All others	64	12	0.73	0.17	−0.10	1.90	4.3	0.23	3.3	1.6
Totals	756	116	1.30	0.08	−0.13	3.72	4.1	0.16	6.2	0.6

TABLE 3. A comparison of the treatment components associated with the prolonged speech and gentle onset techniques. Scaling: 0 = not used: 1 = minimal component; 2 = important component: 3 = principal component.

Component	Prolonged speech	Gentle onset
Airflow	0	0
Assertive training	0	0
Attitude therapy	1	1
Behavioral rehearsal	0	0
Biofeedback	0	0
Densensitization	0	0
Easy stuttering	0	0
Gentle onset	2	3
Negative practice	0	0
Prolonged speech	3	2
Reinforcement	2	0
Relaxation	0	0
Rhythm	0	0
Self control	1	1
Self report	0	0
Shadowing	0	0
Slow speech	2	2
Social support	1	0
Psychotherapy	0	0
Transfer	2	2
Maintenance	2	1
Form of Treatment		
Duration (hrs)	135	96
Intensity (hrs per wk)	40	23
Daily practice required	2	1
% group setting	80%	40%
Pearson Correlation	0.65	

an individual patient. Speech pathologists, psychologists, and physicians reported equally good results; similarly, private and public practice appeared equally likely to benefit subjects. Of the stutterers' characteristics studied, only youth had a positive relationship with effect size. Milder stutterers have often been reported as doing well in therapy. The present analysis was based on grouped data and this may have inhibited that relationship from appearing.

The major question remains: Can one use these data to determine how an effective treatment program should be designed? The predictors of treatment effect size for these data were obtained by a hierarchical stepwise multiple regression analysis (Table 4). Groups of features were entered in the following blocks: principal treatments, ancillary treatments, format of treatment, and outcome measures. The following constraints were used: only features present in at least 5 percent of the studies were included, F to enter was set at 1.0, and tolerance to enter was greater than 0.4.

Principal Treatments. Prolonged speech was the first of the principal treatments to enter the equation, and it accounted for 15 percent of the variance in effect size. Rhythmic speech and attitude were the other specific treatments to enter, bringing the variance explained by specific treatments to 21 percent. Airflow and gentle onset did not enter the equation.

Ancillary Treatments. Five ancillary treatments were included in the second block in the hierarchy. They were, in order of importance, the presence of a reinforcement program, transfer activities, maintenance activities, emphasis on slow speech in the training phase, and recruitment of social support to potentiate improvement. When these variables were added to the regression equation, the explained variance rose to 30 percent.

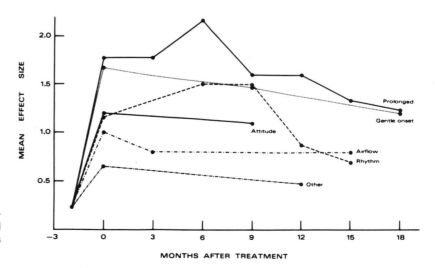

Figure 3. The average effect sizes for six treatments from 0–18 months after treatment, classified in blocks of 3 months. The scales and conventions are the same as in Figure 2.

TABLE 4. Results of hierarchical stepwise multiple regression analysis used to predict effect size. All treatment variables scored by at least 5% of the studies were included. Variables were entered sequentially in four sets: principal treatments, ancillary treatments, format of treatment, measurement criteria. F to enter was set at 1.0 and tolerance greater than 0.4.

Variable	Variance explained by variable	Variance explained by set	Variables not entering equation
Principal treatments			
Prolonged speech	15.1%		Airflow
Rhythmic speech	4.8%		Gentle onset
Attitude therapy	1.3%		
		21.2%	
Ancillary treatments			
Reinforcement to defined schedule	4.1%		
Slow speech during instatement	1.5%		
Transfer program	1.0%		
Maintenance program	1.2%		
Social support	1.3%		
		9.1%	
Format of treatment			
Hours of treatment	9.7%		Hours per week
		9.7%	
Characteristics of outcome measurement			
Treatment to assessment interval	1.3%		Outcome measure
Percentage clients lost	1.2%		
Reliability of measures	0.8%		
		3.3%	
Total Variance Explained	43.3%	43.3%	

Format of Treatment. Effect size was linearly related to the hours spent in treatment. In fact, the simple correlation between effect size and hours of treatment was 0.58, and it was the best single predictor of outcome. If one considers stuttering to be due primarily to a physiological dysfunction, just as regular jogging makes for fitness or length of dieting for weight loss, length of rehabilitation should have a direct relation to improvement. However, hours of treatment may be confounded with treatment type. The most effective treatments (prolonged speech, gentle onset, and rhythm) used longer and more concentrated periods, and part of the simple correlation between hours of treatment and outcome might be due to this association. These effects had been removed earlier in the regression analysis, and hours of treatment contributed a further 9.7 percent of the variance to that explained by the specifics of treatment. Thus the present conclusion is secure—training helps stutterers. The possibility that hours of contact without technique might be beneficial has not been an issue since Rousey (1958), using continuous speaking for 10 hours per day for 5 days, found no change in rated stuttering severity in 18 stutterers. Obviously, if you have an effective treatment technique, it pays to spend time training clients in its use. Intensity of treatment did not enter the equation, perhaps because all the longer treatments were delivered intensively. The three groups of treatment features, principal, ancillary, and format, accounted for 40 percent of the variance in effect size.

Characteristics of Outcome Measurement. The last question to be dealt with is whether reliability and the nature and timing of outcome measures are related to effect size. In the Smith and Glass study (1977), effect size differed markedly depending on the sensitivity of the measures. Because of the importance of outcome measurement, this matter will be explored in depth.

Effect size varied with type of outcome measure. Fifty-three percent of the measures were of frequency of stuttering (mean effect size 1.25 ± 0.1), 25 percent were of rate of speech or other observed aspects of speech (mean effect size 1.6 ± 0.2), and 22 percent were of attitude or other measures of the stutterer's self-concept (mean effect size 1.1 ± 0.2). As might be expected from the standard errors, these effect sizes were significantly different at the $p < 0.05$ level in a one-way analysis of variance. Scrutiny of the data suggests that measures of rate of speech would generate larger effect sizes because of the relatively small standard deviations in the original distribution. In contrast to the Smith and Glass (1977) findings, this variation in effect size did not appear related to particular outcome measures associated with any particular treatment. Indeed, the type of outcome measure did not enter the regression equation as a predictor of effect size; however, the time of the measurement did. The relation between effect size and treatment to assessment interval is illustrated in Figure 2.

Another variable often associated with inflated effect

sizes is the percentage of clients lost to follow-up and not recorded as treatment failures. Sixty percent of the studies examined lost no clients, and three-quarters reported on at least 85 percent of the original group. Not surprisingly, in the face of such diligent follow-up, there was only a small relationship between wastage and effect size.

The last variable, reliability of the measure, should be associated positively with effect size, if only because reliable measurement reduces error variance. In the raw data, reliability of measures correlated 0.38 with effect size. This association could have been an artifact because the more reliable measures of percentage of syllables stuttered and syllables per minute were used frequently in studies of prolonged and rhythmic speech, two of the more powerful treatments. Accordingly, a partial correlation of effect size with reliability was obtained to control for the effects of these treatments. The resulting partial correlation of 0.19 is probably a better estimate of the gain one obtains by using more reliable measures of outcome. When the effect size is regressed onto these three characteristics of outcome measurement (treatment to assessment interval, percent of clients lost, and reliability of measures) with the influence of the treatment variables removed, an additional 3 percent of the variance in effect size is accounted for (Table 4).

Summarizing the regression analysis as a whole, one may conclude that the principal and ancillary treatments, the format of treatment, and the characteristics of outcome measures accounted for nearly half the variance in improvement in these 756 stutterers. The unexplained remaining variance is customarily attributed to individual clinician and client differences, error variance, and Brownian movement.

DISCUSSION

What Is the Validity of This Meta-Analysis?

A number of methodological issues should be discussed. In some meta-analyses, doubt has been expressed about the wisdom of combining data from unpublished material, book chapters, and reviewed journal articles because of the possibility of introducing error-prone data to the matrix. In this study, publications are listed in Table 1 and readers can make their own decisions about which may be error-prone. Analysis of studies by publication mode revealed no discernible differences in effect sizes; mixing different outcome measures together in the analysis can be defended on the basis that all relate to a general improvement in well-being. Moreover, the extent to which treatment improves one measure as compared to another is of interest. To have calculated only an average effect size for each study would have resulted in the loss of much potentially valuable information, even though including more than one effect size for each study permits dependence in the errors and violates some assumptions of inferential statistics. To control for this possibility, the regression analysis was repeated using one outcome measure from each study, the immediate post-treatment measure of the frequency of stuttering. The results were similar to the full analysis.

The second problem concerns the meaning of the results. For some conditions, such as lung cancer, a treatment-induced improvement in symptoms may be clinically meaningless because the growth of the life-threatening cancer will continue. In stuttering, however, the fewer the symptoms, the less severe the disorder, and while total removal of the stutter would be an ideal outcome, an 80 percent reduction in stuttering a year after treatment is clinically meaningful, even if not ideal.

A third problem is that data that are heavily skewed may give a distorted effect size. To illuminate this matter, the distributions of stuttering frequency, speech rate, and attitude scores of 132 patients awaiting treatment in our clinic were examined. The distribution of pretreatment measures of stuttering frequency proved to be skewed to the right (skew = 1.14) and the pretreatment mean was only 1.4 times. as great as the standard deviation. Since stuttering frequency following treatment will shift away from the tail of this distribution, there is a lower limit (zero stuttering) beyond which treatment effects cannot extend even if all clients achieve complete fluency; this lower limit represents only 1.4 standard deviation units. Assuming a normal distribution, an effect size of 1.4 implies that after treatment the average client is more normal-speaking than 92 percent of pretreatment clients, rather than the 100 percent that would be the case if all clients had zero stuttering. Thus, effect sizes in the present study that were based on stuttering frequency will give conservative estimates of the improvement actually occurring.

By contrast, the pretreatment speech rate scores of the same 132 subjects were normally distributed, and therefore effect sizes based on speech rate should not be distorted. In the case of attitude questionnaire data, the distributions varied considerably. In this meta-analysis, half the measures were of frequency of stuttering, a quarter of speech rate, and a quarter from questionnaires, and therefore most of the resulting effect sizes are expected to be conservative estimates of improvement. As a check on this, the data from the 132 untreated subjects were used to generate a distribution of a composite score weighted according to the frequency of the three types of measures. The distribution of these scores was a flat-topped, quasi-normal distribution with a slight positive skew, and the expected treatment shift was away from the distribution tail. Overall then, most effect sizes would be conservative estimates of improvement. The results of this meta-analysis similarly may be a conservative estimate of the outcome of stuttering therapy.

There is another possible source of effect size bias. As seen in Tables 1 and 2, the more effective treatments tend to be associated with larger groups of subjects. In a normal distribution, variations in the standard deviation will lessen as the number of subjects increases, which may have influenced the effect size in some treatments. Accordingly, a correlation between effect size and number of clients measured was calculated for the 116 measurement occasions. There was no significant relationship ($r = 0.06$, $p = 0.27$).

The last problem concerns the future. Because meta-analysis is a new technique, none of the studies reviewed could have biased their results either by selecting which outcome variables to report or by selecting a statistically homogeneous group of stutterers to maximize effect size. In the future, however, this may not be the case: a *minimum* set of measures that could be agreed upon when reporting effects of stuttering treatment would be helpful. The measurement of frequency of stuttering and rate of speech and the use of a speech attitude scale, before, at the end, and 6 months after treatment, is suggested as the minimum assessment to circumvent this problem. Mean, range, standard deviation, and skew of pretreatment scores should also be reported.

How Effective Is Stuttering Therapy?

The average effect size of the 42 studies was 1.3 standard deviations, and some classes of treatment had mean effect sizes as high as 1.5 and 1.6. In Smith et al.'s (1980) meta-analysis of 475 controlled studies of psychotherapy and behavior therapy, the average effect size was only 0.85, yet they concluded, "Psychotherapy is beneficial, consistently so and in many different ways. Its benefits are on a par with other expensive and ambitious interventions, such as schooling and medicine. The benefits of psychotherapy are not permanent, but then little is" (chap. 9).

In medicine, data rarely are presented in the form of means and standard deviations of symptoms or test abnormalities. Therefore, effect sizes frequently cannot be calculated. Data available to the authors show an effect size of 1.0 for the treatment of asthma and 0.6 for the effect of patient education in arthritis. With education, radical changes in the system of instruction give effect sizes of 0.5, and when changes to classroom size and environment are conducted, 0.4 (Kulik, Kulik, & Cohen, 1979). By any of these criteria, stuttering therapy is effective, particularly as the results appear more stable, less influenced by choice of outcome measure, and less likely to decay with the passage of time.

What Types of Treatment Produce Best Results?

The rank order of effectiveness of the different treatments, based on average effect size, is displayed in Table 2. Their effectiveness over time is displayed in Figure 3. Validity of these results may be further assessed by examining the five same-experiment studies that compared one treatment with another. In each, the results are consistent with the meta-analysis results. Helps and Dalton (1979) compared prolonged speech with rhythm and found that the former was consistently more effective. The average observed differences in effect size between the two treatments was 0.34, close to the 0.38 expected from the meta-analysis results.

Azrin, Nunn, and Frantz (1979) found the airflow technique superior to a brief desensitization regime. The effect size difference in their study was 0.79, larger than the 0.38 expected from the meta-analysis result. The poor showing of desensitization, as these authors acknowledged, was probably due to the brevity of their desensitization procedures. Öst et al. (1976) compared rhythm with shadowing and found an effect size superiority of 0.54 for rhythm. Peins et al. (1972) compared attitude treatment with instruction to speak slowly and found no significant difference. Martin and Haroldson (1969) investigated two brief treatments, attitude and reinforcement, neither treatment incorporating transfer activities. In both these treatments, effect size failed to exceed 0.22, the change likely to be observed with repeated measurement in the absence of treatment, and therefore neither treatment appeared beneficial.

Both the meta-analysis and individual comparison studies show prolonged speech and gentle onset techniques to be better in the short and long term than either attitude or airflow treatment. These four, except for rhythm, are better than any of the other reported treatments and certainly are better than no treatment. For an individual client, however, there can be no predictable "best treatment." What is best in a particular case depends on the values and symptoms of the client, the specific skills of the clinician, and the treatment alternatives available.

What Are the Implications for the Treatment of Stuttering?

The results of the multiple regression analysis describe the currently used, well established, more effective programs well. Before detailing those features of treatment that emerge from the meta-analysis as predictive of good treatment outcome, some comment on rhythmic speed is called for. This treatment technique produces a good initial effect size, but deterioration over time is considerable. Stutterers dislike the cadence of rhythmic speech, and when they begin to stutter again, they commonly experience a return of the complicated secondary stuttering (Andrews & Ingham, 1972b). Rhythm is an unloved treatment.

Rhythm apart, many of the features that were associated with large effect sizes in the regression analysis are contained in most prolonged speech and gentle onset programs. The similarities between these two treatments were described earlier (Table 3); the overlap of features may have precluded the gentle onset technique from entering regression analysis as a significant predictor of effect size.

Using the information provided by the meta-analysis (Table 4) on the effective features of stuttering treatment, what kind of program would one develop? The data suggest that substantial improvement needs at least 100 hours of treatment in which a varient of the prolonged speech technique is used at a slow rate to establish control over stuttering, with the resulting fluent speech shaped to normal speech by a defined schedule. Systematic transfer of the new speech into the real world appears beneficial, and some clients may need counseling to improve their attitudes. Some may benefit if their family and friends offer support as they seek to generalize their fluent speech. Finally, the clinic may need to offer a planned maintenance program to consolidate all these activities. Using such a treatment approach, the effect size should approximate 1.6; the average stutterer could be more normal-speaking than 95 percent of the untreated group, and a few may cease to stutter. Howie, Tanner, and Andrews (in press) describe the results of a program that contains these characteristics.

The prolonged speech and gentle onset techniques have produced similar results when used by different therapists in different clinics, and the former, since its introduction into clinical practice by Curlee and Perkins (1969), has proved equally effective for American, Australian, and English stutterers. Such stability of results could hardly reflect a spurious finding or be the result of some methodological flaw. The airflow and attitude techniques have been less well researched, need further replication, and may not prove effective when used by other therapists or in other settings. Nevertheless, one conclusion is sure—some stuttering therapies are sufficiently effective to be useful.

Two areas in the literature lack research data. First, there are no results of treatment designed specifically for younger children, and thus it is not clear whether any of the four preferred techniques are applicable to children under eight years of age. Second, there are no analyses of the essential components of these relatively complex treatments and no research on why they work. Each treatment may well contain unnecessary and irrelevant features. Gottman and Markman (1978) have stressed that as well as a need for the usual program development studies there is a need for dismantling programs step by step and evaluating the effects of removing each step.

Granted that published results of treatment will be better than the results obtained with the same treatment in routine clinical practice, there is little need for pessimism regarding the treatment of stuttering. The standard of research in studies reporting data is good, and reliable measures and adequate follow-up periods are common. The evidence suggests that treatments based on training the stutterer in prolonged and gentle onset techniques are superior to other types of treatments. Relapse over time is slow, certainly slower than with some other treatments for chronic conditions. Some stuttering treatments are clearly beneficial and their effects are comparable with treatments for other chronic problems in the health sciences.

ACKNOWLEDGMENTS

This work was completed while the senior author was on study leave at the Social Ecology Laboratory (Professor R.H. Moos), Stanford University. He was grateful to receive practical support and editorial comments from Drs. R. Cronkite, J. Finney, W. Fowkes, G. Glass, H. Kraemer, R. Moos, and W. Perkins. Requests for reprints should be sent to Dr. G. Andrews, Prince Henry Hospital, Sydney, N.S.W., Australia 2036.

REFERENCES

Andrews, G., & Harris, M. (1964). *The Syndrome of Stuttering*. Clinics in Developmental Medicine. London: Heinemann.

Andrews, G., & Ingham, R.J. (1972a). Stuttering: An evaluation of follow-up procedures for syllable-timed speech/token system therapy. *Journal of Communication Disorders, 5*, 307–319.

Andrews, G., & Ingham, R.J. (1972b). An approach to the evaluation of stuttering therapy. *Journal of Speech and Hearing Research, 15*, 296–302.

Azrin, N.H., & Nunn, R.G. (1974). A rapid method of eliminating stuttering by a regulated breathing approach. *Behavior Research and Therapy, 12*, 279–286.

Azrin, N.H., Nunn, R.G., & Frantz, S.E. (1979). Comparison of regulated breathing versus abbreviated desensitization on reported stuttering episodes. *Journal of Speech and Hearing Disorders, 44*, 331–339.

Bloodstein, O. (1975). *A Handbook on Stuttering*. Chicago: National Easter Seal Society for Crippled Children and Adults.

Boberg, E., & Sawyer, L. (1977). The maintenance of fluency following intensive therapy. *Human Communication, 2*, 21–28.

Boudreau, L.A., & Jeffrey, C.J. (1973). Stuttering treated by desensitization. *Journal of Behavior Therapy and Experimental Psychiatry, 4*, 209–212.

Brady, J.P. (1971). Metronome-conditioned speech retraining for stuttering. *Behavior Therapy, 2*, 129–150.

Burgraff, R.I. (1974). The efficacy of systematic desensitization via imagery as a therapeutic technique with stutterers. *British Journal of Disorders of Communication, 9*, 134–139.

Culatta, R.A., & Rubin, H. (1973). A program for the initial stages of fluency therapy. *Journal of Speech and Hearing Research, 16*, 556–568.

Curlee, R.F., & Perkins. W.H. (1969). Conversational rate control therapy for stuttering. *Journal of Speech and Hearing Disorders, 34*, 245–250.

Cypreanson, L. (1948). Group therapy for adult stutterers. *Journal of Speech and Hearing Disorders, 13*, 313–319.

Daly, D.A., & Darnton, S.W. (1976). *Intensive fluency shaping and attitudinal therapy with stutterers: A follow-up study*. Paper presented to the Annual Convention of the American Speech and Hearing Association, Houston.

Frayne, H., Coates, S., & Marriner, N. (1977). Evaluation of post treatment fluency by naive subjects. *Australian Journal of Human Communication Disorders, 5*, 48–54.

Glass, G.V. (1976). Primary, secondary and meta-analysis of research. *The Educational Researcher, 5*, 3–8.

Gottman, J., & Markman, H.J. (1978). Experimental designs in psychotherapy research. In S.L. Garfield & A.E. Bergin (Eds.), *Handbook of psychotherapy and behavior change*. New York: John Wiley.

Gregory, H.H. (1972). An assessment of the results of stuttering therapy. *Journal of Communication Disorders, 5*, 320–334.

Guitar, B.E. (1975). Reduction of stuttering frequency using analog electromyographic feedback. *Journal of Speech and Hearing Research, 18*, 672–685.

Guitar, B.E. (1976). Pretreatment factors associated with the outcome of stuttering therapy. *Journal of Speech and Hearing Research, 19,* 590–600.

Helps, R., & Dalton, P. (1979). The effectiveness of an intensive group speech therapy programme for adult stammerers. *British Journal of Disorders of Communication, 14,* 17–30.

Howie, P.M., Tanner, S., & Andrews, G. (1980). Short and long term outcome in an intensive treatment program for adult stutterers. *Journal of Speech and Hearing Disorders,* in press.

Ingham, R.J., & Andrews, G. (1973). Behavior therapy and stuttering therapy: A review. *Journal of Speech and Hearing Disorders, 38,* 405–441.

Ingham, R.J., Andrews, G., & Winkler, R. (1972). Stuttering: A comparative evaluation of the shortterm effectiveness of four treatment techniques. *Journal of Communication Disorders, 5,* 91–117.

Ingham, R.J., & Lewis, J.I. (1978). Behavior therapy and stuttering: And the story grows. *Human Communication, 3,* 125–152.

Kondas, O. (1967). The treatment of stammering in children by the shadowing method. *Behavior Research and Therapy, 5,* 325–329.

Kulik, J.A., Kulik, C-L.C., & Cohen, P.A. (1979). A meta-analysis of outcome studies of Keller's personalized system of instruction. *American Psychologist, 34,* 307–318.

Lanyon, R.I. (1978). Behavioral approaches to stuttering. In M. Herson, R.M. Eisler, & P.M. Miller (Eds.), *Progress in behavior modification* (Vol. 6). New York: Academic Press.

Martin, R.R., & Haroldson, S.K. (1969). The effects of two treatment procedures on stuttering. *Journal of Communication Disorders, 2,* 115–125.

Öst, L., Götestam, K.G., & Melin, L. (1976). A controlled study of two behavioral methods in the treatment of stuttering. *Behavior Therapy, 7,* 587–592.

Peins, M., McGough, W.E., & Lee, B.S. (1972). Evaluation of a tape-recorded method of stuttering therapy: Improvement in a speaking task. *Journal of Speech and Hearing Research, 15,* 364–371.

Perkins, W.H. (1974). *Behavioral Management of Stuttering: Final Report.* Social and Rehabilitation Service. Research Grant No. 14-P-55281.

Rosenthal, R. (1979). The "file drawer problem" and tolerance for null results. *Psychological Bulletin, 86,* 638–641.

Rousey, C.L. (1958). Stuttering severity during prolonged spontaneous speech. *Journal of Speech and Hearing Research, 1,* 40–47.

Ryan, B.P. (1974). *Programmed therapy for stuttering in children and adults.* Springfield, IL: Charles C. Thomas.

Schwartz, D., & Webster, L.M. (1977). More on the efficacy of a protracted precision fluency shaping program. *Journal of Fluency Disorders, 2,* 205–215.

Smith, M.L., & Glass, G.V. (1977). Meta-analysis of psychotherapy outcome studies. *American Psychologist, 32,* 752–760.

Smith, M.L., Glass, G.V., & Miller, T.I. (1980). *The Benefits of Psychotherapy.* Baltimore: Johns Hopkins.

Thompson, J. (1977). Suggestions for research: Young stutterers. *Journal of Fluency Disorders, 2,* 45–52.

Van Riper, C. (1973). *The treatment of stuttering.* Englewood Cliffs, NJ: Prentice-Hall.

Webster, R.L. (1974). A behavioral analysis of stuttering: Treatment and theory. In K.S. Calhoun, E.E. Adams, & K.M. Mitchell (Eds.), *Innovative methods in psychopathology.* New York: John Wiley.

Webster, R.L. (1979). Empirical considerations regarding stuttering therapy. In H.H. Gregory (Ed.), *Controversies about stuttering therapy.* Baltimore: University Park Press.

Weiner, A.E. (1978). Vocal control therapy for stutterers: A trial program. *Journal of Fluency Disorders, 3,* 115–126.

Wingate, M.E. (1971). The fear of stuttering. *Asha, 13,* 3–5.

Yin, R.K., Bingham, E., & Heald, K.A. (1976). The difference that quality makes: The case of literature reviews. *Sociological Methods and Research, 5,* 139–156.

APPENDIX

Features of Studies Coded as Independent Variables

Author characteristics:
> level of qualification; private or non fee paying patient; profession; speech pathology, psychology, or medicine.

Client characteristics:
> mean age; mean intelligence; percent male; mean severity; possibility of spontaneous remission accounting for improvement; were subjects regular clients or experimental subjects?

Principal treatments:
> airflow; attitude; biofeedback; desensitization; gentle onset; prolonged speech; reinforcement; rhythm; self control; shadowing; slow speaking.

Ancillary treatments:
> assertive training; attitude therapy; behavioral rehearsal; biofeedback; desensitization; easy stuttering; gentle onset; negative practice; prolonged speech; reinforcement; relaxation; rhythm; self control; self report; shadowing; slow speech; social support; psychotherapy; transfer; maintenance.

Format of treatment:
> duration of therapy; intensity of therapy; requirement of daily practice; group or individual therapy.

Characteristics of outcome measurement:
> type of outcome measure; reliability of measure; treatment to assessment interval; percent of clients lost to follow-up; internal validity of research design; number of clients in study when measure taken.

Treatment of Disfluency: Future Trends

Eugene B. Cooper

INTRODUCTION

To discuss the problem of stuttering with a claim of understanding the enigma is presumptuous. To predict the future of its treatment is not only presumptuous, it is preposterous. Nevertheless, having never allowed the lack of data to muzzle my speculations, I am delighted to have this opportunity to describe what I think the future holds with respect to the treatment of stuttering.

I doubt if there is an individual present who does not feel we need, for the sake of those who stutter, to make significant improvements in our treatment of these individuals.

I will begin this brief statement concerning the future of stuttering by being critical of several concepts that continue to influence significantly our thinking and our therapy for stutterers. I hasten to add, however, that I think very highly of the efforts made by the many creative and caring clinicians who have contributed to enhancing the lives of individuals who stutter. I am proud of my work in developing procedures and materials to help clinicians help clients. There is much to praise in such efforts, and I would be doing us all a disservice not to acknowledge the contributions of those who have gone before us as well as those still toiling, as our beloved Charles Van Riper might say, "in the vineyards of fluency."

I see my role, however, as that of stimulating affective as well as cognitive responses in you, the readers. Thus, I begin by cursing the darkness with the very good chance that I may offend some. I beg their forbearance. As I curse the darkness, please be sensitive to the fact that I speak only of stuttering therapy practices in the United States. I am not familiar with the course the treatment of stuttering has taken in other countries. I will allow others to determine the extent to which my criticisms are relevant to other countries. I will conclude my remarks by attempting to light a few candles. They may not be new ones, but they may assist in lighting our way as we strive to improve our services to those who stutter.

Reprinted from *Journal of Fluency Disorders*, vol. 11, 317–328. Copyright © 1986 by Elsevier Science Publishing Co., Inc.

THE LEARNING MODEL TRAP

For too long, we in the United States have sought answers to the enigma of stuttering from the frameworks of learning theorists. Learning theorists and their descendants, the behaviorists, have dominated our thinking about stuttering too long. One of my favorite sayings is "By our frameworks, we are hung." Too many of us have allowed ourselves to be hung too long by simplistic learning paradigms. Since the late 1940s and the early 1950s when Wischner (1950) and others began to apply learning paradigms to stuttering, we have been obsessed with explaining the onset as well as the maintenance of stuttering on the basis of one learning model or another. Since the 1960s, the obsession has been with applying these simplistic constructs to the treatment of stuttering. I wonder how many college sophomores, after grasping the concept of the operant model, have grown to maturity believing they possess the key to modifying all human behavior?

Enough, I say! It is 16 years since Siegel (1970) concluded, after reviewing 20 years of research on stuttering and the learning models, that we need to look elsewhere if we wish to understand stuttering. It is 16 years since the meaningfulness of such a conceptualization was challenged when we found the words "wrong," "right," and "tree" had the same effect on the frequency of stuttering (Cooper et al., 1970). I think it is time we escape from the parameters dictated by frameworks that have proven so barren in their usefulness. I join with Wingate (1983) in concluding, and I quote, "Speech-language pathologists should know better; they should have learned that speech is not so simply conceived" (p. 261).

THE FREQUENCY FALLACY

The obsessive application of learning models to the treatment of stuttering leads to abuses in our treatment practices. I am about to discuss one abuse I believe harms many clients. I refer to practices stemming from what I call "the frequency fallacy." The frequency fallacy is the belief that the frequency of stuttering is the single most valid measure of stuttering severity.

In our rush to identify things to count so we could apply our chosen learning model, we fixated on the frequency of stuttering. Despite our knowledge of the unreliability of such measures, not to mention their obvious lack of validity in indicating the significance of the problem to the individual, authors continue to perpetuate the obsession. How many currently popular treatment programs measure progress in therapy by frequency counts? How many therapy programs use the frequency criterion for moving from one therapy activity to another on the assumption that a change in a frequency count indicates the client's readiness to undertake more complex tasks? How can anyone argue such assumptions are valid? Again, we are "hung by our frameworks."

In addition to leading clinicians to the frequency fallacy trap, the proliferation of simplistic, behaviorally oriented therapy procedures resulted in a generation of clinicians coming to maturity believing that the treatment of stuttering involves only the manipulation fluency and that any concomitant behavioral, cognitive, and affective problems the client might have will resolve themselves once the frequency of fluency is adjusted. I agree with Van Riper (1984) in questioning the quality of help being offered by the typical clinician in the United States today. I hold the behavioral bandwagon that rolled unchecked for too many years responsible for the present questionable state of the treatment of stuttering in our country. Happily, more than a few of us are seeing that the emperor, to use an old fairy tale, is without his clothes. In reporting in the *Journal of Fluency Disorders* our 10-year study of clinicial attitudes toward stuttering, my wife and I noted a significant decline over the past decade in the number of clinicians who believe operant therapies to be the most effective form of treatment (Cooper & Cooper, 1985a). Fortunately, an increasing number of clinicians recognize the inadequacies inherent in programs failing to address the stutterer's feelings, attitudes, and beliefs. It is time to put treatment traps created by blinded behaviorists behind us.

THE FEAR OF EARLY INTERVENTION

It also is time to bury the notion that we should avoid early intervention with the young disfluent child. For too long, we have been intimidated by, at best, an unsubstantiated theory. For 40 years, the prevailing practitioner's notion in the United States, without the support of compelling data (Wingate, 1976) has been that most chronic stuttering results from normal disfluent behavior being labeled stuttering by overanxious parents (Prins & Ingham, 1983). Generations of clinicians were trained under this belief, and its influence continues in the professional community (Cooper & Cooper, 1985a).

On the basis of our studies concerning recovery from stuttering (Cooper, 1972; Lankford & Cooper, 1974; McLel-

observations, I came to believe over a decade ago that early intervention by concerned parents is the single most significant factor in the high incidence of spontaneous recovery from stuttering (Cooper, 1977, 1979a, 1979b). I am convinced of the efficacy of early intervention with very young stutterers, and I can think of no one better suited to direct those early intervention strategies than speech-language clinicians. Thus, I was pleased to find such distinguished colleagues as Costello, Ingham, Perkins, Prins, and the Rileys concluding their recent text on the treatment of stuttering in early childhood with the plea that clinicians put behind them unsubstantiated fears and embrace early intervention activities with the very young disfluent child (Prins & Ingham, 1983). Let us hope the professional community of practitioners hears and heeds such a challenge, belated though it may be.

THE FUTURE

I have indicated that a brighter future awaits as more of us break away from the limiting frameworks of narrowly defined learning paradigms. Wall and Myers' (1984) recent text *Clinical Management of Childhood Stuttering,* written from the language perspective, is one example of the kind of new perspectives we need if we are to escape the learning model web entrapping so many of our colleagues. I am confident other equally refreshing perspectives will be generated as those in neurolinguistics and neurogenics continue to expand our understanding of the bases of language behavior. I wish I could foresee what the future holds with respect to developments in these exciting areas. Although I cannot, I can, with some confidence, make predictions with respect to the following issues: therapy goals, early intervention programs, metalinguistics and early intervention, commercially produced therapy materials, short-term intensive versus long-term nonintensive therapy programs, the life-long chronic stutterer, and support systems for the adult stutterer.

Therapy Goals

One encouraging development I see in the treatment of stuttering is a change with respect to the goals of therapy. As clinicians born and bred in the golden age of behaviorism adopt more productive models to guide their therapy behavior, the currently popular focus on stuttering frequency will shift to a focus on the client's ability to identify and reinforce his or her own fluency-enhancing attitudes, feelings, and behaviors. The goals of therapy will deal with assisting clients in developing the feeling of fluency control rather than in achieving, as is too frequently the practice today, an arbitrarily predetermined level of fluency in arbitrarily selected, unrealistic speech situations. I know behavioral purists shrink at the thought of measuring such hypothetical constructs. Nevertheless, I suggest that those who shrink from the difficult task of quantifying the uncountable begin to do so. The evidence is overwhelming that it is in those constructs where we shall find the coin of fluency we seek. I cannot count how many times I have been advised by my behaviorally oriented colleagues that constructs such as the feeling of fluency control cannot be measured, whereas the number of disfluencies can be heard and counted with precision. Those continuing to seek fluency in frequency counts remind me of the story of the man who was searching beneath a street lamp for a coin he had dropped half a block away. When asked why he was searching at that spot for a coin he had dropped down the block, he replied, "The light is better here." It is time we abandon such reasoning.

Early Intervention Programs

I noted previously the reluctance of clinicians in the United States to embrace early intervention programs. I also noted the current trend towards a greater acceptance of early intervention, even with the 2½-year-old disfluent child. I see this trend continuing. More disfluent children than at present will learn techniques for altering their fluency before the struggle and stigma associated with a communicative disorder adversely affects their chances for a normal youthful development. I take joy in this change. I am confident that we will assist more disfluent individuals, for whom fluency is a realistic goal, to achieve that goal than we are presently helping.

Metalinguistics and Early Intervention

Twenty-five years ago, the new term thrust upon us was "psycholinguistics." The age of language assessment and language intervention had arrived. Ten years ago, the new term thrust upon us was "pragmatics." Today, the new term is "metalinguistics," and it refers to an individual's ability to talk about language (Blodgett & Cooper, 1983; Kamhi & Koenig, 1985). It took some time before I grasped its relevance to the treatment of stuttering. Now, I am caught up in measuring the ability of our very young clients to talk about their speech. As I began to focus on the very young disfluent child and as I attempted to instruct them in altering various aspects of their speech, I found myself becoming an instructor in the language of fluency. As I did so, I began to appreciate the significance of the development of metalinguistic abilities to our intervention activities for these preschool children.

I am confident that as we increase our understanding of the development of metalinguistic skills, we will increase our efficiency in instructing children in the language of fluency. Before we ask children to use slow speech, easy speech, deep breath, or easy onset, we will ascertain if the child has sufficient metalinguistic skills to process such a request. My colleague, Dr. Elizabeth G. Blodgett, and I have been involved during the past 3 years in the development of the "Metalinguistic Abilities Checklist" (Blodgett & Cooper, 1983). A revised and standardized version of this metalinguistic abilities assessment instrument is scheduled for publication in 1987. I am hopeful that by its publication, we will be adding a useful assessment instrument to the armamentaria of clinicians working with the 3- to 8-year-old disfluent child.

Commercially Produced Therapy Materials

I am proud of the fact that our Personalized Fluency Control Therapy Program (Cooper, 1976; Cooper & Cooper, 1985b) was the first comprehensive treatment program for children and adults made commercially available to clinicians in the United States. I was criticized by some for venturing into the commercial arena, and was accused of being nonprofessional and practicing opportunism. At professional meetings I was referred to derogatorily as being of the "kit mentality." Having been advised by my father early in life that if I found myself in favor with most, I should know at best I was mediocre, such criticism became my badge of honor. I wear it more proudly today, now that I have lived for more than 10 years in the "tainted world," as my critics would call it, of commercialists. I have learned the power the commercial world has to assist articulate and creative individuals in communicating effective and efficient therapeutic strategies to practicing clinicians. Many fine procedures and techniques would most likely never have been developed if it had not been for resources put to the task by commercial publishers.

Most practicing clinicians are confronted daily with a full schedule of clients to serve. They do not have the time or perhaps the ability to develop their own therapy strategies, materials, and techniques. Because of the commercial world, they now have access to comprehensive treatment programs with attractive and stimulating materials to assist them in providing their clients with an effective and efficient treatment program. I say "Poo" on my critics for their pseudointellectualism. Our profession's past failure to capitalize on the willingness of publishing firms to assist in the development of therapy programs and materials for the practicing clinician is criminal.

Two publishing firms with which I have been associated conducted independent marketing research to determine what stuttering treatment strategies practicing clinicians in the United States were using. Both of their reports were disturbing to me and confounding to them. In essence, they found that most clinicians were unable to articulate what approach they were using with their stuttering clients. In addition, they found that clinicians who did describe what they were doing with their stuttering clients indicated that they were using a variety of specific fluency-enhancing techniques for which they had no underlying rationale. The market researchers were puzzled by these results. I was not surprised.

Practicing clinicians need help. In some countries, stuttering therapy is the province of the stuttering specialist. Such is not the case in the United States, although there appears to be an increase in the number of individuals calling for the education of such specialists. I am one of them. However, I am also a realist. I know that it will be at least a decade before we can hope to see any significant number of specialists entering the field. In the meantime, individuals capable of developing worthwhile therapy procedures and materials suitable for commercial distribution should be encouraged to do so. They will provide a valuable service in helping clinicians serve those who stutter. It is exciting to contemplate what might be achieved with the resources major publishing firms can bring to the task. The future is bright in this area, and I see continued growth in the number of worthwhile therapy programs commercially available to practicing clinicians.

Short-Term Intensive versus Long-Term Nonintensive Treatment Programs

The popularity of short-term intensive programs will wane as it becomes more evident that, for the large majority of stutterers, long-term nonintensive educative and rehabilitative programs are more effective. During the past several years, we have witnessed a rebirth in the popularity of short-term intensive stuttering therapy programs reminiscent to us in the United States of such programs as that offered by the Benjamin N. Bogue Institute of Indianapolis or the Lewis School for Stammerers of Detroit, both well known stuttering clinics in the United States early in this century (Wingate, 1976). Having directed short-term intensive stuttering programs myself over a 20-year period, first at Pennsylvania State University and then at the University of Alabama, I am more than a little familiar with the advantages and disadvantages of such programs.

Anyone having conducted short-term intensive programs using any one of the myriad of available fluency-eliciting techniques knows the exhilarating feeling of seeing disfluent individuals of all ages and with varying degrees of stuttering severity achieve fluency with a seemingly miraculous rapidity. Anyone having participated in any kind of intensive, short-term, away from home group endeavor (be it a religious retreat, a sales seminar, or a personal growth experience) is not surprised by such results. Unfortunately, too many of our colleagues without such experience, finding themselves conducting short-term intensive stuttering programs, have jumped to the conclusion that the particular fluency-facilitating techniques they happen to be using are responsible for their clients' flight into fluency. They are unaware of the power that short-term intensive experiences possess in bringing about abrupt changes in complex behavioral patterns. They erroneously attribute their clients' increased fluency to the particular speech modification procedures they are teaching rather than to the multitude of unique factors present in such artificial environments.

Potentially more detrimental to the stutterers involved, however, is the naive leader's belief or hope that the fluency being observed during the program will persist when the client goes home. They are unaware of or do not acknowledge the ephemeral quality of most behavioral changes achieved under such circumstances.

I am hopeful we will see a decline in quick-fix programs. I am also hopeful we will see an increase in the development of educative and rehabilitative stuttering therapy programs that capture the dynamic aspects of short-term intensive programs by successfully stimulating and motivating rapid behavioral and attitudinal changes without forcing clients into artificial environments away from home.

The Life-long Chronic Stutterer

Progress will be made in differentiating between stutterers who can conquer their stuttering with or without professional assistance and those individuals for whom the control of stuttering will require a lifetime of vigilance.

Some years ago during my brief tenure as a Washington bureaucrat, I was shocked to see a national organization for the hearing-impaired launch a nationwide bumper-sticker campaign with the slogan "Deaf Children Can Speak." This campaign appalled me. I immediately thought of the thousands of nonspeaking adult deaf individuals and their parents who would experience a sense of loss, if not guilt, from such a campaign. I protested to the leadership of the organization, and the slogan was changed to a less dramatic but more accurate phrase indicating that deaf children can learn speech. I find myself with similar feelings when I hear colleagues suggesting that all stutterers can be fluent. I do not believe all stutterers can be fluent.

My research as well as my 30 years of experience with hundreds of stutterers of all ages convinces me that a significant number of disfluent stutterers will remain disfluent despite anything they might do or have done to them. Certainly, we all hope that the day will arrive when we have the ability to cure stuttering in everyone. Realistically, however, we know that such a time may never come. Until it does, I trust that our practitioners will communicate to those for whom normal fluency is an unrealistic goal the real sense of success that comes from being able to modify fluency. I have never known disfluent individuals unable to alter their fluency.

At a recent stuttering conference sponsored by the Speech Foundation of America, David A. Daly (1985) spoke compellingly and movingly of the danger of destroying stutterers' dreams of being fluent and of many stutterers' life-fulfilling quests for fluency. We need to be sensitive when that dream and that quest are present in the clients we serve. Our clinical skills will be challenged as we make difficult decisions regarding how we should respond to such clients. Nevertheless, we must not reinforce clients making unrealistic demands of themselves when our clinical judgement is that normal fluency, for whatever reason, is beyond their grasp.

Support Systems for the Adult Stutterer

Another positive development I forsee with respect to the treatment of stuttering in the United States is the development of cooperative efforts between existing self-help groups and professionals in creating networks of support groups for those chronic adult stutterers seeking such support. I understand many cooperative endeavors of this nature already exist in Europe. As charter president of the National Alliance on Stuttering, a recently incorporated nonprofit alliance of groups and individuals in the United States committed to encouraging cooperative activities between professional and self-help groups, I hope to learn of these successes. In the United States, the development of self-help groups has been largely ignored by the professional community. Many self-help groups have been formed by professionals who stutter, but the movement has never received the active or organized support of the general professional community.

Many factors might be cited to explain the typical professional's lack of enthusiasm for self-help groups. I suspect that one of those factors is the professional's failure to accept the fact, as noted, that some individuals will continue to stutter no matter what they may do or have done to them and that even some successfully controlled stutterers need such continuing support to maintain their control. Clinicians may be uncomfortable with the existence of groups of individuals who may or may not continue to experience disfluencies but who appear to benefit from the association with others with similar experiences. Perhaps professionals experience discomfort believing that they or their colleagues have failed if former clients seek such support.

On the other hand, some self-help group participants have actively spurned the support of professionals when help has been offered. Such occurrences are understandable if the stutterers involved have been led by clinicians from whom they sought help to believe that all stutterers can be fluent. The stutterers' reluctance to embrace the professional is equally understandable if, again, they have been led to believe their inability to achieve or maintain lasting fluency is because of their failure in the vigilant application of the techniques that the clinician has taught them rather than in the techniques themselves. Hopefully, the National Alliance on Stuttering can change attitudes such as I have been describing by encouraging cooperative endeavors between self-help groups, support groups, and professional groups.

I am encouraged by the responses I have received by our professional community to the development of the National Alliance. As our practitioners adopt more realistic goals in their treatment of the chronic adult stutterer and as they come to value the role that support groups can play in enhancing the quality of life for adult stutterers, be they fluent or not, I am confident we will add a significant new dimension to our treatment programs for those who stutter.

SUMMARY

The United States clinicians' obsession with learning paradigms was suggested as being a major obstacle in the development of more effective treatment strategies. The perpetuation of the frequency fallacy, which suggested that disfluency counts are the single most significant measure of stuttering, was described as being one result of this fixation on learning models. The fear of early intervention was another. Future trends were suggested as being the adoption of more meaningful therapy goals, an increased emphasis on early intervention, an increasing awareness of the significance of metalinguistic skills to early intervention, the valuing of commercially produced therapy programs, an increased awareness of the limitations of short-term intensive treatment programs, the recognition and acceptance of the existence of the life-long chronic stutterer, and the development of support systems for the adult stutterer.

The problem of stuttering has fascinated me since the first day I became conscious of its existence. I would have left the discipline of human communication sciences and disorders many years ago if it were not for the fascination that this particular problem holds for me. I want to be around another 50 years to see how much validity, if any at all, there is in what I have just described.

REFERENCES

Blodgett, E.G., & Cooper. E.B. (1983). *Metalinguistic abilities checklist: A preliminary report*. Paper presented at the annual convention of the American Speech-Language-Hearing Association, Cincinnati.

Cooper, E.B. (1972). Recovery from stuttering in a junior and senior high school population. *Journal of Speech and Hearing Research, 15,* 632–638.

Cooper, E.B. (1976). *Personalized fluency control therapy*. Allen, TX: DLM Teaching Resources.

Cooper, E.B. (1977). Controversies about stuttering behavior. *Journal of Fluency Disorders, 2,* 75–86.

Cooper, E.B. (1979a). Intervention procedures for young children. In H.H. Gregory (Ed.), *Controversies about stuttering therapy*. Baltimore: University Park Press.

Cooper, E.B. (1979b). *Understanding stuttering: Information for parents*. Chicago: National Easter Seal Society.

Cooper, E.B., Cady, B.B., & Robbins, C.J. (1970). The effect of the verbal stimulus words "wrong," "right," and "tree" on the disfluency rates of stutterers and nonstutterers. *Journal of Speech and Hearing Research, 13,* 239–244.

Cooper, E.B., & Cooper, C.S. (1985a). Clinician attitudes toward stuttering: A decade of change (1973–1983). *Journal of Fluency Disorders, 10,* 19–33.

Cooper, E.B., & Cooper, C.S. (1985b). *Cooper personalized fluency control therapy-Revised*. Allen, TX: DLM Teaching Resources.

Daly, D.A. (1985). *Intensive versus conventional treatment for stutterers*. Unpublished paper presented at Speech Foundation of America sponsored conference, Champaign, IL.

Kamhi, A.G., & Koenig, L.A. (1985). Metalinguistic awareness in normal and language disordered children. *Language, Speech, and Hearing Services in Schools, 16*, 199–210.

Lankford, S.D., & Cooper, E.B. (1974). Recovery from stuttering as viewed by parents of self-diagnosed recovered stutterers. *Journal of Communication Disorders, 7*, 171–180.

McLelland, J.K., & Cooper, E.B. (1978). Fluency-related behaviors and attitudes of 178 young stutterers. *Journal of Fluency Disorders, 3*, 253–263.

Prins, D., & Ingham, R.J. (1983). *Treatment of stuttering in early childhood: Methods and issues*. San Diego: College-Hill Press.

Siegel, G.M. (1970). Punishment, stuttering, and disfluency. *Journal of Speech and Hearing Disorders, 13*, 677–714.

Van Riper, C. (1984). On stuttering. *The National Council on Stuttering Journal*, (Spring), 12.

Wall, M.J., & Myers, F.L. (1984). *Clinical management of childhood stuttering*. Baltimore: University Park Press.

Wingate, M.E. (1976). *Stuttering: Theory and treatment*. New York: Irvington.

Wingate, M.E. (1983). Speaking unassisted: Comments on a paper by Andrews et al. *Journal of Speech and Hearing Disorders, 48*, 255–263.

Wischner, G.J. (1950). Stuttering behavior and learning: A preliminary theoretical formulation. *Journal of Speech and Hearing Disorders, 15*, 324–335.

CHAPTER 5 ADDITIONAL READINGS

Adams, M.R. (1983). Learning from negative outcomes in stuttering therapy. I: Getting off on the wrong foot. *Journal of Fluency Disorders, 8*, 147–154.

Adler, L., Leong, S., & Delgado, R. (1987). Drug-induced stuttering treated with propranolol. *Journal of Clinical Psychopharmacology, 7*, 115–116.

Andrews, G., & Craig, A. (1982). Stuttering: Overt and covert measurement of the speech of treated subjects. *Journal of Speech and Hearing Disorders, 47*, 96–99.

Andrews, G., & Feyer, A.M. (1985). Does behavior therapy still work when the experimenters depart? An analysis of a behavioral treatment program for stuttering. *Behavioral Modification, 9*, 443–457.

Andrews, G., & Tanner, S. (1982a). Stuttering treatment: An attempt to replicate the regulated-breathing method. *Journal of Speech and Hearing Disorders, 47*, 138–140.

Andrews, G., & Tanner, S. (1982b). Stuttering: The results of 5 days of treatment with an airflow technique. *Journal of Speech and Hearing Disorders, 47*, 427–429.

Azrin, N.H., Nunn, R.G., & Frantz, S.E. (1979). Comparison of regulated-breathing versus abbreviated desensitization on reported stuttering episodes. *Journal of Speech and Hearing Disorders, 44*, 331–339.

Beaty, D.T. (1980). A multimodal approach to elimination of stuttering. *Perceptual and Motor Skills, 50*, 51–55.

Blaesing, L. (1982). A multidisciplinary approach to individualized treatment of stuttering. *Journal of Fluency Disorders, 7*, 203–218.

Boberg, E., Howie, P., & Woods, L. (1979). Maintenance of fluency: A review. *Journal of Fluency Disorders, 4*, 93–116.

Bowman, S. (1987). Support for those who stutter needs support. *Asha, 29*, 55–56, (April).

Burley, P.M., & Morley, R. (1987). Self-monitoring processes in stutterers. *Journal of Fluency Disorders, 12*, 71–78.

Cooper, E.B., & Cooper, C.S. (1985). Clinician attitudes toward stuttering: A decade of change (1973–1983). *Journal of Fluency Disorders, 10*, 19–33.

Coppola, V.A., & Yairi, E. (1982). Rythmic speech training with preschool stuttering children: An experimental study. *Journal of Fluency Disorders, 7*, 447–457.

Craig, A.R., & Andrews, G. (1985). The prediction and prevention of relapse in stuttering: The value of self-control techniques and locus of control measures. *Behavior Modification, 9*, 427–442.

Craig, A.R., & Cleary, P.J. (1982). Reduction of stuttering by young male stutterers using EMG feedback. *Biofeedback and Self-Regulation, 7*, 241–255.

Craig, A.R., & Howie, P.M. (1982). Locus of control and maintenance of behavioral therapy skills. *British Journal of Clinical Psychology, 21*, 65–66.

Craven, D.C., & Ryan, B.P. (1984). The use of a portable delayed auditory feedback unit in stuttering therapy. *Journal of Fluency Disorders, 9*, 237–243.

Dopheide, W. (1987). Competencies expected of beginning clinicians working with children who stutter. *Journal of Fluency Disorders, 12*, 157–166.

Eversham, M., & Fransella, F. (1985). Stuttering relapse: The effect of a combined speech and psychological reconstruction programme. *British Journal of Disorders of Communication, 20*, 237–248.

Ham, R.E. (1988). Unison speech and rate control therapy. *Journal of Fluency Disorders, 13,* 115–126.

Howie, P.M., Tanner, S., & Andrews, G. (1981). Short- and long-term outcome in an intensive treatment program for adult stutterers. *Journal of Speech and Hearing Disorders, 46,* 104–109.

Howie, P.M., Woods, C.L., & Andrews, G. (1982). Relationship between covert and overt speech measures immediately before and immediately after stuttering treatment. *Journal of Speech and Hearing Disorders, 47,* 419–422.

Ingham, R.J. (1980). Modification of maintenance and generalization during stuttering treatment. *Journal of Speech and Hearing Research, 23,* 732–745.

Ingham, R.J. (1982). The effects of self-evaluation training on maintenance and generalization during stuttering treatment. *Journal of Speech and Hearing Disorders, 47,* 271–280.

Ingham, R.J., Gow, M., & Costello, J.M. (1985). Stuttering and speech naturalness: Some additional data. *Journal of Speech and Hearing Disorders, 50,* 217–219.

Ingham, R.J., Ingham, J.C., Onslow, M., & Finn, P. (1989). Stutterers' self-ratings of speech naturalness: Assessing effects and reliability. *Journal of Speech and Hearing Research, 32,* 419–438.

James, J.E. (1981). Behavioral self-control of stuttering using time-out from speaking. *Journal of Applied Behavior Analysis, 14,* 25–37.

Johnson, G.F. (1987). Ten commandments for long-term maintenance of acceptable self-help skills for persons who are hard-core stutterers. *Journal of Fluency Disorders, 12,* 9–18.

Maxwell, D.L. (1982). Cognitive and behavioral self-control strategies: Applications for the clinical management of adult stutterers. *Journal of Fluency Disorders, 7,* 403–432.

Metz, D.E., Samar, V.J., & Sacco, P.R. (1983). Acoustic analysis of stutterers' fluent speech before and after therapy. *Journal of Speech and Hearing Research, 26,* 531–536.

Miller, S. (1982). Airflow therapy programs: Facts and/or fancy. *Journal of Fluency Disorders, 7,* 187–202.

Moore, M.S., & Adams, M.R. (1985). The Edinburgh masker: A clinical analog study. *Journal of Fluency Disorders, 10,* 281–290.

Nittrouer, S., & Cheney, C. (1984). Operant techniques used in stuttering therapy: A review. *Journal of Fluency Disorders, 9,* 169–190.

Perkins, W.H. (1981). Implications of scientific research for treatment of stuttering—a lecture. *Journal of Fluency Disorders, 6,* 155–162.

Perkins, W.H. (1983). Learning from negative outcomes in stuttering therapy. II: An epiphany of failure. *Journal of Fluency Disorders, 8,* 155–160.

Prins, D., Mandelkorn, T., & Cerf, F.A. (1980). Principal and differential effects of haloperidol and placebo treatments upon speech disfluencies in stutterers. *Journal of Speech and Hearing Research, 23,* 614–629.

Prosek, R.A., & Runyan, C.M. (1983). Effects of segment and pause manipulations on the identification of treated stutterers. *Journal of Speech and Hearing Research, 26,* 510–516.

Ramig, P.R. (1984). Rate changes in the speech of stutterers after therapy. *Journal of Fluency Disorders, 9,* 285–294.

Rousy, C.G., Arjunan, K.N., & Rousy, C.L. (1986). Successful treatment of stuttering following closed head injury. *Journal of Fluency Disorders, 11,* 257–261.

Rustin, L., & Kuhr, A. (1983). The treatment of stammering: A multimodel approach in an in-patient setting. *British Journal of Disorders of Communication, 18,* 90–97.

Ryan, B.P., & Van Kirk, B. (1983). Programmed stuttering therapy for children: Comparison of four established programs. *Journal of Fluency Disorders, 8,* 291–321.

Saint-Laurent, L., & Ladouceur, R. (1987). Massed versus distributed application of the regulated-breathing method for stutterers and its long-term effect. *Behavior Therapy, 18,* 38–50.

Salend, S.J., & Andress, M.J. (1984). Decreasing stuttering in an elementary-level student. *Language, Speech, & Hearing Services in Schools, 15,* 16–21.

Samar, V.J., Metz, D.E., & Sacco, P.R. (1986). Changes in aerodynamic characteristics of stutterers' fluent speech associated with therapy. *Journal of Speech and Hearing Research, 29,* 106–113.

Silverman, F.H. (1980). The stuttering problem profile: A task that assists both client and clinician in defining therapy goals. *Journal of Speech and Hearing Disorders, 45,* 119–123.

Starkweather, C.W. (1984). A multiprocess behavioral approach to stuttering therapy. In W.H. Perkins (Ed.), *Current therapy of communication disorders: Stuttering disorders.* New York: Thieme-Stratton.

Stocker, B., & Gerstman, L.J. (1983). A comparison of the probe technique and conventional therapy for young stutterers. *Journal of Fluency Disorders, 8,* 331–339.

Williams, D.E. (1982). Stuttering therapy: Where are we going and why? *Journal of Fluency Disorders, 7,* 159–170.

Yeakle, M.K., & Cooper, E.B. (1986). Teacher perceptions of stuttering. *Journal of Fluency Disorders, 11,* 345–359.

Zibelman, R. (1982). Avoidance-reduction therapy for stuttering. *American Journal of Psychotherapy, 36,* 489–496.

Author Index

Subject Index